ALZHEIMER'S DISEASE

ALZHEIMER'S DISEASE

What If There Was a Cure?

The Story of Ketones

MARY T. NEWPORT, M.D.

Basic
Health
PUBLICATIONS, INC.

The information contained in this book is based upon the research and personal and professional experiences of the author. It is not intended as a substitute for consulting with your physician or other healthcare provider. Any attempt to diagnose and treat an illness should be done under the direction of a healthcare professional.

The publisher does not advocate the use of any particular healthcare protocol but believes the information in this book should be available to the public. The publisher and author are not responsible for any adverse effects or consequences resulting from the use of the suggestions, preparations, or procedures discussed in this book. Should the reader have any questions concerning the appropriateness of any procedures or preparation mentioned, the author and the publisher strongly suggest consulting a professional healthcare advisor.

Basic Health Publications, Inc.
28812 Top of the World Drive
Laguna Beach, CA 92651
949-715-7327 • www.basichealthpub.com

Library of Congress Cataloging-in-Publication Data is available through the Library of Congress.

ISBN: 978-1-59120-293-6

Editor: Cheryl Hirsch
Typesetting/Book design: Gary A. Rosenberg
Cover design: Mike Stromberg

Printed in the United States of America

10   9   8   7   6   5   4   3

Contents

This book is dedicated to my husband, Steve,
who says that taking care of our girls was the best
job he ever had. He made it possible for me to fulfill
my two dreams of becoming a doctor and having
children, and he was always right there behind
me with his love and support. Now it is
my turn to take care of him.

This book is also dedicated to the millions of other
caregivers who are fighting hard for their loved ones
with Alzheimer's and other tragic neurodegenerative
diseases; may it offer a glimmer of hope. So many
of you have shared your stories with me, real people
who want nothing more than to keep their loved ones
with them for as long as possible—a goal that I fully
understand because we are on this journey together.

Acknowledgments

This book would not exist if not for the many years of dedication on the part of Richard L. Veech, M.D., D. Phil., to learning what ketone bodies can do and to applying this knowledge for the betterment of the millions of people who suffer from Alzheimer's disease, Parkinson's disease, and a host of other neurodegenerative diseases. His work has personally affected my own family, giving us hope for the future, and for this I am extremely grateful. I also want to thank Dr. Veech for reviewing the chapters on ketones and providing me with many of the historical details. I would also like to express my gratitude to the other people who have worked side by side with Dr. Veech in this pursuit of knowledge to help others: M. Todd King, M.S.; Yoshihiro Kashiwaya, M.D., Ph.D.; Monica Skarulis, M.D.; Christian Bergman, B.S.; Shireesh Srivastiva, Ph.D.; Robert Pawlosky, Ph.D.; and Calvin Crutchfield.

I want to acknowledge the decades of work dedicated to researching and improving human nutrition by Theodore B. VanItallie, M.D., who worked out many details of the important metabolic principles discussed in this book. His article, "Ketones: Metabolism's Ugly Duckling?" provides a foundation for much of the discussion in Part Two of the book. I greatly appreciate his continued interest and involvement in ketone research and his keen review of the chapters on ketones and medium-chain triglycerides for this book.

I wish to acknowledge George F. Cahill, Jr., M.D., for his discovery that ketones can provide an alternative fuel for the brain, the fundamental principle underlying the dietary intervention discussed in this book. I also greatly appreciate his efforts in accompanying Dr. Veech and me to Capitol Hill to bring attention to the urgent need for funding for mass production of the ketone ester and clinical trials.

I want to acknowledge Beverly Teter, Ph.D., lipid biochemist from the University of Maryland, for her friendship as well as her extremely helpful, critical review of the sections on cholesterol and saturated fats.

I want to express my love and deepest appreciation to my sister, Angela Bertke, for her immense moral support and the innumerable hours she has spent helping me to get the message out, directly through her own efforts and by making herself available to take care of Steve so that I could get the message out. I want to recognize the endless hours she has spent reading my book, which have helped me stay on track with my goal of making the book readable for the nonscientist, and for her keen eye in proofreading the book. I also want to thank her husband, John Bertke, for going out of his way to spend time with Steve while I attended conference lectures.

I also want to express my love and gratitude to our daughter, Joanna Newport, not only for her day-to-day help with her father, but also for her assistance with some of the more tedious typing, for her expertise in creating diagrams for the book, and for the many hours she spent setting up our website www.coconutketones .com. I also want to recognize the love and support of our daughter, Julie DiPalo, and our many other family members.

I want to thank Lois Walsh for allowing me to share her poignant poetry that captures the very essence of caregiving for a loved one with Alzheimer's disease.

I would also like to acknowledge the following: Eve Hosley-

Moore, Steve Nohlgren, and their editors at the *St. Petersburg Times* for their efforts in writing and publishing their stories about Steve and ketones; the many people who have invited me to give interviews and lectures to further my cause of getting the message out to others; Tom Sokoloff for introducing me to Norman Goldfind, the publisher; and the editor of this book, Cheryl Hirsch, for her expertise in helping me bring our story and the story of ketones to the public.

Most importantly, I want to thank my husband, Steve, for his love, support, and patience and for being the kind of person whom you want to fight for.

Preface

Like millions of people in this country and around the world, my sixty-one-year-old husband, Steve, suffers from the nightmare that is Alzheimer's disease. Alzheimer's is the most common form of dementia in the United States. Many other people suffer from Parkinson's disease and less common forms of dementia and neurodegenerative conditions. These diseases take their toll not only on the victim but on their loved ones as well. No matter how young or old a person is at the onset of these diseases, the diagnosis is a devastating, life-altering blow. The future, once rosy and full of promise, takes on a different set of colors, bleak and gray.

How sad and cruel is the disease process known as dementia, that so many people finish out their lives without memories of what they have accomplished, unable to recognize the people they loved and who loved them, and finally unable to remember how to perform the simplest physical maneuver such as standing up and sitting down. How sad and cruel that people have to watch their beloved spouse or parent slowly slip away in this manner, and then worry that they will suffer the same fate.

Presently, there is no cure for Alzheimer's disease. After decades of study and many billions of dollars spent on research, the causes of Alzheimer's disease are still mostly unknown, and pharmaceutical companies have yet to find a treatment that will stop, much less reverse, its downward spiral.

A recent campaign by a national Alzheimer's organization pronounced that this disease "has no survivors," a message intended, no doubt, to promote contributions for research, but also a message that conveys a sense of hopelessness to the very real people and their families who are dealing with Alzheimer's disease now. In March 2009, Steve and I attended a conference presented by this organization in Washington, D.C., where they proudly announced the "good news" that a cure is on the horizon, probably within five years. This was not good news to us and to the many others who are dealing with this disease in the here and now. This was the same message we had heard five years prior when Steve was in the early stages of this disease. At that time, we were so very hopeful that, if he took his special medications to "slow the decline of the disease," he would survive in a meaningful way, long enough to enjoy the benefits of the promised cure.

When you are a relatively young couple such as us, it is quite a shock when it becomes apparent that we will not get to enjoy the "golden years of retirement" that most people look forward to. Like many others contending with the disease, we often talk about the fact that, if Steve could just stay the way he is now, we could still live with this disease. The cold reality is that neurodegenerative diseases, such as Alzheimer's, are relentless, and hope fades with each passing year until it is finally extinguished. We cannot wait five more years, because we don't have five more years.

This book is about ketones—tiny molecules of organic fuel that have been around since the beginning of life on this planet and have insured our survival as a species. These are molecules of "hope" for those suffering from Alzheimer's and other degenerative brain diseases. A drinkable form of ketones can be made now in the National Institutes of Health lab of Richard Veech, M.D., D. Phil., a world-renowned researcher who has been working with ketones for decades. But it will take substantial money and several years of clinical trials after the money comes through to be available to the millions who need this. Sadly, competition is fierce for research dollars, and the money to mass-produce this ketone ester has not come through as of this writing. As it often does, politics has gotten in the way of true progress.

My primary goal in writing this book is to draw attention to the existence of ketone ester, get the mass production of ketone ester funded, and get clinical trials of ketone ester on the fast track toward Food and Drug Administration approval. I hope this book will increase awareness in such a way that the powers-that-be can no longer overlook ketone ester and will be pushed to fund its production. I also hope that an explosion of ketone research will occur. For those dealing with dementia and other neurodegenerative diseases, this cannot happen soon enough.

We need this miracle now, but it is not here yet. While we are waiting, we can take advantage of a metabolic miracle that occurs in our bodies when we eat certain foods that contain medium-chain fatty acids. These fats found primarily in coconut and palm kernel oils are converted in the liver to ketones, which can be used by the brain and most other organs as fuel. The levels of ketones we can expect from consuming these fats are relatively low compared to the lab-made ketone ester; however, many people can expect a "reprieve" from the downward spiral of this disease. This reprieve may come in the form of improved memory, a return of personality and sense of humor, greater social interaction, resumption of daily activities, and/or relief from certain physical symptoms. These effects are very real and very meaningful, not only to the people suffering from the disease, but also to their caregivers and other loved ones who are suffering with them.

For many people, the difference after beginning this dietary intervention is readily apparent and can even be dramatic, as it was in my husband's case. For others, the reprieve may come in the form of stabilization rather than obvious improvement. For this reason, I encourage caregivers to keep a journal so that several

months later they can look back to decide if this dietary intervention is helping to at least stall the disease process. How long we
can expect this reprieve to last is uncertain since this discovery is
so new. At the time of this writing, it has been nearly three years
since we found and instituted this dietary intervention for Steve.
He has often told me that the light bulb came back on the day he
started consuming medium-chain fatty acids. Some of the changes
were fairly obvious during the first few days, and others took
many months to become apparent.

Compared to early in 2008, Steve is no longer depressed. He is
happy and feels that he has a future. His personality and sense of
humor are much more like the sweet husband I had ten years ago,
before all this happened. He is sociable, laughs, participates in
conversations (even in a large group), and contributes with jokes
and comments of his own creation. He no longer has any of the
physical symptoms that were affecting him before the dietary intervention, such as tremors, a weird gait, inability to run, a visual
disturbance that interfered with reading, and sudden episodes of
faintness. His ability to stay on task improved to the point that he
was able to take on a volunteer job at the hospital where I work.
His short-term and recent memory is far from normal, but they are
much improved. A magnetic resonance image (MRI) showed considerable shrinkage in Steve's brain before we began this dietary
intervention, meaning that much of his brain tissue has died. So we
know there are limits to how much improvement we can expect. In
April 2010, two years into this intervention, his MRI was reported
as "stable."

The road to recovery has not been free of some serious bumps.
Steve had one major setback in the summer of 2009, lasting several
weeks. He became more "dazed and confused" during an illness,
and some new problems popped up that have not completely gone
away. However, with patience and persistence, we have seen a
return to his previous baseline in most respects.

This dietary intervention may offer even more hope in the form of prevention for those of us who are at risk of developing Alzheimer's and other neurodegenerative diseases. The more I learn about ketone bodies, the more I conclude that short- and medium-chain fatty acids may be "essential fatty acids" for some, and perhaps all, of us. If we incorporate these essential fats regularly into our diet, we may be able to avoid some of the damage to our brains and other organs related to the aging process.

After Steve improved in response to medium-chain fatty acids, I made considerable effort to get the leaders of a national Alzheimer's organization and the Alzheimer's Study Group to investigate this and make the public aware of it. I was told that extensive clinical trials are needed before they would go out on a limb to help get the message out. One group even took measures to suppress my efforts to get this message out. All this will be recounted in detail in this book.

Clinical trials can take fifteen years from the time the first applications are made for funding until they are completed. Most of those currently suffering from Alzheimer's disease don't have years to wait. They may not be with us in five or even three years. Oils and other foods with medium-chain fatty acids are not dangerous drugs. They are foods that have been consumed on a regular basis for millennia or longer in other parts of the world where people first evolved as a species. These are foods that are available on the shelf in nearly every natural food store and many grocery stores.

We can take advantage right now of the metabolic miracle that happens when we eat foods with medium-chain fatty acids to try to get a reprieve from the nightmare that is Alzheimer's. I don't know how long this reprieve will last, or even if it will happen for you and your loved ones, but what do you have to lose?

Introduction

More than 5 million Americans are believed to have Alzheimer's disease, a degenerative brain disease. The number of people with Alzheimer's doubles roughly for each five-year interval over age sixty-five, so that people who live beyond eighty-five years of age have a nearly fifty-fifty chance of developing the disease. As the generation of Baby Boomers reaches their mid-sixties and beyond, unless a medical breakthrough identifies ways to prevent or treat the disease, by 2050, the number of Alzheimer's victims is predicted to triple to a staggering 15 million people in the United States alone and over 100 million worldwide.

According to the national office of the Alzheimer's Association, this disease is the sixth leading cause of death overall in the United States and the fifth leading cause for people over age sixty-five. The National Center for Health Statistics reported that, while the rates of deaths related to stroke, heart disease, and certain cancers declined between 2000 and 2006, deaths from Alzheimer's disease increased by 47.1 percent. In addition, at least 30 percent of people with Alzheimer's die of other causes, so the actual number of people with the disease may be grossly underestimated.

The annual costs of caring for people with Alzheimer's to Medicare, Medicaid, and U.S. businesses are currently estimated at an astounding $148 billion. In addition, the Alzheimer's Association estimates that 9.9 million people provide unpaid caregiving for people with Alzheimer's and other dementias that is equivalent to about $94 billion if such care was provided by paid attendants. Eighty-seven percent of caregivers are relatives of the person with dementia, so many people caring for their loved ones must watch them slowly and painfully deteriorate, at first forgetting little things such as where they placed their wallet or keys and, ultimately, forgetting how to do the simplest things they have done for a lifetime, such as getting out of bed, and worst of all, failing to recognize the people who love and care for them, the child they gave birth to, the spouse they married many years earlier.

Alzheimer's is a progressive brain disease that is considered to be irreversible, a mysterious process that causes brain cells to lose their connections with one another and subsequently die. In spite of intense worldwide research since the early 1970s, the exact cause of the disease is still unknown in 2011. The first case was described by Alois Alzheimer (1864–1915), a German psychiatrist and neuropathologist, during a lecture in 1906 and published in detail in 1911. His patient was a fifty-one-year-old lady, Auguste Deter, who presented with symptoms of "impaired memory, aphasia (difficulty speaking), disorientation, and psychosocial incompetence" and died at age fifty-five after gradual worsening of the disease, including loss of other cognitive functions and hallucinations. After her death, when Dr. Alzheimer performed an autopsy on her brain, he found that nearly one-third of the cells of her cerebral cortex (portions of the brain related to higher functions) had died off and, in their place, were large numbers of what are now called amyloid plaques and neurofibrillary tangles, the hallmarks of the disease that bears his name. He called this disease "presenile dementia" because of her age; now she would be considered to have early onset Alzheimer's disease.

When someone younger than sixty-five develops this type of dementia, it is called "early onset Alzheimer's disease," and an estimated 200,000 people, about 3.8 percent of the 5.3 million affected in the United States, fall into this category. Alzheimer's disease has even been described in people in their thirties and forties. People sixty-five and older are considered to have "later onset Alzheimer's disease" and represent the vast majority of cases. Dr. Alzheimer's first patient also had signs of hardening of the arteries at the time of her autopsy, indicative of the overlap with other conditions that is often seen with the disease. Alzheimer's is the most common form of dementia, representing 50 to 80 percent of cases, with vascular dementia the next most common. Many people have evidence of both of these types of dementia.

Recent advances in imaging technologies have made it possible to detect subtle changes in the brain a decade or more before a person develops obvious symptoms of the disease. Such advances will make it possible for people who are known to be at risk to take preventive measures, such as stopping smoking, controlling blood pressure, increasing exercise, treating sleep apnea, adopting a healthier diet, and taking measures to prevent or reverse the effects of impaired insulin-related conditions. While the cause of Alzheimer's is not known, such lifestyle changes, particularly if adopted sooner than later, could potentially prevent, delay the onset, or otherwise alter the course of the disease.

Only a handful of drugs have been approved by the U.S. Food and Drug Administration to treat Alzheimer's disease, and none of them stop or reverse the course of the disease. They have been shown to slow the worsening of the disease, but only for about six to twelve months on average, and only in about half the people who take them. Hundreds of drugs are currently in development for Alzheimer's, but it takes many millions of dollars and an average of thirteen years to bring a single drug from the concept stage to the market.

Even though the exact cause, or causes, of Alzheimer's is unknown, many details of the pathology have been worked out. The brain that allows us to breathe and move and think, and defines who we are as individuals, is an incredibly complex machine, made up of a vast network of cells that interconnect with one another as well as to the other types of cells in the body. Hundreds of chemical reactions take place within each cell and cell membrane and in the spaces between the cells where they connect and communicate with one another. These reactions are in delicate balance, and an excess or deficiency of one substance can upset this balance in such a way that the entire organ is affected. Insulin is one of those substances for which either an excess or deficiency can have profoundly negative effects on the organ or organs involved.

One of the prominent known features of Alzheimer's disease is the problem of insulin deficiency and insulin resistance in the brain. Just six years ago, in 2005, the term "type 3 diabetes" to describe Alzheimer's disease was coined by Suzanne de la Monte, M.D., of Brown University. Glucose is the primary fuel for our cells, including the cells of the brain, and insulin is required to allow glucose to enter our cells. As the ability to make insulin and use insulin becomes defective in the brain, cells malfunction and die off as the connections between these cells disintegrate, a process that appears to begin one or more decades before symptoms, such as memory loss and poor judgment, become apparent.

Glucose is in rather short supply in our bodies and should we go without food for more than a day, there is a backup plan to ensure we will not quickly die. Our brains and most other organs have the ability to use certain alternative fuels if glucose is not available. Without this capability, we would not exist today as a species. During starvation, we begin to tap into our stores of fat and release fatty acids, some of which are converted to ketone bodies that can cross the blood/brain barrier and provide an alternative fuel for our brain cells. Short of starving ourselves, there are other ways to provide ketone bodies. One way is to adhere to a strict ketogenic diet, a diet that is high in fat and relatively low in carbohydrate and protein. Another less challenging way to provide ketones is to consume foods that contain medium-chain fatty acids, which are easily absorbed from the intestine during digestion and are partially converted to ketone bodies in the liver. Even better, a doctor at the National Institutes of Health has developed a ketone ester that, when available, will make it simple to provide this precious fuel.

What all of this means for someone with Alzheimer's disease, or any number of other diseases that involve insulin deficiency and insulin resistance, is that a simple dietary intervention could bypass this fundamental problem and provide fuel to energy-starved cells, thereby keeping the brain alive and functioning.

My husband, Steve Newport, has early onset Alzheimer's disease. We were living with this disease for nearly seven years, and hope was fading when everything turned around. Since our lives changed for the better in May 2008 when Steve began consuming medium-chain fatty acids, I have communicated with a multitude of people dealing with Alzheimer's and other neurodegenerative diseases. One of the most distressing comments I have heard is that, upon relaying a diagnosis of probable Alzheimer's disease, some physicians will tell the person and his or her family that nothing can be done, that they should "go home and have a good life." Too many people take this kind of advice at face value and truly believe that there is nothing they can do. So they go home and cope the best they can with what appears to be a hopeless situation—a situation that is anything but good.

At the opposite extreme, knowing that doctors are human and don't have all the answers—I can say this because I am a doctor—there are people who refuse to accept a course of action that involves giving up. I am one of those people. The Internet makes it possible to look for answers to this complex disease, and I know of many people, some with no previous background in the sciences, who spend hours on the Internet nearly every day trying to learn whatever they can to help their loved one.

Were it not for the Internet, I wouldn't be writing this book. It was the "perfect storm" of my background as a physician, specifically one who cares for premature infants, having a husband with Alzheimer's, and a chance encounter with a press release on the Internet that led me to the discovery that changed our lives. This is our story and the story of ketones.

PART ONE

Falling into the Alzheimer's Abyss and Climbing Out

1

Steve Before the Fall

S teve is the love of my life. We have known each other for more than forty years and have been married for thirty-nine. For the first three decades, when I thought about our future, I always pictured that we would live long, full lives and grow very old together. Alzheimer's disease changed all of that, and much sooner than I would ever have expected.

We met in 1968 when he was eighteen years old, a freshman at Xavier University in Cincinnati, Ohio, and I was sixteen years old, a high school junior, on a snowy evening in the parking lot of Good Samaritan Hospital. He was working full-time on the evening shift in the housekeeping department to pay for college and was the first member of his family to graduate from college, receiving a bachelor of science and business administration (BSBA) in accounting. He tells everyone that he chose accounting because, during career day at his high school, a counselor asked him if he could count to ten. When Steve said yes, the man said, "Well, then you should be an accountant; you will make a lot of money." So for Steve it was accounting (he didn't make a lot of money!).

I grew up in a middle-class family in a suburb of Cincinnati, the oldest of five girls. My father was a machinist and roundhouse foreman for the Baltimore and Ohio Railroad (eventually Chessie System), while my mother stayed home with the children.

I first thought of becoming a doctor when I was ten years old after spending a night in that same hospital with a broken arm and "making rounds" on all the other children on the wing to find out why they were there. I saw children in traction and in wheelchairs with urine bags clipped to the side. A few months later, I found a biography in our school's bookmobile about Dr. Elizabeth Blackwell, the first American woman physician. Until then, I did not know women could be doctors, and after that, I knew what I wanted to do with my life.

THE PEACEFUL, EARLY YEARS

At the point in time that Steve and I met, I was working on the pediatric unit as a part-time nurses' aide after school and on weekends. I was very pleased to have such a job that would give me the opportunity to make sure that medicine was my calling, before embarking on the many years it would take to complete my education.

After my shift was over that life-altering evening, my friend Kathy and I arrived in the snow-covered parking lot to find a dead battery in my dad's Volkswagen Beetle. Kathy went inside to call for roadside assistance and came out with Steve. Steve was just a little taller than me and had a crew cut with honey blond hair and large, dark-rimmed glasses. He showed us how to kick-start the car and we were on our way.

About a year later, Steve invited me to share some pizza while I waited in the break room for my father to pick me up. It was the first time we had a real conversation, and I was struck by how comfortable I was speaking with him. A week later, he asked me to go to Xavier's Victory Dance. Of course, I said yes. We hit it off and were married in March of 1972. Steve had completed his bachelor's degree and found full-time employment in his field at the Comprehensive Care Centers of Northern Kentucky. By that time, Steve was twenty-two and I was twenty, a sophomore in the honors bachelor of arts program, majoring in pre-medicine, at Xavier. My advisor warned that getting married at that point could interfere with acceptance into medical school. However, I continued to work hard and, in many ways, found it easier to concentrate on my studies as we settled into married life.

We lived on the first floor of a 100-year-old "cracker box" house in Covington, Kentucky, across the Ohio River from Cincinnati, paying eighty dollars per month for rent, including utilities. We had three rooms with the entrance in the kitchen. The only way to get to the living room was through the bedroom. We lived across the street from a railroad track and a church with a bell tower that played the "Angelus" at 6 A.M., noon, and 6 P.M.

The first six months of our marriage were a challenge, as we found out how very differently we did things. Eventually we settled into a relationship in which we treated each other as equal partners. We took long walks around our neighborhood and car rides through the country and always had plenty to talk about.

Steve enjoyed his job at Comprehensive Care Centers, and as an accountant and office manager, he picked up a number of new skills, such as using a printing press and videotaping special events. One of his favorite tasks was managing the school buses for children with special needs. He stayed with this job for nine years as I completed medical school at the University of Cincinnati and the first two years of my pediatric residency at the Cincinnati Children's Hospital Medical Center. We had some rough times while adjusting to the extreme hours I had to spend in the hospital during my training, but managed to get through it with our marriage intact.

Some of Steve's most amazing qualities are his creativity and ability to fix almost anything. If we needed something and it didn't exist, he would "invent" it. My first experience with this was about a year after we began dating. I lived in a dormitory at Xavier University during my freshman year and continued to work two eight-hour shifts each weekend as a nurses' aide at Good Samaritan Hospital. After walking in fear to the bus stop in the very early morning for a few weeks, I used my accumulated savings to buy a used Chevy sedan for $110. Shortly thereafter, it became apparent that I had bought a lemon. There was a problem with the ignition, and it sometimes stalled and would not start up again. Steve taught me how to hot-wire the ignition, which was acceptable for a while, until I found myself on a steep hill in serious traffic under the hood of my car with a screwdriver. At the next opportunity, he connected the wires to a toggle switch, so that I could push a button to start my car instead of using a key. Nearly forty years later, this is standard on some new cars!

All the stories about how much study is required during medical school are absolutely true. I had thirty-five hours of classes per week and an extreme amount of reading to do every evening. It was difficult to concentrate on reading with a television in the room. So that we could spend more time together, Steve devised a precursor to the headset of today, a rudimentary earphone attached to the television with a wire so that we could sit side by side as he listened to TV while I studied.

Steve loved to fish and boat at that time. One of our first purchases as a married couple, even before buying a living room couch, was a ten-year-old, red and white, fifteen-foot runabout, with a fifty-horsepower engine and fold-down seats that we bought for $500. We spent many weekends on Lake Cumberland in southern Kentucky, and Steve reconstructed the canvas, windows, and zippers of an old tent into an amazing snap-down tent to cover our little boat. We spent days exploring the many inlets of the sixty-mile lake, and we spent nights anchored in a cove, sleeping in the boat on the gently rocking water. We awoke each morning to a quiet, glassy lake. These were the most peaceful years of our marriage and so special because of the time we spent together, leading the simple life.

HEADING SOUTH ON A NEW ADVENTURE

As an outdoor person, Steve tended to become depressed in the wintertime in Cincinnati with its gray skies. My father planned to move Florida when he retired, and Steve and I would often say to each other, "Why wait until we retire?" After the blizzard of 1978, with six straight weeks of snow and freezing rain on the ground, we were ready to leave Cincinnati for a warmer climate at the first opportunity. After vacationing in Charleston, South Carolina, and experiencing its beautiful beaches and historic charm, a position became available at the hospital for a third-year pediatric resident, and so we moved to Charleston in the summer of 1980. The ensuing year of training would give us an opportunity to decide if this was an area where we would like to settle before making a long-term commitment to a medical practice.

Leaving our families to go off on our new adventure was much harder than we expected. To further complicate things, Steve was not able to find a job in Charleston before the move. As we loaded up the rental truck, Steve became ill and I found myself driving the van down the steep incline from North to South Carolina. Steve often had fever blisters on his mouth, but along with this illness, he developed similar blisters around his eye, probably related to the extreme stress of leaving home. This type of infection is usually caused by herpes simplex type 1 virus. Little did we know at the time that these repeated infections might have consequences which would affect him profoundly later in life. Ruth Itzhaki, Ph.D., a researcher in Great Britain, and her associates have found evidence of the herpes simplex type 1 virus in the brains of people with Alzheimer's disease. This will be discussed in more detail in Chapter 15.

Discovering My Specialty

Charleston was a world apart from Cincinnati. As we arrived in the dark by rental van, we experienced a side of Charleston we missed on our prior idyllic visit. There were rundown tenements, deteriorating shacks side by side with larger newer homes, and the sickening smell of paper factories. Medical University Hospital was old and had ineffective window air conditioning and stifling elevators that moved at a snail's pace. Trying to get some sleep while on-call was a challenge, since four pediatric residents shared a co-ed sleep room with two rickety bunk beds. I was assigned to a parking lot five blocks from the hospital and, on several occasions during the monthly high tide, I had to wade into work, as the downtown area of Charleston, just a few feet above sea level, flooded. On the other hand, I had wonderful physician teachers and have never regretted changing programs. Above all, I learned that there may be more than one successful approach to treating the same disease. Patient management was sometimes very different in Charleston than in Cincinnati, but both approaches produced the same good outcome. I believe that the opportunity to witness this firsthand has helped me be more open-minded than the average physician, who completes the training process entirely in one facility.

I did some moonlighting, performing physical exams for the Head Start program in rural locations occupied by the very poor. I was dumbfounded to find one of these programs operating in an old house with holes in the floor and inoperable plumbing. Many of the tiny children had never been seen by a physician since leaving the hospital after they were born. It was common in Charleston County to see people of color occupying the roadsides, weaving and selling their beautiful handmade baskets.

When we first arrived in Charleston, Steve was in the running for a management job in the city's department of recreation. He was highly disappointed when he did not get that job or any other in his field. Our real estate agent suggested that he get a license and join his office, though at the time mortgage rates were peaking at 17 and 18 percent. Steve had no closings, and therefore no income, for eight months. He is an honest man who felt that it was only fair to point out the defects in a potential home. He had more success when he began to sell new condominiums on the Isle of Palms, a barrier island on the South Carolina coast, but he was not happy with his new career. We spent some of our leisure time on our little runabout, shrimping with a "cast net" and fishing for crab with chicken necks tied to a string. When we returned home, we boiled the shrimp and made a crabmeat and Swiss cheese quiche, one of the many Southern recipes we came to enjoy.

During our first year in Charleston, I realized that neonatology was my calling. There is nothing comparable to the experience of attending deliveries of fragile premature newborns, helping them take their first breaths, and then caring for them over the course of weeks, and even months, until they are big and strong enough to go home with their families. It took all the courage I could muster to tell Steve that I wanted to spend two more years in training as a neonatology fellow, instead of going into practice. He was surprised and somewhat disappointed, since the light at the end of the tunnel grew dim again, but as always, he told me to go for it and continued to provide the emotional support I needed.

Stay-at-Home Dad

One glitch in our relationship was our disagreement about having children. I fought the urge, believing that it would be best to finish my training first. However, Steve did not believe we should have children at all. He was concerned that my hours would be very unpredictable (he was right!) and this would make for a very unsettling home for small children. Neither of us wanted to use day care for the children we might have. In the fall of 1981, I was less than a year from completing my fellowship, and we had been married for nine years. I was dying to have my own baby and painfully aware that Steve was not feeling the same way. Much to my surprise, he came to me one day and said that he thought we should have children after all. We could provide stability for our children if he was a stay-at-home dad. This was a wonderful turn-about, and Julie was conceived shortly thereafter. Steve spent his last day as a real estate agent the day before Julie was born, and thus he embarked on a new path. He fully embraced his new job and had a maternal instinct that is foreign to most men. I remember sitting in the hospital bed with Julie the morning after her birth, and Steve came bouncing into the room, beaming, with a bag full of clothes for the baby. Joanna followed three and a half years later. Steve tells everyone that taking care of our little girls was the best job he ever had.

Just before Julie's first birthday, I finished my neonatology fellowship, and we decided to move to the even warmer climate of south Florida. I took a position with a group at Memorial Hospital in Hollywood, Florida, just north of Miami. The position required that I stay in the hospital for twenty-four-hour shifts every third night. As the group took on more hospitals and did not have sufficient numbers of doctors to cover all of them, I found myself staying in the hospital every other night for weeks on end. Within three years, the group grew to fifteen members covering five hospitals. I felt like a ping-pong ball bouncing from hospital to hospital and found very little satisfaction with my work, due to the lack of continuity with the little patients and their families and serious sleep deprivation.

Joanna was born in January 1986, and a year later we moved to the west coast of Florida, where I took a position as medical director of a brand new neonatal intensive care unit at Mease Dunedin Hospital near Clearwater. I was the first and only neonatologist for the next fifteen months. The job was very unpredictable and demanding during this period. I took care of the girls when I was home, but Steve had to be available every minute of the day and night should I receive an emergency call. Every minute counts when a baby is born and isn't breathing. When this happens, I literally have to drop everything to get to the hospital as soon as possible while the staff does their best to care for the little one until I arrive.

"Mr. Steve"

It is not easy having a spouse or a parent who is a neonatologist. It definitely takes a toll on family life. Steve and I were both on a very short leash, and when my partner joined me in 1989, it was a tremendous relief for both of us. We eventually added nurse practitioners to our practice as it grew. Steve began to work from home as the accountant, bookkeeper, and billing manager for our practice, often toiling well into the night after the girls were sleeping. He designed very detailed forms on the computer that were letter perfect. He made trips to the bank and post office every day and took care of whatever problems we had. He used an accounting program on his computer and completed the quarterly and annual tax returns and financial statements every year for many years without a hitch. In 1992, we decided to get help for him with the billing, and he built an office inside our three-car garage, complete with air conditioning. He screwed the walls and ceiling together, rather than using nails, to make it easier to dismantle down the road.

We built our home in Dunedin less than a block from Garrison-Jones Elementary School, and Steve became involved as the coordinator for volunteers in the school clinic, often filling in when someone could not make it. He designed and built several unique and fun games that were a hit at the annual Pioneer Day fundraiser. The children called him "Mr. Steve" and so that is a nickname I call him even now.

Steve loved to garden and had a knack for landscape design. He planned and planted the landscape and installed sprinkler systems at three homes we owned over the years, complete with special bubblers and other devices to make sure each plant got its share of water.

Around 1998, Steve developed an interest in kayaking and spent many afternoons rowing out to the small barrier islands. He usually took off from Honeymoon Island and kayaked out to the surrounding islands. He invented a device that he could attach to the kayak to keep it going straight while paddling on alternating sides and another device to hoist it up onto the back of his truck with ease.

> STEVE: "I was totally free. With my kayak, I would paddle as fast as my arms would go. I could stop to get a tan or take a walk on one of the little nearby islands. The first time, I went about three miles from the starting point. On the way back, a storm came up suddenly and there were big waves crashing over the kayak, capsizing the boat. I felt like Superman as I finally felt the sand under my feet and I literally dragged myself back on shore. I had to get back to pick Joanna up from middle school, and was late at this point. I called Mary, while I was on the ground for several minutes and out of breath."

After that, kayaking was a breeze.

When our older daughter became involved in music, Steve again became a volunteer, helping the youth symphony with their accounting and in any other way that he could. He was the kind of person you could ask to do something and know that it would get done. That held true for the work he did for our practice as well . . . at least before the effects of Alzheimer's disease set in.

2

Steve's Descent

STEVE: "I felt like I was diminishing somehow. Things were getting worse already, and I felt like I was unfulfilled. I felt that I was coming to an end, and there was nothing else there to fill in the empty parts. The job started being less important to me, as well as other matters, such as getting things done on time, and deadlines for tax reports. I feel like I would have been fired somewhere along the line, if I were working for anyone but my wife."

Flashback to 1980, Steve at age thirty:

"I felt like I was in a box and that everything had to be done 'just this way,' and it wasn't enough for me. Getting the reports done just didn't mean that much anymore. I did what I could do, but I was happy to quit Comprehensive Care Center. I think that they were saying, 'Good! He is going away.' I was free of the everyday stuff and happy to leave."

In retrospect, there may have been signs of memory issues as far back as age fourteen. Steve wanted to play football but couldn't catch on to the rules. He remembers the coach yelling at him, "Get in there; get in there!" He had no idea what he meant, so he quit. Steve also recalls, "I wanted to be an altar boy in the worst way, but couldn't get it right. I just couldn't remember the routine of what I was supposed to do after several Masses, and so the priest 'fired' me!"

In the early years of our marriage, Steve had terrific difficulty catching on to the simplest card or board games, and he would avoid playing whenever possible. If he was my partner in a game, I would have to help him with every move. I was mystified that someone who was otherwise so intelligent could have trouble playing cards. Were these very early signs that something was wrong? A recent study suggests that some people who develop dementia have a lifelong problem with memory (Flory, 2000). Another study showed that people who are at risk for Alzheimer's based on family history may have an abnormal PET (positron emission tomography) scan as early as twenty years of age (Reiman, 2004).

When we were in the process of moving to Charleston, Steve applied for a job as a manager in the city's recreation division with high hopes, which were dashed when they chose someone else.

STEVE: "I felt like this 'Yankee boy' was never going to fit in. I put an ad in the paper to do personal taxes and had two responses. I felt like I botched both of them. I took a job as a real estate agent, and that was a disaster."

Considering that this was 1980 and the mortgage interest rates were at an all-time high of up to 18 percent, it was no surprise that real estate didn't pan out for him. There were no commissions, no pay for eight months, but then he had some modest success selling condominiums on the Isle of Palms.

STEVE: "I saw no future in real estate for me. I was in the wrong job."

FREEFALLING

A few years later, Steve had some difficulty remembering to take the girls to various appointments and lessons while I was working. I often called to remind him of a specific appointment, and even then, a mere half hour later, he would sometimes forget. To remind himself, he began to hang notes on long pieces of tape in the doorway to his office, a tactic that was effective for several years. I thought this was just a "guy thing."

Then, between 2001 and 2002, he began having trouble with the payroll. Mistakes became more frequent, and I began to sit down with him to double-check his calculations. I thought it was simply that our practice was more complicated, with more employees, and he had managed to get it right for the previous twelve years.

> STEVE: "Thank God, there was someone else who could figure this out. I was just lost, freefalling. I think I knew I was lost by then. I should never have been an accountant anyway!!"

Steve used stalling tactics to avoid completing tax reports, spending time organizing his desk and shuffling things around in his office for several days before buckling down to get the job done. With his love of the outdoors, he often said he should have been a forest ranger.

As he was losing his accounting skills, Steve gradually taught me to use his computer program to write checks, do payroll, and print out various reports. At first, I learned all of this to help him, later to double-check and correct his work, and eventually to do the work myself. At that point, my practice was smaller, with just a few employees, so it was easier and less time-consuming for me to cut four checks or print out a 941 quarterly report than take records to another accountant to do.

Part of Steve's job routine was to go to the bank to make deposits and pick up the mail from our post office box every weekday. But then the mail, including collections from our medical billing, began turning up in odd places. When asked if there was any mail on a given day, Steve began to have difficulty remembering if he had even gone to the post office, which seemed rather odd.

Around the same time in 2002, Steve sunk into a severe bout of depression, another early sign that something was amiss. Our younger Joanna was a temperamental teenager at that point, and it seemed logical that his depression was somehow connected to a change in their relationship and behavior toward one another.

> STEVE: "I lost a lot of my confidence for doing everything. I had given up on having anything better. I was lost and basically became a cripple, because nothing was working."

Steve and I talked many times about what other job he might pursue, the possibility of going back to school, and other options, but by that time he could not garner the interest or energy to make such a change in his life. Even our once beautifully landscaped yard became overgrown and out of control.

We engaged in family counseling, and the psychiatrist evaluated Steve specifically with regard to his memory issues. He explained that it could be dementia, but that depression can also be the cause of memory issues. He prescribed antidepressants for Steve, who found some help with individual counseling. However, over the next year or so, it was apparent that depression was not the whole story.

SIGNS AND SYMPTOMS

In 2003, our lives took an unexpected turn as we made a very complicated decision to move from our home of sixteen years to Spring Hill, Florida, two counties north. Hospital mergers were affecting my practice in such a way that I would soon be expected to cover several hospitals, one more than an hour away. Spring Hill Regional Hospital had built a newborn intensive care unit (NICU) but didn't have a neonatologist to provide the necessary physician services. By taking this position, I would once again have the opportunity to open a new NICU and bring desperately needed services to a semi-rural community. Our daughters could continue to attend their respective schools. With deeply mixed emotions, we uprooted our family to move to Spring Hill.

Within months of moving, it became apparent that Steve was suffering from more than depression. I called our local Alzheimer's Family Organization and asked them to recommend a neurologist who cared for people with memory issues. We made an appointment, and the doctor evaluated Steve for various conditions that might cause his symptoms. He had blood work, an EEG (electroencephalogram), and an MRI (magnetic resonance imaging) study, all of which were normal at that time. The doctor performed a Mini-Mental Status Exam (MMSE), a 30-point memory test (Folstein, 1975). Nearly everyone who is normal scores a 29 or 30 on this very simple test; however, Steve only scored 23. The doctor advised us that this was consistent with possible Alzheimer's disease, but didn't want to put this label on Steve's condition just yet. To make such a diagnosis, it is important to see worsening over a period of time. The doctor was also reluctant to start a dementia medication such as Aricept at that point because it would mean a lifetime commitment to taking the drug. He explained that if a drug such as Aricept is started and then stopped, the person could experience a sudden deterioration from which he might not recover, even if the drug is restarted.

The doctor reevaluated Steve every six months, and in 2005, as his symptoms worsened and his MMSE score dropped to 21, the doctor decided to place him on Aricept, a cholinesterase inhibitor. Cholinesterase inhibitors slow the metabolic breakdown of acetylcholine, an important brain chemical involved in nerve cell communication. In 2006, after an evaluation at the Johnnie Byrd Alzheimer's Institute in Tampa, the drug Namenda was added to Steve's growing list of medications. Namenda appears to protect the brain's nerve cells against excess amounts of glutamate, a messenger chemical released in large amounts by cells damaged by Alzheimer's disease.

The following are some of the signs and symptoms that developed over the several years leading up to Steve's diagnosis of probable Alzheimer's disease.

Hoarding

Steve began to lose things in his garage and would spend hours looking for a tool or other object. You need to understand what his garage was (and still is) like! It is overwhelming to open the garage door to the disheveled mess. To start with, as you enter the doorway, there is an obstacle course. No matter how often we work together to create logical pathways, they disappear within a few days. There is no rhyme or reason to where items are located, as they are piled miscellaneously into giant heaps. Steve cannot part with anything, believing that someday he will need it. The problem is, when we do need one of these treasures, we can't find it, or if we do find it, it is rusted and nonfunctional or missing an important part. There are duplicates and triplicates of tools, many in their original wrapper or box.

Bringing all this "stuff" to Spring Hill was an expensive and very time-consuming nightmare, but Steve could not part with it. We stored it in the three-car garage of our temporary home and three-storage units, eventually moving it into the garage of our new house. We built a home with a separate detached garage for Steve and his things and an attached garage that was supposed to be for cars only. It was six months before there was room to put even one car in the attached garage. That is a lot of stuff! I have talked to others who have a spouse with dementia who have experienced a similar problem with hoarding, and I often wonder if this is a symptom of the disease for some people.

When Steve decided that he wanted to tow a trailer behind his truck to take things to the dump, he would spend hours looking in the garage for the hitch.

> STEVE: "'I've got to find it, dammit, where is it, why are you doing this to me? I've got to find it,' would go through my head the whole time. And that didn't help. It was the angry me. I was yelling at myself. Fatigue would finally make it stop and get the demons out of my head."

Sometimes he would go out and buy a duplicate of the item he couldn't find, and at other times, he would just give up doing the job. He would sometimes begin to look for "something" before I left for work and would still be searching when I came home much later in the day. At that point, he could not even remember at times what the "something" was that he was looking for, and he was extremely anxious and ready to pull his hair out. I told him repeatedly that he should just move on to something else instead of wasting so many hours looking for "something." On one occasion, I found the hitch he was looking for all day, disguised in green bubble wrap on the back seat of his truck—a logical place to keep it, but not a logical way to disguise it.

Losing his keys and wallet became a frequent occurrence. Steve would often unload his pockets in the garage, and his wallet and keys would disappear for days to weeks at a time. We could never be sure if they were simply lost or stolen. After moving to our newly built house, Steve lost his wallet three times in just over a month. The one credit card he still carried had to be cancelled three times, and we decided that it was time for him to give up the card. He carried a debit card while he was still driving so that he could purchase gas or stop at the grocery store, but when he stopped driving, it was time to retire that card as well.

> STEVE: "I couldn't find anything. I was so stymied, I didn't have a clue."

Attempting to organize his garage and searching for tools and other items became Steve's full-time job.

Kayaking

After moving to Spring Hill, Steve bought himself a second, longer, sleeker kayak that he ordered from a catalog, with all intentions of exploring the new waters. But he began to spend a lot more time reading magazines about kayaking, and talking about kayaking, than actually getting out and doing it.

Driving

Before Alzheimer's disease set in, Steve could find any place almost by instinct; he could "follow his nose," as we often said. When we moved to Spring Hill in June 2003, a small town with just a few main arteries in an easy-to-learn north/south and east/west pattern, Steve had tremendous difficulty finding his way around. He was often confused about whether we were heading north or south and which street we were on. He did manage to learn the way to his favorite places—Home Depot, Sam's Club, and a few others—but if he had to go a little beyond familiar territory, he panicked.

We discovered that Steve could no longer read a map when he had to drive himself to see an endodontist about thirty minutes away. The office staff had to "talk him in" after he drove around randomly in the general area, hoping he would find the office, and he was forty-five minutes late. I was at the hospital that day, and when he left the office, I stayed on the phone with him to help him get home.

After that episode, Steve limited how much driving he did by himself, even to familiar places. When we were riding together, he continued to drive most of the time for a while, though he often forgot where we were headed and asked me which way to turn. I began to call him "Mr. Opposite" because he would turn left if I told him to turn right. This phenomenon occurred with other situations in which he would do the opposite of what he meant to do. It was as if he figured he had a fifty-fifty chance of getting it right, and he would take that chance, rather than endure the embarrassment of asking again what he was supposed to do. I began to drive if we were headed anywhere that was the least bit complicated. Finally, it was a relief to both of us when I decided to take over all the driving.

One of the most frightening things that happened as the disease worsened led to the decision that Steve must stop driving. Joanna took a road trip by herself to visit a girlfriend in Tallahassee and broke down by the side of the expressway, about four hours away from home. The car was towed to a nearby gas station. A friend, who was a car mechanic, volunteered to ride with Steve to help her repair the car. I was on call at the hospital and couldn't ride along. After the job was completed, Joanna's friend jumped in the car with her, leaving Steve alone in his truck to follow her. About the time I expected to hear him pull into the driveway, I received a phone call from Steve advising me that he was in Jacksonville, several hours in the wrong direction on the opposite coast of Florida. It was about 9:30 P.M. and dark. I asked why he hadn't gotten off and turned around sooner. He said that he "couldn't get over" and missed each of the exits the entire way to Jacksonville.

I stayed with Steve on the cell phone until I was sure he was headed west on I-10 and then called him about an hour later to make sure he headed south on I-75, fearing that my next call would be from Cincinnati! He managed to exit in the wrong location again, and we decided that he should spend the night in a hotel that he spotted. He started out at daylight the following morning and stayed with me on the phone until he arrived in our driveway, just before I needed to leave for the hospital. I was very happy to see his face and wondered what would have happened if he did not have a cell phone. I think about how many families lose their loved ones this way, with no cell phone available, and the extreme panic they must endure until they are found.

When Steve arrived home, he handed me the keys, and we mutually decided that driving was no longer an option for him.

STEVE: "So they got one more bad driver off the road!"

The decision to stop driving affects not only the victim of the disease, but also the spouse and/or other members of the family, who must pick up additional driving responsibilities, take over errands, and get the person to wherever he or she needs to go. I remember thinking about the ramifications of how I would be affected when Steve could no longer drive and dreading that day. Every errand would now become my job, I would have to take him to all of his many appointments, and this would all have to happen on my relatively few days off, contributing even more to the general overload I was already experiencing. For this reason, I can understand why it is often so hard for the family to take the keys away. It is even considerably more difficult when the person is oblivious to their illness and doesn't comprehend why driving is no longer a viable option. Fortunately, we did not have that problem with Steve. He didn't like it, but he knew that he had to give up driving for his safety and that of everyone else on the road.

Reading

An avid reader, Steve often spent time in the sun, reading one novel after another. His favorite authors over the years were Stephen King and Clive Cussler. He read through the newspaper every day and never missed the comic strips, a common topic of discussion at the breakfast table. As he began to have difficulty remembering the day of the week and the date, he used the newspaper as a reminder, until eventually that didn't help and he no longer cared.

Until a couple of years ago, I bought novels for him for Christmas and his birthday, but they began to pile up unread. At first I thought he had simply lost interest or perhaps had too much trouble retaining the plot line or comprehending what he was reading. Even with the comics, he would pick up the paper, look at it for a few seconds, and then put it down. He said they just weren't funny anymore, and so he stopped reading even the simplest material.

I assumed for a long time that it was a problem of comprehension, but eventually I learned that there was a physical reason for this problem. I had a brief insight into Steve's visual disturbance during a return visit to the Johnnie Byrd Alzheimer's Institute in May 2008. He was waiting in a hallway for me to come out of the lady's room, and when I joined him, he pointed to a thermostat on the wall and told me that it was "jumping around."

Steve tells me now that he could not read because the words appeared to be moving around erratically. It was impossible to read anything with so much movement when he tried to focus on the words.

> STEVE: "The words would become little squares, like pixels on a TV screen, and move rapidly in all different directions. I would see the word in a block and then it would go someplace else. It was not under my control at all. I don't think people would notice that my eyes were moving. It was just inside of me. It was four, five, or six blips or blocks. This would happen and then suddenly it would stop. There is no name to describe it."

The closest comparison I can think of would be during bad weather, when the picture on a digital TV breaks up, like a cubist painting, and the blocks rearrange. We visited an ophthalmologist and were reassured that there was no anatomic reason related to Steve's eyes for his reading problem.

Conversation

As the disease progressed, Steve found it more and more difficult to have an ordinary conversation, even with me. His jaw would often tremor as he tried to find the words.

> STEVE: "I would stumble over words. I couldn't get the words out. I would stumble over finding the words to make some sense, and I just gave up. I don't think I could remember what I was trying to say for more than twenty seconds. I was probably able to retain a little bit more of what someone was saying to me, but it didn't stay with me. I would get out the first few words, then I would say, 'What was I saying?' and it would be gone, like chasing a rabbit."

Steve participated less and less in conversation. He did not like being in a situation with a lot of people.

> STEVE: "Who in the world would want to talk to me? I was not comfortable with speaking to adults in those situations."

I am the kind of person who needs to ventilate when I get home from work, and at the beginning of our marriage, Steve would cut me off and tell me he wasn't really interested in hearing all of that. However, I convinced him that I needed this time from him to help reduce the stress, and Steve agreed to put up with fifteen minutes of a nonstop rundown of my day, after which I could let it all go and move on. I am sure he sometimes tuned me out while pretending to listen, but nonetheless, it was very therapeutic for me. On the other hand, Steve would often listen intently, make appropriate comments, and provide good advice about various problems. As the Alzheimer's disease worsened, his comments often did not relate to the conversation, and I felt like he was on a different wavelength. At that point, I began to feel a sense of loneliness. His personality was fading, and he was going away. He seemed more and more like a stranger to me, and I felt like I was slowly, but surely, losing my husband.

Listening

When I would say something to Steve, even a short sentence, as clearly as possible, he would often cup his ears and say, "Blah, blah, blah, blah, blah?" which indicated that I needed to repeat, sometimes more than once. I do not think he had an actual hearing problem, but rather a problem with comprehension. He doesn't remember doing this, and so he can't explain now what was going on in his mind, but this rarely happens now.

It can be very stressful on a spouse to repeat virtually everything you say. At first I thought Steve was deliberately ignoring me or simply not paying attention, but eventually I learned to accept that the words were just not sinking in. I also came to realize that it helps to get his attention, make eye contact, and keep it simple. Now, if I need Steve to do a series of things, such as getting dressed to go out, it helps to suggest he do one thing, such as picking out a shirt, and when that is done, suggest the next step—picking out a pair of pants—and then help him find a good match.

A recent study showed that people with dementia do not like to be spoken to as if they are children and are more likely to resist assistance if approached in that manner (Williams, 2008). However, it is not easy to keep it simple and still speak to someone at an adult level.

Cooking and Eating

Steve was a creative cook and frequently made meals for our family for many years. In the beginning of our marriage, he bought an encyclopedia of Chinese cooking and learned to use a wok in a skillful manner. He liked to make a breakfast of eggs and add whatever was leftover from the day before. He often added ingredients that weren't in the recipe, and his experiments were nearly always successful.

After we moved to Spring Hill, he cooked less and less often. When I was working, he sometimes put a boxed meal into the microwave and forgot it was there. I would find it much later when I got home or even the following day.

Our temporary home in Spring Hill had an electric stove, but after experiencing a three-day blackout related to a tropical storm, we decided to put a gas stove into our new home, so that we could continue to cook should a similar situation occur. In the summer of 2005, when we were building, it was becoming more obvious that Steve's memory problems were progressing. Shortly after we moved in, I came home late one evening and noticed an unusual odor. Steve had turned the knob off in the wrong direction, and with the stove on the lowest setting, propane was leaking. As we aired out the house, I wondered about the wisdom of installing a gas stove.

Fast forward to two years later, early in the summer of 2007, after another long day at work, I arrived home in the late evening to the odor of something rotting. This time, it smelled as if something died in the attic above the kitchen. Our kitchen and family room are one large area, where we spend most of our time in the mornings and evenings. A pest-control technician, who came into our house for an unrelated reason, concurred that something must have died, but stated that, worst case, it should dry up in a week. About thirty-six hours later, I decided to cook something on the stove and realized that, once again, Steve had used the stove and turned the knob off in the opposite direction (Mr. Opposite!), allowing the gas to leak. Fortunately, our bedroom is on a separate air conditioner zone. Since then, Steve rarely cooks and never without direct, by-his-side supervision. His "cooking" is limited to cutting things up for me and stirring the pot while I'm beside him working on something else.

Late that summer, we were into one of our busiest months ever with deliveries and admissions to the NICU. We had taken a very nice vacation to California, but as is often the case with hospital-based physicians, if you take time off, you have to make up the days later in the month. For the next twenty-one days, I had only three nights off, and virtually every day, I worked late into the evening or was called back before I could get dinner ready. Prior to our vacation, Steve was usually capable of putting a meal together for himself. When I finally arrived home, I would ask if he had eaten, and his answer was always in the affirmative and that he wasn't hungry. However, at the end of August, he began to look rather thin, and we discovered that he had lost ten pounds over three weeks. I started looking for evidence that he had eaten dinner, and finding none, I realized that he was no longer cooking for himself for lunch or dinner.

Sudden weight loss can signal the beginning of a serious decline in Alzheimer's disease from which the person never recovers. Steve had been placed on Aricept and Namenda several years earlier, with the hope that these medications would slow his decline and eventually something better would come along. It seemed like new drugs to treat Alzheimer's were just over the horizon, with so very many drug studies in progress. Steve's doctor changed him from Aricept to Exelon, another cholinesterase inhibitor, to see if it would make a difference, but there was no noticeable effect.

With Steve's ten-pound weight loss, I began to lose hope that a medication would come along that would hold off the inevitable decline. At age fifty-five, I fully expected to be a widow by sixty. I tried to mentally prepare myself that I would very likely spend the later years of my life without Steve, whom I naturally expected to grow old with. We often talked about traveling, as many do, when they retire. But I know that, if I am fortunate enough to have Steve still with me when I retire, travel will be virtually impossible. One's vision of the future changes rather significantly when Alzheimer's disease enters the picture. Lois Walsh, a caregiver of a spouse with Alzheimer's, expresses that so well in the following poem:

LOSSES

I am lying here crying, alone with you beside me.
Crying for that little girl and the woman I am.
Covered with years and weighted down with words.
The little girl was happy, believing in Santa,
Til death do us part, and words like forever and always.
I am crying for her losses: Lost dreams, lost love, lost time,
    lost health, but most of all lost hope.

Thereafter, I made sure Steve had a very good breakfast and prepared a lunch that could sit out on the table, with the hope that he would notice it and eat it. Sometimes he did and sometimes he didn't. He had a habit of peeking into the refrigerator to nibble, so I kept plenty of fruit and yogurt available to tide him over until I was home and could cook. I had to work out a plan to have someone stop by when I was at the hospital, usually our younger daughter, to make sure he had his lunch.

During the last couple of years before starting the coconut oil, Steve often ate ten to twelve pieces of fruit throughout the evening. Since learning about the possible problem of glucose (blood sugar) uptake into neurons that occurs with Alzheimer's disease, I wonder now if his consumption of so much fruit was the result of a craving for glucose (Klein, 2008; Zhao, 2008; de la Monte, 2005). Steve had normal fasting blood sugars on several occasions, ruling out diabetes as the source of his weight loss and fruit consumption.

The reason I bring this up now is that the intense craving for something sweet, in this case fruit, could be a symptom of Alzheimer's disease and other neurodegenerative diseases that share this pathology. My maternal grandmother died at age ninety-three of "senile dementia," which was most likely Alzheimer's disease. She would put multiple layers of clothes on and then complain that it was hot! Like Steve, she seemed to have a craving for sweets. She would drink many cups of tea in a day's time and would add as many as a dozen teaspoons of sugar to each cup, complaining that it wasn't sweet enough. Another relative in my family, who also died with dementia, had a problem with alcohol, drinking at least a gallon of beer a day and an unknown quantity of whiskey. It has occurred to me that perhaps some cases of alcoholism could be more about a craving for the sugar in the wine, beer, or hard liquor than the alcohol. The alcoholic beverage just happens to be the source of the "carbohydrate of choice" that person has latched on to.

I came across a study showing that people who drink alcohol to excess develop dementia seven years sooner than those who don't. Could it be that the craving for alcohol is an early symptom of, and not necessarily a causative factor for, the onset of the disease? Of course, the excess alcohol wouldn't be beneficial to the neurons—quite the contrary.

Wondering if this sugar craving is a common symptom for Alzheimer's disease, I started a thread on one of the Alzheimer's message boards, asking if others noticed this about their Alzheimer's disease loved ones, and sure enough, many responded in the affirmative:

TR: "My loved one never ate sweets, but craves them now . . ."

SC: "Sweets are the food of choice for Charlie . . . who has been diagnosed with garden-variety Alzheimer's disease. He grazes on them throughout the day but finds additional room for three small-ish meals. The number of calories he consumes in a day must be astronomical."

SN: "My mother died weighing eighty-five pounds. Toward the end, her doctor told us anything we could get her to eat was fine.

We concentrated on sweets as she loved them and, in fact, the last thing I fed her the night before she died was a bowl of ice cream . . . Mom loved candy bars, ice cream, cookies, sweet and sour chicken, and her wine at night."

TL: "OMG [Oh, my God]!!! My mother is a junk-food junkie . . . I have never seen anything like it . . . Mom has vascular dementia and is in the sixth stage . . . My mom will eat between a half and one gallon of ice cream in a day. No lie! Then she will eat pastries and cookies and whatever else she can get her hands on . . . One day mom bought four boxes of Edy's coconut ice bars that come six to a pack. She ate three boxes for a total of eighteen ice bars in about four hours . . . My mother would never eat that way before vascular dementia . . . Oh, my mom weighs 145 pounds and she never gains weight."

CJC: "My mom, age eighty-five, cannot get enough sweets. I bake dozens and dozens of cookies every other day and she eats them as fast as I bring them. At first, I thought she just liked my baking . . . Now I can't keep up with her. She will sit by the kitchen table for hours on end, eating cinnamon rolls, donuts, cookies, cake . . . and everything has to have butter on it. I mean everything! She eats all this and I still can't get an extra pound on her."

DS: "My husband has vascular dementia and will eat two to three dozen cookies a day and one to two bowls of ice cream at night. He demands sugary cereal for breakfast and peanut butter and jelly sandwiches for snacks in addition to regular meals. He never gains a pound. It seems pointless to me, but he also takes Lipitor for his cholesterol. Can't imagine why he has high cholesterol!"

GT: "Boy, does she [crave sugar], ice cream, cinnamon rolls, waffles with syrup, anything sweet! Maybe it's the calories to compensate for the endless wandering and nervous rubbing and the chewing she does all the time."

YH: "I have FTD [frontal temporal lobe dementia] and crave sweets 24/7! No matter how hard I try not to eat them, I have to find something, even if it is a can of cake frosting."

TC: "My mom never ate sweets. She's Italian and the sweetest thing she ever enjoyed was anise! About six or so years ago she started buying and hoarding candy bars. Now, she will eat as many as I let her. I understood it to be the taste buds going and sweets being the easiest thing to taste."

And on and on! I was surprised at how many people responded in the affirmative to this question about craving sweets. The problem involving the use of glucose in the brain by people with Alzheimer's disease will be discussed at length in Chapter 14.

Life in Slow Motion

There is a book called *The 36-Hour Day* (2001) by Nancy Mace and Peter Rabins. When a family member has Alzheimer's disease, at some point life goes into slow motion. Things that most of us do without thinking can require an extreme amount of time for someone with Alzheimer's, and the designated caregiver also begins to spend an exorbitant amount of time helping that person accomplish the smallest of tasks. You no longer have to worry about just dressing yourself, for example, but you have to guide the other person to find appropriate clothing and make sure each piece of clothing is put on successfully.

As hard as Steve tries to get his underwear on, even after carefully studying the clothing, more than half the time, items will end up backwards. Then he may decide that is not okay, take them off, and try again; or after several attempts with the same outcome, he will give up and decide that it is okay to just have them on backwards. He may or may not be in the mood to let me help him. If it is a situation in which it really doesn't matter, then I can let it go. If we are going out of the house, I know that it will cause a problem when he has to use a public restroom, so I have to intervene and convince him to let me help.

After the underwear is in place, the next undertaking is to get his shirt on. Once again, the first attempt is usually unsuccessful; the shirt goes on backwards or an arm lands in the neck hole. As he pulls the shirt off, he turns it inside out; then I take it and turn it right side out; and he tries again, sometimes more than once, until he finally gets it on right. The same process happens with the pants, the socks, the shoes. I want to let him do as much for himself as possible, and yet it is agonizing to watch this process and not intervene, not try to speed it up somehow, particularly when there is a deadline to get out the door and be somewhere.

On several occasions I thought I would be very efficient and get Steve completely dressed and ready to go out the door before taking care of myself. I took a quick shower and exited the bathroom, only to discover that he had completely undressed himself in the interim, and the best laid plans had once again gone astray. It is very much like taking care of a young child, except that, over time, the child learns how to take care of him or herself, but the person with Alzheimer's disease will become even less capable of doing so. The worst part is that Steve is fully aware that he was able to do all of this at one time and now he cannot. I can only try to imagine how humiliating and frustrating this must be for someone who was so competent in the past and now is so dependent. Another Lois Walsh poem perfectly sums up the caregiver's quandary.

LIFE ON HOLD

Dum da da dee dum. Diddle diddle de dum.
Thank you for your patience.
Life on hold.
Waiting.
There are 1,646 people ahead of you.
Estimated wait time is four years.
Thank you for your patience and have a nice day.

As the disease evolves, a time comes when the caregiver has to keep a constant lookout for the person with Alzheimer's and often has to think for them: about what they are trying to do and how to do it, what they want and how to get it. I try to get up a couple of hours early to have some time to myself and get some important, or not so important, things done before Steve wakes up. I do this because, from the moment he enters the kitchen, the gears shift and it becomes all about him and what he needs. He cannot simply pour himself a cup of coffee and get himself something to eat, no matter how simple the meal would be, much less find his medication and take the right pills. So this has now become my job.

Steve wants so much to help me, and yet, when he does, it takes considerably more time to get the job done. For example, he likes to help with the dishes, but gets confused about whether the dishes in the dishwasher are clean or dirty. He will decide that it is time to work on the dishes when I am not ready to get involved. Even with a sign on the counter above the dishwasher that says "Clean," he will pick up dirty dishes from the sink and add them to the dishwasher instead of clearing out the clean dishes first.

Steve wants to take the garbage out, but needs my help to complete the task, since he can't remember where the replacement bags are for the cans and how to get them back on the liners and the liners back into the kitchen garbage cans. Inevitably, this doesn't happen when I would like it to happen. He decides he wants to do it and I must stop short with whatever I am working on to get involved in his project. If I let him try to carry this out on his own, I will witness his frustration with trying to figure out this task that should be so simple and yet is so complex for him. It becomes easier for me to "help" him, so that he can feel like he is doing something to "help" me.

In the spring of 2008, Steve and I were driving to Tampa for an appointment and he turned to me and asked, "Who sired Julie?" I asked what he meant, "Who was Julie's father?" He said, "Yes." I said, "Who do you think it was, the milkman? You are her father, Steve." He told me that he had no recollection of Julie as an infant or of taking care of her, even though he was her primary caretaker when I was working. This was a startling revelation to me and the first hint of a time, possibly in the not-too-distant future, when he might not recognize Julie or her sister, and perhaps not even recognize me. Lois Walsh expresses this anguish so eloquently in this poem.

FAILURE

I am learning there comes a time when you can no longer
Reason, argue, teach, correct, or explain.
A very hard lesson when I have worn many hats of a very
    independent woman:
Wife, mother, nurse, artist, poet.
It is my nature to fix things, make things right, keep everything
    on even keel.
Impossible then and even more so now.
The journey started ten years ago, it's just now getting difficult.
I will forgive myself for seeking perfection.
I am swimming against the tide, trying to keep my head above
    water
But drowning in pools of sadness.
Trying to keep normalcy but failing,
Still wanting to reason, argue, teach, correct, or explain.

Gait

Steve was on the wrestling team in high school and has always been very strong physically. In the summer of 2007, he remarked that he was no longer able to run, and by winter of 2008, his walking gait had become slow and deliberate, as he picked his feet up higher than normal. A nurse practitioner remarked at one of his evaluations that this gait was typical of many people with Alzheimer's disease. It is a sign that the disease process is affecting the areas of the brain that control movement. As Steve "worked" around the yard, he often seemed to be in slow motion with a lack of energy, accomplishing very little. He spent a great deal of time trying to "organize" his collection of garden hoses and left a snaky mess covering the walkways around the garden, making it difficult to navigate for anyone and even more so for someone in his condition.

Whistling

While many people like to sing, Steve enjoys whistling and actually can carry quite a tune. He likes to talk to the birds, often trying to mimic their calls. For many years, he had medleys of songs that he whistled while working. It made me happy to hear him whistling because I knew that he was feeling good.

As Alzheimer's set in and worsened, his repertoire diminished to the point where he would often whistle the same eight notes over and over and over from the Johnny Cash song "Because you're mine, I walk the line." I thought I was going to go out of my mind listening to these same notes, now more like a nervous tic than a happy tune.

We recently rediscovered how much Steve loves music when I overheard him whistling along to a Barry Manilow song. Almost daily now, he spends time listening to one or more of his favorite artists or sound tracks, such as *Fiddler on the Roof* or *South Pacific,* and it is amazing how many of the tunes he can whistle along to. If he is in a bad mood, putting on the music will nearly always bring him around to a happier place.

Dealing with Shoes

Some things that happen when a person has Alzheimer's disease are funny and seem inexplicable. For well over a year, Steve often walked around with just one shoe on, usually the left shoe. Sometimes it was just one sock and no shoes. There would often be a pile of all left shoes in the closet or by the door to the garage, with no right shoe in sight. I would point this out to him, but he didn't care enough to correct the situation. When we shopped and he spotted the shoe department, he would ask to buy another pair or two of flip-flops and I would usually humor him. We would also buy four or five pairs of the same shoe style at the same time. I thought that, if we had enough of the same type of shoe, we would be able to find a match when we needed to, as when we were walking out the door to go somewhere, right? Wrong! This was not quite so funny when we had a deadline to get somewhere and we could not find a match in the house, even with so many pairs of shoes.

Where were all the right shoes? Apparently, when he was "organizing" out in his garage, he would take off the right shoe and sock and leave them there. So, periodically, when there were no more pairs left in the house, I would send him deep into his garage, and if he spotted a shoe, I would tell him to throw it out to me. We would find six or seven shoes, and then we were all set for a while.

There is a phenomenon in which people with more atrophy on one side of the brain than the other will begin to ignore the non-dominant side. Since Steve is left-handed, he ignored the right side. On his last MRI, he did have more severe atrophy in the hippocampus and the amygdala on one side of the brain compared to the other. The hippocampus is important for its role in the formation of long-term memories, one of the first areas affected by Alzheimer's disease; the amygdala is involved in many brain functions, including emotion, learning, and memory. One physician told me about a lady who put lipstick on just one side of her mouth. Strange things happen with this disease!

These days, Steve keeps his pairs of shoes together most of the time and wears two shoes nearly all the time. However, we still aren't perfect. Recently, he put on two different colors of socks and two different shoes. One could say it was my fault because there were two pairs of each to choose from where he was dressing. I find that if he sits on the edge of the bed and two different pairs of shoes are available, he will inevitably mix and not match. It helps to have only one pair of shoes available when he is dressing.

Taking Things Apart and Losing the Pieces

Steve used to fit the definition of Jack-of-all-trades, able to fix almost anything with little or no instruction. For many years, he did much of the work on our cars, and he could perform most of the repairs around the house. He even had the nerve to open the computer when it stopped functioning and was usually able to figure out what was wrong and get it working again, to my utter amazement.

Steve told me early in our marriage that this was his method for fixing things. This habit became a problem a few years ago when he could perfectly well take things apart, but would then become distracted, put them aside, and misplace one or more of the pieces. They would find their way into a pocket or some container of odds and ends, and were later deposited in a peculiar location, never to be found again.

We have gates leading out of our courtyard that have special locks. When Steve had trouble getting the key into the lock, he decided, instead of spraying a lubricant into it, to remove the entire lock from the gate. He put the pieces into a small container, which also contained parts from the tracks for the cover of our small exercise pool. The container mysteriously disappeared. Steve insisted that it was "stolen," even after I suggested that, if someone was going to steal something, they would be more likely to go for something valuable. A common symptom of Alzheimer's disease is to believe that misplaced items have been stolen. The person does not remember moving the items, and the idea that they were stolen somehow seems more logical to them. Even now, as of this writing, if something is missing, Steve will tell me that "they" are stealing us blind! But he cannot tell me exactly who "they" are.

On one of those long workdays in August 2007, Steve began to vacuum the bedroom carpet for me as I left for the hospital. I arrived home at about 8 P.M. after a very difficult day. It was raining, I was hungry, and my mind was focused on what to make for dinner. As I pulled into the garage, I noticed the purple parts of my Dyson vacuum cleaner distributed around the garage. I hate to use the word "love" in reference to a household appliance, but if it is possible to love an appliance, then I love my Dyson! I must admit that, with the perfect storm of fatigue, hunger, and the sight of my vacuum cleaner in that condition, I lost it.

I know that Steve can't help doing these things. I have been told and have read that I need to maintain patience for this reason, but there are times when it is virtually impossible for me to be a saint, and this was one of them. His explanation for this tragedy was that the inside of the canister looked grimy and he decided to clean it. He said he would put it back together tomorrow, but fearing that pieces would be misplaced and knowing that he would not be able to figure it out, I began to reassemble the vacuum. It did not take long to realize that the canister itself was completely missing. It was not unusual for things to disappear to the yard or to Steve's chaotic garage. It was raining and getting dark, so I spent the next hour (still very hungry) searching every conceivable location indoors and out. At last, the canister was found, enclosed in a tall metal cabinet out in his garage. Steve had no recollection of putting it there, much less could he explain why. Lois Walsh's poem expresses the caregiver's yearning for patience.

MY PRAYER

I feel I am losing both the battle and the war,
Trying to keep things normal but nothing's normal anymore.
Trying to live in the present with a willing heart but
Feeling myself slowly falling apart.
Crying and screaming then walking away.
Taking deep breaths, stopping to pray.
Please God give me strength to continue on this day.

In the end, the pieces all came together, and, voila, the vacuum was back in service. It was many months before I could look back at that day and smile, not only because of what happened to the vacuum, but also because of the way that I lost it with Steve. That is definitely not the only time I've lost it, but the intensity was such that it sticks in my mind. Part of this phenomenon of losing it for me has to do with thoughts about how I have lost the man who was my partner for so many years, who could do so much, so well, replaced by someone who takes things apart when I am not looking. I become obsessed with the additional cost of my time, when my time is already so stretched to the max. I expect to come home, make dinner for us, eat, relax together for a short time, then go to sleep, and instead, I find myself on a hunting expedition in the rain, dinner delayed, and no time to relax afterward because it is now time to go to bed and sleep is more important.

But by that point, sleep was no longer simple. I began having difficulty getting to sleep and staying asleep, often waking at 5 A.M., thinking about how our lives had changed, how bleak the future appeared, going over and over all of this in my mind, reviewing the past, looking for a reason. Was it something Steve had done or not done? Was it something I had done wrong, something I could have changed if I had only recognized the illness soon enough?

Managing the Yard

Steve has always loved gardening, and he designed and planted some very beautiful, unique landscapes at several of the homes we lived in. He even installed sprinkler systems with special gizmos for the various types of plants. My favorite spot was at our home in Dunedin, where he planted red bromeliads around a very old oak tree and the ring of plants slowly spread over the years we were there.

If he spotted bulbs sitting by someone's garbage cans, he would ring the doorbell and ask if he could have them. When we visited amusement parks, he would pocket seeds that he found on the ground. He would plant these in plastic pots, make them grow, and use them in various gardens around the house. He kept the grass neatly trimmed and edged and the gardens nicely weeded and mulched.

As Alzheimer's disease set in, Steve began to lose interest, and the grass grew too tall, the edging went by the wayside, and the gardens became overgrown. I suggested that we get help with this, but he insisted he could handle it. So we began to work together on the yard, and I found that I actually enjoy gardening, even if my hands do get dirty.

By the spring of 2007, Steve was no longer able to design a layout, so that became my job, and we shopped together at the garden store to pick out plants that we both thought would work well together. I put the plants in pots in the spot they were to be planted and Steve dug the holes, put the plants in, and added mulch around them. It wasn't the neatest garden, but we both felt good about it. On the other hand, Steve wanted to cut and trim the grass. He decided to get his John Deere tractor up and running, and instead, pieces, such as the air filter and gaskets, went missing and the grass kept growing. We hired a lawn service "temporarily." Steve was very critical of their work and was certain he could do it better; however, the tractor sat in the garage unused.

In 2008, we quickly learned that Steve needed significantly more supervision with planting the courtyard. This time, I had to tell him exactly where to dig the hole and stay with him to complete the digging of even one hole, since he would become distracted midway through and wander away. I would suggest that he make the hole deeper or wider, and instead he would begin to fill the hole in. He couldn't seem to see the plant right in front of him to put into the hole, and couldn't see the gaps around the plant when he tried to fill in around it. We were both frustrated and very sad, since this brought home the magnitude of the deterioration that had taken place in the intervening year. Needless to say, it was my turn to pick up the shovel.

After the dietary intervention, Steve wanted to cut the grass again himself. We stopped by a nearby mower shop, and I asked if they made house calls to fix tractors. They took the tractor to their shop, replaced the missing parts, and found that Steve had put the gasoline in the oil tank and the oil in the gasoline tank. Once it was home, Steve proudly got on the tractor and cut the yard on his own for the first time in several years. The grass may be at several levels and the trimming could be neater, but he is doing something that he enjoys and can do to contribute to the upkeep of the house. And he has stopped tinkering with the parts.

Dealing with Depression

By the winter of 2008, Steve had been living with depression for at least eight years. His early memory problems were attributed to depression, but antidepressants didn't take away the problems that led to depression, nor did his memory improve. In fact, the problems continued to worsen, and he also had to endure the side effects related to the medication. He was first placed on Zoloft and then Wellbutrin, but in the summer of 2005, when we were building our new home and in the months following, the depression clearly worsened. By this time, Steve was no longer capable of doing anything but the simplest accounting work. He spent an exorbitant amount of time in his garage, accomplishing nothing. He was sad most of the time.

When he didn't know I was watching, he would often talk to himself and it did not sound like happy talk. When we sat down to discuss this, he told me there was a voice in his head that was constantly berating him, much like his father had berated him as a child. He said this voice was his own voice, but sometimes felt like his father's voice. This voice was telling him that his life was pointless and we would all be better off if he did himself in. He finally admitted that he was so obsessed that he had thoughts of suicide at least sixty times a day. As soon as possible, I got him to his psychiatrist, who added a second antidepressant. With the new medication and regular counseling, his mood improved, and he said "the voice" was gone, but he was still far from happy.

By the winter of 2008, his depression was growing worse again. Steve told me that he felt like he was dying and had no future, so "why bother." He promised that he was not going to try to kill himself, but he was sad much of the time, and became quiet and bland, rarely laughing or even smiling. We had a Christmas party at our home for the nurses I work with, and some of them commented later that he seemed lost and aloof. He avoided conversation and even avoided being present in the room where the party was going on.

3

Looking for Clinical Trials

In March 2008, we returned to the Johnnie Byrd Alzheimer's Institute in Tampa to have Steve evaluated and to find out if there were any new studies on the horizon that he could participate in. At that time, there were no drug studies. However, we enrolled him in a study that included an annual evaluation with extensive memory testing, an assessment of activities of daily living, an evaluation for depression, and a physical examination, blood work, and an MRI scan—all part of an Alzheimer's Disease Research Center study funded by the National Institutes of Health (NIH). While there, we were also approached about donating Steve's brain, which would be beneficial from a scientific point of view, since they could correlate his clinical condition with the condition of his brain at the time of his death. Steve told them he wasn't ready to give it to them yet, but agreed to think about it.

We left somewhat dismayed, since once again it looked like the future was grim and there was little hope that a drug would come along in time for Steve. The results of his MRI from the evaluation were even more depressing. His previous MRI several years earlier was normal, but this time he had considerable shrinkage of the brain in the areas (hippocampus and amygdala) associated with Alzheimer's disease. These two areas were moderately affected on one side and severely affected on the other. He also had atrophy (shrinkage) of the cerebral cortex (portions of the brain related to higher functions), and the ventricles (areas that contain cerebrospinal fluid deep inside the brain) were enlarged, in this case replacing areas previously occupied by normal brain tissue that had now atrophied. Atrophy can occur in any organ of the body when areas of cells die due to lack of circulation, lack of energy to the cells, or lack of use.

It was clear that Steve was "going down the tubes," as we often say in the medical world. He seemed less and less like the Steve I had married and more like a cross between a frail elderly man and a two-year-old, but without the energy. I had to constantly worry about where he was and what he was doing. If he disappeared from the room for too long, I looked for him, and more often than not, found him rummaging through his closet, the garage, or the drawers of his vanity, looking for what he did not know. This poem by Lois Walsh describes "trying to live with ambiguity" that accompanies Alzheimer's.

ALZHEIMER'S DISEASE

I have found an unwanted guest inhabiting our home.
Oh, at first she was sly like a fox,
Showing up briefly but with slow determination.
Then little by little snatching away what was ours.
Now I find myself alone with you beside me
And this uninvited guest.
You are with me, but I miss you, alive but not here.
Here but gone at the same time.
Such an ambiguous loss.
There is no closure like in death.
Each day I grieve over another loss and your former self.
Then feel guilty because it is not all about me.
I am letting go, hanging on,
And at the same time, trying to live with ambiguity.

TWO NEW DRUG TRIALS

A couple of months later I saw an ad in the paper for a clinical trial for the ICARA (Investigational Clinical Amyloid Research in Alzheimer's) study of a new vaccine called bapineuzumab by Elan Pharmaceuticals and learned that the Johnnie Byrd Alzheimer's Institute would be participating. I looked it up on www.clinicaltrials .gov (a registry of federally and privately supported clinical trials conducted in the United States and around the world) and found out that Steve should meet all the criteria. In contrast to the previous trials I had seen, this one did not have an exclusion criteria for a history of depression or use of antidepressants. On May 9, 2008, with hopeful anticipation, we made the hour drive to the University of South Florida for the screening.

We were met by a research assistant named Laura, and she made us feel very comfortable with the screening process. We were told all about the new medication, a vaccine that would be given intravenously at various intervals. A previous vaccine drug trial was discontinued because some of the subjects developed inflammation in the brain. This was a different type of vaccine that also removes beta-amyloid from the brain but by a different mechanism. Beta-amyloid is a protein normally made in the body whose function is not completely understood. When it accumulates in excess in brain tissue, it forms dense plaques, a hallmark of Alzheimer's disease. These plaques appear to be toxic to nearby brain cells and to interfere with communication between brain cells. We also learned that about 40 percent of the people in the study would receive a placebo instead of the vaccine, which is typical of drug studies, so that researchers will be able to determine if the drug is effective and safe. We were given consent forms for the screening process. Steve needed to initial and date each page, but could not remember what he was supposed to do and where to sign from page to page, much less remember the date. He needed to be shown exactly what to do each time and talked through each entry.

Some basics were done to determine if he qualified, such as taking a medical history and checking a list of his medications. Steve was taken to another room for the Mini-Mental Status Exam, or MMSE, and when he returned, we received the shocking news that his score was quite a bit lower than on his previous visit two months earlier. He needed at least a score of 16 to qualify for the study, since they wanted to investigate the drug using people with mild to moderate Alzheimer's. Steve only scored a 12, indicative of a more advanced stage of Alzheimer's, and he was not accepted. This was a serious blow to both of us. The physician came to speak with us and advised us that we could schedule another visit to try for a better score, since he appeared to qualify in every other respect. We left quite devastated, back to square one. It seemed that this disease was going to take Steve from me after all.

A few days after I discovered the ICARA study, I read about another new drug trial, this one at the Comprehensive Neuro-Science Center (CNS) in St. Petersburg, Florida, for a drug semagacestat by Eli Lilly & Company. Once again, it appeared that Steve should qualify for the study. Semagacestat is an oral medication, a gamma-secretase inhibitor that is intended to decrease substances in the bloodstream that become beta-amyloid plaque in the brain. It was not known if this drug would actually decrease the beta-amyloid in the brain, but it would hopefully keep more from accumulating. One exciting aspect of this study was that, after a year, people who were given the placebo during the study would be switched to the actual medication. I had two days off coming up and had scheduled screenings for the ICARA study vaccine and the Eli Lilly drug on back-to-back days.

A few days before the discovery discussed in Chapter 4, Steve came out to the kitchen for breakfast in a fog, as usual, barely talking. I put a bowl of cereal at his place at the table, and he sat down and said, "Oh, I need a spoon." He turned around to the buffet behind him, opened the drawer, looked and looked, and picked up a small knife. He turned around to the cereal and said once again, "Oh, I need a spoon." He repeated this process four more times, finally coming back with a spoon on the final attempt. I offered to help him find it, but he said, "No, I need to do this." It is so much easier to do these things for him, but whenever possible, painful as it is to watch, I try to respect his wishes and just let him try to figure it out, no matter how long it takes. That particular episode of "slow motion" stuck in my mind because just a few days later, life was about to change so that such episodes would become a thing of the past.

4

A Chance Discovery

I stumbled upon it completely by accident.

The evening before the first screening, I began to think about what would happen if Steve qualified for both the ICARA and Eli Lilly studies. Which should we choose? I got on the Internet to learn as much as I could about both drugs, including the potential risks and benefits. While searching, I came across a press release for a third promising drug called AC-1202. The company making the medication, Accera, a small biotech firm, was working toward Food and Drug Administration approval. They reported that AC-1202 actually improved memory in a significant number of the people with Alzheimer's disease.

PRESS RELEASE:

ALTERNATIVE ENERGY SOURCE FOR THE BRAIN MAY HELP TREAT ALZHEIMER'S

A sugar called glucose is the primary energy source for brain cells. In people with Alzheimer's, scientists have detected a dramatic decrease in glucose use in certain brain areas that begins ten to twenty years before any visible symptoms appear. Deprived of their primary energy source, neurons [brain nerve cells] suffer irreparable damage. The cause of decreased glucose metabolism remains uncertain.

Scientists at Accera have developed a compound called AC-1202 that provides these glucose-deprived neurons with an alternative energy source known as ketone bodies, which can be metabolized even when glucose cannot. Accera's hypothesis is that increased availability of ketone bodies will improve memory problems and other functional losses that occur in Alzheimer's.

At the Alzheimer's Association Prevention Conference, Lauren Costantini, Ph.D., vice president, clinical development, at Accera, reported results of a double-blind, placebo-controlled Phase IIb clinical trial with 152 subjects with probable mild to moderate Alzheimer's. AC-1202 was taken as a drink each morning (20 grams). Most study participants continued to take other Alzheimer's drugs such as acetyl-cholinesterase inhibitors, so this study was measuring the effectiveness of AC-1202 on top of existing therapy.

Treatment lasted for three months, followed by a two-week washout, then an additional six-month follow-up where all subjects, including both placebo- and AC-1202-treated patients, were given the opportunity to receive AC-1202 in an open-label extension study. The main outcome for efficacy was improvement in the ADAS-Cog [Alzheimer's Disease Assessment Scale–Cognition, a popular 75-point test of cognitive function used in clinical trials to detect changes in the core symptoms of Alzheimer's].

The researchers found that, after forty-five days of treatment, participants who took AC-1202 showed statistically significant improvement compared with placebo with the highest response in subjects not carrying the E4 variant of the apolipoprotein gene (ApoE4-), which occurs in half of all Alzheimer's patients. These effects on ApoE4- subjects were maintained for the duration of the initial study period (ninety days). In contrast, patients carrying the E4 variant of the APOE gene (ApoE4+) showed no differences between AC-1202 and placebo.

Forty-nine study participants entered the six-month open label extension; thirty-four completed the study. According to the researchers, subjects taking AC-1202 for nine months showed very little disease progression (mean change in ADAS-Cog score from baseline to day 294 = 0.8). From "A Possible Alzheimer's Blood Test and Two Trials of Innovative Therapies" presented at the Alzheimer's Association International Conference on Prevention of Dementia, 11, 2007.

Since we never hear the phrase "improves memory" associated with the current drugs for Alzheimer's, I was very curious about how this treatment might work. At present, the FDA-approved drugs for Alzheimer's disease claim at best to slow down the decline of the disease. The press release did not say what kind of drug this was or how it worked, so I performed an Internet search for AC-1202.

PATENT APPLICATION #20080009467

The first item to pop up was a 2008 patent application (U.S. Patent #20080009467) on www.freepatentsonline.com. This was a continuation of a patent application that was originally submitted by Samuel Henderson, Ph.D., executive director of research at Accera, in May 2000. I printed out the seventy-five-page document and began to read it. After several pages of legalese, there was a well-written summary of what was known about Alzheimer's disease at that time in relation to their invention. It talked about beta-amyloid plaques and neurofibrillary tangles, but also about a problem with glucose transport into neurons. It said that researchers have discovered that neurons in certain areas of the brain in Alzheimer's disease are unable to use glucose and that this same problem occurs in other neurodegenerative diseases, including Parkinson's disease, Huntington's disease, and Lou Gehrig's disease (amyotrophic lateral sclerosis, or ALS), but in different parts of the brain.

This rang a bell because I had previously come across research about the problem of glucose transport in Alzheimer's patients by William Klein, Ph.D., and others (Klein, 2008). Researchers described a problem with the location of insulin receptors, which would normally be found on the surface of the cell membrane but are not. The hormone insulin is needed for glucose to enter cells. Insulin attaches to the receptor on the cell membrane, initiating a chain of metabolic events that allows glucose into the cell where it is converted eventually into the energy molecule adenosine triphosphate (ATP). ATP is necessary for the cell to function and maintains its very life. Some scientists had even begun to call Alzheimer's disease a "type 3" diabetes (de la Monte, 2005), a concept that will be discussed at length in Chapter 13.

The patent application then described the "invention," which was based on the known fact that neurons can use a type of fuel other than glucose called ketones or ketone bodies. Ketones are transported into the cell by a different mechanism than glucose and therefore, if available in the bloodstream, can bypass the glucose/insulin transport problem and provide fuel for neurons and other brain cells, potentially keeping them alive.

The Body's Back-Up Fuel

Ketones are fundamental to the evolution of human beings. Without ketones, humans as a species would not have survived. Our ancient ancestors, and even people living in our world today, have endured periods of feast and famine. When food is available, we lay down stores of glucose (from ingested carbohydrates) and fat for future use as fuel and then tap into them when food is unavailable. When the stores of glucose in the body are used up, which happens after twenty-four to thirty-six hours, the body turns to burning fat and releases ketones (small carbon-containing fragments), which are then used as the primary fuel by the brain and other organs until food is once more available. This protective process is called ketosis.

Most of us these days in the United States do not have to struggle with the problem of feast and famine. As a result, there is not much ketone circulating in the bloodstream, since plenty of glucose fuel is available.

The body shifts its main fuel supply from glucose to ketones under several other conditions. Consuming a ketosis-inducing diet, an extremely high-fat, low-protein, low-carbohydrate diet that is sometimes used to treat severe childhood epilepsy, is one way. The Atkins and South Beach diets, which promote cutting carbohydrates, are less restrictive forms of the ketogenic diet and may result in mild ketosis. Diabetic ketoacidosis is a serious complication of type 1 diabetes that occurs when the levels of ketones become dangerously high, as much as five to ten times higher than one would have during starvation or on a ketogenic diet.

There is yet another way that ketones become available to brain cells. When a person eats foods with medium-chain fatty acids, they are partially metabolized in the liver to ketones and enter the bloodstream. According to one study, circulation to the brain increases by as much as 39 percent during ketosis (Hasselbalch, 1996). Ketones readily cross the blood/brain barrier and can be used by brain cells as fuel. Ketones are a more potent fuel than an equivalent amount of glucose, producing nearly twice as much ATP inside the cell. The levels of ketones from consuming medium-chain fatty acids would never come remotely close to reaching the levels of diabetic ketoacidosis.

Medium-Chain Triglyceride Oil

The inventor of AC-1202 (now known by the brand name Axona), Dr. Samuel Henderson, applied for the patent to market medium-chain triglyceride (MCT) oil for people with Alzheimer's disease. (MCT oil consists of 100 percent medium-chain fatty acids.) This was based on the company's research showing that the mild ketosis produced by ingesting MCTs appears to improve cognitive ability in a significant number of people with Alzheimer's disease.

When Dr. Henderson and his colleagues conducted studies of people with Alzheimer's and mild cognitive impairment, they found that by ingesting 20 grams (about four teaspoons) of AC-1202 (which we know from the patent application is MCT oil), nearly half the subjects showed significant improvement within forty-five days as measured by the ADAS-Cog exam compared to the people taking a placebo, who declined more significantly as people with Alzheimer's disease normally do. People who did not have the harmful ApoE4 gene, which increases the risk of developing Alzheimer's, improved more significantly than those who had the ApoE4 gene. The researchers also found that the higher the beta-hydroxybutyrate level (the primary ketone used by neurons), the greater the improvement. In addition, people who were taking Alzheimer's related medications—Aricept, Namenda, Exelon, or Razadyne (formerly known as Reminyl)—appeared to particularly benefit from taking MCT oil, with the greatest improvement in people taking Razadyne. A subgroup of these subjects continued the study for an additional six months, and those who were receiving MCT oil showed very little disease progression over that time period.

I later learned that MCT oil has been available over the counter for decades and is used by bodybuilders to help increase lean body mass. Some athletes and fitness buffs use MCT oil to increase energy levels and enhance endurance during high-intensity exercise. There have also been studies showing that MCT oil increases satiety and, if substituted for other oils, can result in weight loss.

The patent application made it clear that Accera did not invent MCT oil, or even make the specific MCT oil used in its product, but rather obtained a product called Neobee from the Stepan Company. Neobee is primarily a medium-chain triglyceride known as tri-caprylic acid, or C:8. Accera mixed the oil with whipped cream to conduct its studies, which will be explained in greater detail in Chapter 18.

At some point after my discovery, I was told by a researcher at one test site that when the AC-1202 trials were completed, the participants no longer had access to the product. As the wife of a relatively young man with Alzheimer's, I can only imagine what it must have been like to be a person with Alzheimer's and that person's spouse or children, to see a significant improvement, perhaps a very dramatic improvement, and then to have that taken away.

The patent application further stated that some people improved with the very first dose of MCT oil. In fact, Henderson stated that other combinations of MCT oils could be expected to produce the same effect. Then there were pages and pages of every conceivable formulation of MCT oil in powders, bars, and liquids, with numerous other additives and supplements, singly and in combination, that might improve people with Alzheimer's, and also in various combinations with the standard medications for the disease. However, the application clearly stated repeatedly that the only ingredient tested was MCT oil.

An Epiphany (in Parentheses)

I didn't know while I was reading the patent application that MCT oil was readily available in many natural food stores and could easily be purchased online. But I clearly remembered using MCT oil during my training and in my practice in the late 1970s and early 1980s to supplement feedings for premature newborns. MCT oil is easily absorbed, even by infants, without digestive enzymes, and is still used today in many neonatal intensive care units (Tantibhehyangkul, 1975). The first formulas for preemies were developed thirty years ago, and since then MCT oil has been added to virtually all standard infant formulas.

And then the moment of my epiphany occurred. Just once in the patent application, Dr. Henderson mentioned (in parentheses no less) that MCT oil is derived from coconut oil or palm (kernel) oil. I remembered seeing coconut oil in natural food stores, and I could not imagine what it was doing there, since it has the reputation of being an "artery-clogging oil." I had never taken the time to find out why it might be considered healthy.

After I finished reading the patent application, I went on an Internet frenzy, looking for everything I could find about medium-chain fatty acids, coconut oil, MCT oil, and ketones. I had to relearn biochemistry from my freshman year of medical school about what distinguishes medium-chain fatty acids from short- and long-chain fatty acids and find the fatty acid composition of coconut oil. I learned that coconut oil is nearly 60 percent medium-chain fatty acids. I calculated that about 35 grams of coconut oil (seven teaspoons, or a little more than two tablespoons) is equivalent to 20 grams of MCT oil. If I could give Steve coconut oil, we might be able to produce the same effect. Steve is an ApoE4 carrier so I had to be prepared that he might not respond at all, based on the results of the AC-1202 studies.

It was now after 1 A.M. on May 20, 2008, and Steve's appointment was at 9 A.M. in St. Petersburg. I had to call it quits for the night. There would be no opportunity to give Steve coconut oil before the first screening.

THE TWO SCREENINGS

The following morning, we got up and had breakfast as usual. On the way to the Comprehensive NeuroScience Center in St. Petersburg, I remembered the suggestion from the research assistant at the previous screening to try to prepare Steve for the Mini-Mental Status Exam test. I reviewed the various questions about orientation to time and place, such as where we were going to be, city and county, what was the current year, season, month, day of the week, and so on. I thought he would surely be able to remember the county of Pinellas that we lived in for sixteen years just before moving to our current town. We talked about other things as usual, but from time to time we went over the same questions again.

The First Screening

Steve went through the screening process. He met all the other criteria, but once again he scored a 14 on the MMSE, too low to be accepted into the study. Very disappointed, we sat down with the doctor. Dr. Nunez shared with us that her mother also has Alzheimer's disease and answered our questions. She asked Steve to draw a clock, a test she said was more specific for Alzheimer's disease. When he returned, she showed me his drawing (Figure 4.1).

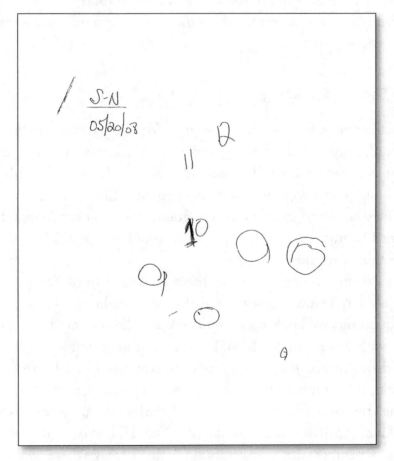

FIGURE 4.1. Clock 1: The day before starting coconut oil.

His clock did not look like a clock at all. There were several random small circles and several numbers with no apparent relationship that did not even remotely resemble a clock. Dr. Nunez took me aside and said this indicated that his dementia was leaning more toward the severe than the moderate range. Surprised and yet not surprised, it was still a shock to hear this, and my thoughts drifted to the road we were heading down, the inevitable decline that no one wants to experience.

On the way home, thinking, "What have we got to lose?" we drove considerably out of the way to a natural food store in Tampa where I had seen coconut oil on the shelf. We purchased a quart and headed home.

The Second Screening

The following day, Steve's screening for the vaccine study was scheduled for 1 P.M. at the Johnnie Byrd Institute. To make sure Steve received at least 20 grams of medium-chain triglycerides, I put more than two tablespoons of coconut oil in his oatmeal with his blessing—and even more for good luck. I added two tablespoons to my oatmeal as well. How could I expect Steve to eat something I wouldn't eat?

Just before noon, we began the hour-long trip to Tampa. Just like the day before, Steve agreed that we should go over some of the questions we knew they would ask and did not mind my obsession with increasing his MMSE score, if at all possible, so that he could qualify for the study. We went over and over the year, the season, the month and day of the week, as well as where we were going, the city, county, and name of the building. He repeatedly confused April for May, Wednesday for Thursday, and couldn't even remember the word "spring," much less where we were going. By the time we arrived, I was quite certain that he would do no better than during the previous visit.

Shortly after arriving, Steve was whisked away to another room for the test. We were told that if he scored high enough, they would continue the screening process. When I pray, it is usually to thank God for what I have rather than asking for favors. I have always believed that most of what happens to us is within our control and that if we want something special we have to use our own resources to get it. When I have a baby in dire straits, I ask God to help me do the right thing to pull the baby through. On this day, while he was gone, I prayed to God to help Steve qualify for this study. I wasn't ready to lose him.

When Steve returned, he said he didn't do very well, so we sat and waited, once again feeling a bit hopeless. The research assistant, Laura, entered the room and began to take Steve's blood pressure and talked about drawing blood. I asked her if this meant Steve had qualified for the study, to which she replied, "Didn't he tell you? He scored an 18! We are going ahead with the screening process." This was 6 points higher than our prior visit there and 4 points higher than the previous day. Laura reviewed the MMSE with us. Steve remembered that it was spring, it was May, and it was Wednesday. He recalled that we were in Tampa, in Hillsborough County, and at the Byrd Institute. We were elated as Laura and the others proceeded with the rest of the screening process.

Was this drastic improvement the result of the coconut oil, the preparation on the way down, the prayers, or just a stroke of good luck? I had read in the AC-1202 patent application that some people improved with the very first dose. Perhaps Steve was one of the fortunate individuals who responded that quickly. According to Accera studies, since he is an ApoE4 carrier, he might not have responded at all.

5

Climbing Out of the Abyss

I felt as if I were living in a parallel universe.

When Steve scored so well on the Mini-Mental Status Exam at the Johnnie Byrd Alzheimer's Institute, I didn't know if it was owing to the coconut oil, a lot of prayer, or just pure luck. At any rate, I decided to continue the coconut oil each day at breakfast. Before we started the coconut oil, Steve would come into the kitchen every morning in a daze, talking very little, and walking very slowly. Eventually, he would find his way to the table and begin to eat very slowly. I continued to add a little more than two tablespoons of coconut oil to his breakfast every morning, which usually consisted of oatmeal. By the third day, Steve began to come to the kitchen alert, smiling, talkative, and generally happy. He seemed to have very little trouble finding his utensils and a glass of water. He spent a considerable amount of time talking at breakfast, and by the fifth day we looked at each other and agreed that our life had changed.

I was accustomed to Steve having fluctuations, sometimes doing better for several days, and then not so well for several more days. But this was different. He said he felt as if a light had switched on, the fog had lifted, and his life had changed for the better. Early on, the most obvious changes were in his personality and in his ability to carry on a conversation. He had more animation in his face, he began to joke, and throughout the day, he became more talkative and appeared to have more energy. In the beginning, he continued to have tremors when he tried to eat and talk, and his gait still looked a little bit weird when he walked, but overall this was a very dramatic improvement compared with the Steve of just a few days earlier.

> STEVE: "It was like a light switch came on and everything came into focus. I felt like I might be able to do something instead of being a 'GOMER.'* It felt brighter inside of me."
>
> *GOMER is an acronym for "Get Out of My Emergency Room;" it's a derogatory term, sometimes used by doctors in training to refer to elderly people with dementia and/or other chronic illnesses.

CAPTURING THE CHANGES

I told my sister Angela, and also my father and his wife, what had happened with Steve. My sister suggested that I start keeping a journal. I found a composition book and began writing down everything I could remember. Here are some excerpts.

May 21 • DAY 1: I put two tablespoons of coconut oil in oatmeal and whey protein for breakfast, then prepped Steve for MMSE on the way to the Byrd Institute. In the car he could not remember it was spring, or May, but repeated reminders at least ten times. He remembered these things for MMSE about four hours after breakfast, scored 18, and qualified for study.

May 22 • DAY 2: We are using coconut oil for breakfast (two tablespoons) and also some later in day for cooking.

May 26 • DAY 6: I put one tablespoon of coconut oil on the sweet potatoes at dinner and—Steve liked it. I also cooked chicken in coconut oil and also found that it works well in smoothies. Steve has been alert every morning so far. He reported a dream one morning that "we did not have enough money." [It had been quite some time since he remembered a dream.] The next day he had a memory from second grade, of a girl he had a crush on and his first grade teacher—he told me this when he came out in the morning. On May 26 he went out in the courtyard and cleaned sides of the pool, then vacuumed the guest room and living room. After that, he got distracted and went outside to work on plants and had some confusion about "critters" digging the bulbs out of planters. I saw him do this earlier and reminded him—he still didn't remember.

May 28 • DAY 8: Steve had another good, alert morning. He had two tablespoons coconut oil with multigrain hot cereal, half of a banana, and one-half scoop of chocolate whey powder. I started adding L-carnitine to his morning and evening meds two days ago. He remembers immediately it is spring and "almost June." He couldn't remember the season or month after multiple prompts a week ago today until mid- to late-afternoon—overall seems more appropriate to his age than that of an eighty-plus-year-old.

May 29 • DAY 9: Steve was alert again today. After breakfast he went out to clean filters for the pool pump. He was able to take all lids off without my presence (before I would have to tell him a few times with each lid what to do). He came in and asked if the pump was set up to turn on automatically (not), and he commented that he would not have thought of that before. Overall, he seems "normal" except some trouble finding words and is completing his thoughts better. He put the filters back together except for one inside cap, which he asked me to check out. I called Stepan Company, the supplier of the Neobee 895 fatty acid product used in Accera's AC-1202 studies. They will send me a quart sample and also e-mailed me a technical bulletin.

May 30 • DAY 10: Steve was alert and frisky today. He cut the grass around the front of house with the small lawn mower.

May 31 • DAY 11: Steve seems "normal"—happy and alert. He went to get the paper, came back quickly, and read part of a magazine. He emptied the dishwasher with a little help and loaded it with help (minimal). He was still very alert in the evening. We are having good conversations, although with some trouble finding all the words.

June 1 • DAY 12: Steve was up and alert early, about 7:45 A.M. We had lots of conversation about things happening, politics (TV on), coconut oil, things he wants to do today. I asked what month it is and he guessed "June?" (Yes!!) He has a good sense of humor and physically looks great with a normal gait.

I wonder if there is a connection between herpes simplex and Alzheimer's. The last time Steve had a bad run, he also had a fever blister on his lower left lip that had trouble healing. I need to check path of the nerves from the lips to the brain. Could this virus travel in through this path to the amygdala and hippocampus?

June 2 • DAY 13: I woke up at 5 A.M. and wrote a three-page letter about AC-1202, Accera, medium-chain triglyceride oil, and coconut oil. Faxed, mailed, and e-mailed the letter to retired Supreme Court Justice Sandra Day O'Connor, the Alzheimer Study Group (ASG), the Alzheimer Association, Senators Hillary Rodham Clinton and Bill Nelson, and heart surgeon Mehmet Oz, as well as to the CNN newsroom and the *Today Show*. Steve woke up around 7:30 A.M. and was still doing well. He went to bed around 10 P.M. I received an e-mail response from ASG; they will investigate the research, report to the study group, and then respond to me.

June 3 • DAY 14: Steve woke up early about 7 A.M., awake, alert, and ready to roll! He drew a clock with a huge improvement from the visit two weeks ago at the CNS (Figure 5.1). He got several things done—he vacuumed all the carpets and floors and also cleaned the pool filters.

June 13 • DAY 24: Monkey man! While I was at work, Steve did a complete load of laundry, washer to dryer, folded and put away without prompting! It has been a very long time since he has been able to finish—usually he forgets to move it from washer to dryer. He was alert all day.

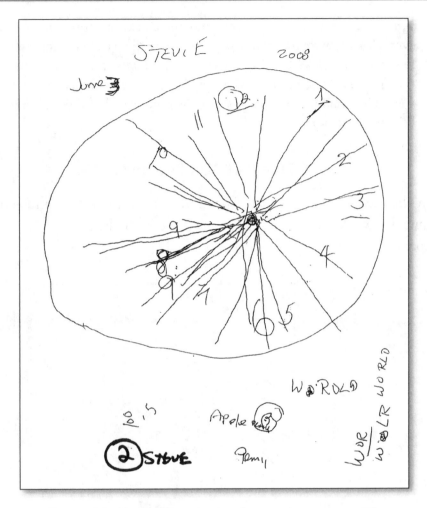

Figure 5.1. Clock 2: Two weeks after starting coconut oil.

Despite these dramatic improvements, not everything went smoothly in the beginning.

June 20 • DAY 31: Steve refused to finish his oatmeal with coconut oil this morning. He wanted to eat a chocolate cookie instead. Last evening I had to convince him to at least take MCT straight to get it in him, since he refused the more pleasant coconut ice cream or other food concoctions. After a lot of cajoling, he finally finished it (breakfast). Aarrgh!

June 26 • DAY 37: Steve drew another clock, and this one was even clearer, with the numbers closer to their usual position and fewer of the spoke-like lines that were part of the prior drawing (Figure 5.2). He continues to gradually improve in other ways as well. His tremor became less and less noticeable, and his gait became more normal.

A FORTUITOUS FINDING

In the meantime, I began to spend almost every waking moment outside work researching ketones, medium-chain fatty acids, coconut oil, and MCT oil.

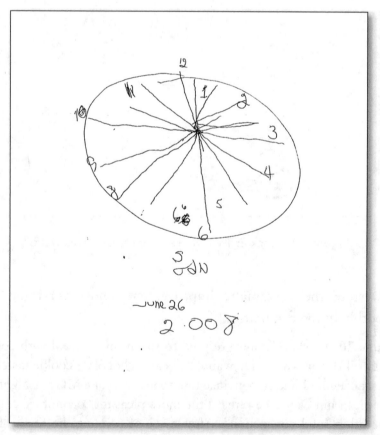

Figure 5.2. Clock 3: 37 days after starting coconut oil.

While researching ketones, I found an entry on www.Wikipedia .com that mentioned the name of Richard L. Veech, M.D., a metabolic specialist at the National Institutes of Health in Bethesda, Maryland and a world-renowned researcher on ketones. I found contact information for him and references for several articles, including one titled "Review: The Therapeutic Implications of Ketone Bodies," published in *Prostaglandins, Leukotrienes and Essential Fatty Acids* (Veech, 2004). In this article, he reviews in detail the science of ketones and how neurons (nerve brain cells) can use ketones instead of glucose as a fuel, particularly in diseases like Alzheimer's and Parkinson's in which the neurons are unable to utilize glucose. He also wrote about their use in diabetes and a variety of other diseases and conditions.

I had so many questions for this physician, not only about the use of ketones for someone like my husband, but also about uses in the newborns I care for. I decided to get up the nerve to contact him by phone and wrote down a list of questions I wanted to ask him:

1. Why not coconut oil instead of MCT oil?

2. Why not use some at every meal rather than just a morning bolus? Wouldn't it be better to try to produce a steady stream of ketone bodies round the clock?

3. Why 20 grams of MCT oil?

4. Would over-the-counter test strips to measure ketones in urine be useful?

5. Are there any studies in newborns regarding the use of ketone bodies from MCT oil to treat problems such as prematurity, hypoglycemia, or birth asphyxia?

In my first phone conversation with Dr. Veech, I did not mention what I was doing with Steve and the coconut oil, but rather asked him my list of questions. He told me about Accera and the Stepan Company (I already knew). He told me he didn't believe that the levels of ketones produced by MCT oil, whether taken at one meal or throughout the day, would be high enough to have an effect. He said he did not know why MCT oil would work. He explained that it shouldn't work, because the blood levels of ketones are one-tenth those needed for transport of ketone bodies into brain cells. But I knew that in Steve's case it did work.

While I knew that Dr. Veech would be skeptical if I told him what had happened with Steve without evidence other than my own impressions to back me up, when asked about using coconut oil to produce ketones, Dr. Veech replied, "Why not?" He also told me about brain-derived neurotrophic factor (BDNF), a substance that can salvage damaged neurons. When asked about over-the-counter test strips for measuring ketones in urine, he responded that they are "worthless." Apparently, they measure only the ketone known as acetoacetate and not beta-hydroxybutyrate (the primary ketone used by neurons for cellular fuel), which are usually present in roughly equal amounts in the bloodstream. Dr. Veech said it would be better to do blood samples. Regarding why Accera would choose a dose of 20 grams, he suggested that most people should tolerate this amount without diarrhea (a sign that the body can tolerate no more). Dr. Veech also said he believes treatment with ketones could be beneficial to premature newborns and those suffering from hypoglycemia or birth asphyxia, and it should be studied.

Lab-Made Ketones

During our conversation, I learned that Dr. Veech synthesizes an ester (a chemical compound made up of an alcohol combined with an acid) of the ketone beta-hydroxybutyrate. This particular ketone ester is a compound in which the alcohol is 1,3-butanediol and the acid is the ketone beta-hydroxybutyrate. This ester combination prevents the blood from becoming too acidic after it is ingested. Ketone ester can be produced in a crystalline form or as a concentrated liquid that can readily be diluted with water. It can be taken orally or given intravenously, and once circulating in the blood, it is taken up eagerly by the brain and other organs and used as fuel. The dosage of ketone ester can be easily adjusted to achieve levels comparable to those that occur during starvation or through the classic ketogenic diet used to treat epilepsy.

Dr. Veech described his ketone ester and how he received initial funding to develop the ketone from the Defense Advanced Research Projects Agency (DARPA). That research and development arm of the U.S. Department of Defense wanted to know whether this "superfuel" might improve the cognitive and physical performance of troops in combat. Dr. Veech had also received some funding from a Parkinson's foundation, but he was very frustrated because he needed an additional $15 million for a larger facility to produce the ketone ester by the ton to test on people with Alzheimer's and Parkinson's diseases. His work was overlooked by the NIH when they were doling out their research dollars. He suggested this might be due to his lack of political savvy and their lack of understanding about the profound potential of ketones to treat disease. He was even more frustrated knowing that other Alzheimer research projects received $75 million, and he was certain, not only as a medical doctor but also as a biochemist, that they would not make a difference with Alzheimer's disease. He e-mailed me two of his articles on the therapeutic uses of ketones.

My Ketone Connections Grow

Fourteen days after Steve had his first "dose" of coconut oil, and much to my amazement and delight had drawn the vastly improved clock in Figure 5.1, I decided it was time to tell Dr. Veech. I told him what I had been doing with the coconut oil and about the clocks Steve had drawn. He suggested that I fax the clocks to him. When he called me back, he said the difference was truly amazing and expressed once again that he didn't think the low levels one could get from coconut oil should be enough to make such a difference.

When Steve drew another clock thirty-seven days after starting the coconut oil (Figure 5.2) that was even clearer, I faxed the new drawing to Dr. Veech as well.

Throughout this time, I continued to read everything I could find about ketones, medium-chain fatty acids, coconut oil, and MCT oil. Dr. Veech continued to e-mail some of the important papers on the subject, and he put me in touch with several of his colleagues who were also involved in ketone research: George Cahill, M.D., Theodore VanItallie, M.D., and Sami Hashim, M.D. (I will discuss more about each of these men and their very important work in Part 2.) I read their papers and took opportunities to pick their brains with my many questions. Dr. Hashim told me that he and Dr. Veech disagreed about how high the levels of ketones would need to be to improve cognitive performance in someone with Alzheimer's. Dr. Hashim believed lower levels would suffice.

Getting the Message Out

As soon as it became apparent that Steve had responded so profoundly to the use of coconut oil, it became my mission to get this information out to as many people as possible. My primary goal was to bring to the attention of high-profile individuals and groups the research related to ketones and how they can provide an alternative fuel for neurons in certain neurodegenerative diseases, as well as the need for funding for production of Dr. Veech's ketone ester. My secondary goal was to make them aware of the research related to medium-chain fatty acids, which are converted to ketones by the liver and can provide this alternative fuel, even if on a more limited basis, until the ketone ester is commercially available.

I believed that if I could get this information to the right person, and that person investigated and understood the scientific basis of how ketones work as an alternative fuel, this message would get out to the general public in a big way.

But who was the right person?

ATTEMPTS TO INCREASE AWARENESS
THROUGH THE MEDIA

My sister Angela suggested that I write a letter to retired Supreme Court Justice Sandra Day O'Connor, whose husband had Alzheimer's disease. This was widely publicized around the time in March 2008 that she testified on Capitol Hill at the annual hearing of the U.S. Senate Special Committee on Aging related to Alzheimer's disease. I also learned that she was a member of the Alzheimer's Study Group (ASG), a government task force created in 2007 that focuses on ways to speed up the development of new medicines and ways to provide better resources and care to families affected by Alzheimer's. I drafted the following letter to her and mailed it in care of the ASG.

LETTER TO SUPREME COURT JUSTICE SANDRA DAY O'CONNOR

To Honorable Sandra Day O'Connor and Other Members
of the Alzheimer's Study Group:

I want to bring to your attention promising research in the area of Alzheimer's disease that needs to be made public urgently, since the premise can be instituted now by a simple change in diet.

I am a full-time working physician in the area of neonatology (critical care of sick and premature newborns). My husband is only fifty-eight and has moderately severe Alzheimer's disease, which became apparent about five years ago. He has gotten considerably worse over the past year but is still able to stay at home. He has been on the usual drugs to slow the decline, and we have been hopeful that, if his progress is slow enough, one of the new drugs will be approved.

Very recently, we learned of two clinical trials recruiting in our area and scheduled him to be screened for both studies. As I researched the two drugs I came upon another study for a therapeutic agent called AC-1202, under development by a company called Accera. In the course of their research, they concluded that persons with Alzheimer's disease overall improved with a daily dose in as little as forty-five days, with even greater improvement if they were also taking one or more of the Alzheimer's medications, such as Aricept or Namenda. The results were more striking for persons who do not carry an Apo E4 gene, which constituted about half of their study participants. In their small preliminary study, some people improved after a single dose.

In trying to further research what is in AC-1202, I located their patent application, which can easily be found on the website www.free patentsonline.com by searching for AC-1202. The application is United States Patent #20080009467, Kind Code: A1. This patent application goes into great detail about Alzheimer's disease and the science behind their "invention." Their original application dates back to 2000. In their studies and news releases related to it, their therapeutic agent is called AC-1202. The therapeutic agent involved is actually MCT oil (medium-chain triglycerides), which they state is commonly derived from coconut or palm kernel oil. There is also a small amount of MCT in butter fat.

If they will take the time to read the patent application, the physicians and other scientists in your study group will recognize the biochemical principles involved and why this should help people with Alzheimer's disease. The application explains their study results using MCT oil. The remainder of the patent application goes into great detail about a vast number of formulations of MCT with other entities, such as vitamins and enzymes that may enhance the performance of the MCT oil. They acknowledge that the exact composition of the MCT oil does not seem to make a difference. The product they used was obtained from Stepan Company, a large supplier for other companies making food and other preparations. I spoke with a sales representative and they sell this to distributors in fifty-five gallon drums, a minimum of sixteen drums per order. It is therefore plentiful.

The references for the other research they have relied upon are included throughout the very lengthy and detailed AC-1202 patent application.

To simply summarize the science, researchers have found that neurons in certain areas of the brain in persons with Alzheimer's disease do not take up and use glucose normally and eventually die, since this is the primary energy that the neurons use. Some [scientists] are now calling this type 3 diabetes. The only other known substrate that neurons can use are ketones. Normally, humans do not produce ketones unless they are in a condition of starvation or [are] on a ketogenic (very low-carbohydrate) diet, such as Atkins. In contrast to the usual fats that Americans eat, medium-chain triglycerides (as in MCT oil) are easily absorbed when taken orally and are metabolized by the liver directly into ketones. Other fats are not processed this way by the body. A 1996 study referenced in the patent application shows that, when this occurs, blood flow to the brain increases by 39 percent. Ketones are known to pass directly into the circulation in the brain, where the neurons can readily take them up for use as an alternative energy to glucose, thereby preserving the life and integrity of the neuron.

Accera states in its patent application that the defect associated with Alzheimer's disease they are targeting may begin to occur decades before there are symptoms, therefore use of MCT oil would be a significant benefit, not only for people who are already suffering from Alzheimer's, but also for prevention for those who are at risk. Most Americans have family members with the disease and may be at risk themselves.

MCT oil is readily available on the open market (I have purchased a one-liter bottle online). It is used for weight loss and to enhance athletic performance due to the type of energy it provides (ketones). In addition, coconut oil contains about 57 percent MCT oil and can be purchased in some grocery stores, Asian markets, and many natural food stores. Coconut milk and many other coconut products now on the market contain a substantial quantity of coconut oil. Larger quantities of coconut oil from 16 ounces to 5 gallons can easily be purchased online. In addition to MCT oil, coconut appears to have other fats that may be very beneficial as well.

The dosage used in the AC-1202 study was a single daily dose of 20 grams of MCT oil, which translates into about four teaspoons of MCT oil or seven teaspoons of coconut oil. This can easily be incorporated into the foods we eat.

My nurse friends from the Philippines have advised me that, in their country of origin (as well as other Asian countries, such as India), coconut and coconut oil are a staple, used on a daily basis, which may explain why there is a much lower incidence of Alzheimer's disease in that part of the world. I have checked out other studies of coconut oil and learned that it does not raise, in fact lowers, "bad cholesterol." Also, areas of the world that primarily use coconut oil as their fat have a much lower mortality related to cardiovascular disease, contrary to myths that have been perpetuated for more than fifty years in our country since the development of the hydrogenated vegetable oils, including those containing trans fats.

If you look at the Accera website at www.accerapharma.com, under "Energy Metabolism," they state that they have developed "novel treatments . . . designed to increase energy to neuronal cells," etc. Nowhere in this website do they mention that this is simply MCT oil that anyone can purchase.

I am the caregiver for my husband. About two weeks ago, I purchased coconut oil and started adding seven teaspoons (equivalent to the amount used in the study) to my husband's oatmeal at breakfast. I have also experimented with a number of recipes that are available in cookbooks and online. Within a few days there was noticeable improvement in his gait, his ability to converse, his sense of humor has returned; he remembers the month and the season immediately, which he could not remember if repeated over and over to him before. He is following through on things that he wants to accomplish during the course of the day. His latest MRI shows extensive atrophy in the amygdala and hippocampus, the areas affected by Alzheimer's. Realistically speaking, I cannot expect him to fully recover, but to see this much improvement in such a short time is very encouraging for both of us. He is well aware that he is suffering from this disease and fully supports and enjoys our dietary change.

Steve is just one person, but his improvement supports the research done by Accera. We hope this improvement will be sustained.

It is disappointing that the people behind Accera have been aware of this science for at least eight years and have failed to provide this information to the medical community and public at large. How many people have deteriorated unnecessarily due to their negligence in this regard? My husband's MRI was "normal" and he could work as an accountant just three years ago.

Accera states in the patent application that there are other entities in which glucose is not used by neurons in different areas of the brain, including Parkinson's, Huntington's disease, and epilepsy. This has treatment implications well beyond just Alzheimer's disease.

I implore the members of the ASG to study this research on an urgent basis and make the findings public knowledge so that everyone who suffers from this disease can potentially benefit. I hope that at least one of you will take the time to read through the AC-1202 patent application that is public record and have your medical experts review this.

I am also sending copies of this letter to important government figures and the media with the hope that someone who is in a position of power to make change will pick up on this, research it urgently, and do something about it for all of us and our families.

I would be grateful for any feedback on this issue.

Sincerely yours,
Mary T. Newport, M.D.
Director of Neonatology
Neonatal Intensive Care Unit
Spring Hill Regional Hospital
Spring Hill, Florida 34609
Cc: Chairperson, Alzheimer's Association (National Office)

While waiting for a response from Justice O'Connor, I developed a list of other high-profile people and organizations and mailed or e-mailed similar letters to them as well. Among them were the Alzheimer's Association (a leading voluntary health organization in Alzheimer care, support, and research) and the Michael J. Fox Foundation; former Senator Hillary Rodham Clinton, Senator Bill Nelson, Ron Reagan (son of former President Ronald Reagan), and Acting Surgeon General Steven K. Galson; television personalities such as Oprah Winfrey and Mehmet Oz; television and print media like CNN, ABC News, CBS News, Fox News, NBC Studios, the *Today Show,* as well as the *New York Times, Washington Post, News & Observer,* and *USA Today.*

This was just the beginning of my campaign to get the message out, and many more attempts were to follow in the ensuing months. I was very well aware that this was just one case study, one man whose wife believed he responded to coconut oil. Why should anyone believe me? Why shouldn't they be skeptical? I was careful to mention the studies performed by Accera, and that this case study was merely further confirmation of its results. My point was that the substance studied was available over the counter and others should have access to this information immediately and not have to wait for a prescription product to become available at some nebulous point in the future.

I thought, at the very least, one of these individuals would contact me for more information, but much to my surprise and chagrin, I heard from none of them. I was far from ready to give up. If I couldn't get the message out by way of the media, it would have to go by way of the grassroots.

ATTEMPTS TO INCREASE AWARENESS THROUGH PHYSICIANS AND RESEARCHERS

A month after Steve's first breakfast of oatmeal and coconut oil, we visited our families in Cincinnati for the first time in a year. It did not take long for my father and his wife, my sisters, and Steve's siblings to notice that Steve was very different, much better, than on the previous visit. They remarked that in May 2007 he seemed lost, didn't remember names of many family members, had no sense of humor, and his responses during conversations didn't make sense. By contrast, on this visit he immediately said hello to nieces and brothers-in-law by name, laughed and joined in, and even made up some of his own jokes. At one point, my sister Rosemary mentioned that, when texting her daughters, she signs off with the numbers "666" because that happens to correspond to "Mom" on the telephone keypad. Steve laughed out loud, immediately understanding the reference to the devil. With Steve's permission, I shared the drawings of the clocks with our families. They all agreed that he was markedly improved from the previous year and that I might be on to something. There were a number of coconut oil converts during that visit.

Encouraged by the reaction of our families to Steve's improvements, and now certain that this was not simply my imagination, it was time to step up my efforts to get the message out to other people who were dealing with Alzheimer's so they could potentially benefit as well. I saw on a news program that there was a conference scheduled for the end of July in Chicago, the International Conference on Alzheimer's Disease (ICAD). I thought this might be a golden opportunity to cross paths with physicians and researchers and increase their awareness of ketone's potential benefits.

The night before we left Cincinnati, I lay awake thinking about what else I could do to get the message out. I could not get the words out of my head, "What if there was a cure for Alzheimer's disease and no one knew?" I quietly got up and found my way to my father's office, where I drafted the foundation for my article, using the words that I couldn't get out of my head for the title. The "cure" I referred to is the ketone ester beta-hydroxybutyrate, derived from coconut oil. Though that is a relatively poor substitute, it's a viable option that can be used immediately for its ketone-producing effect. As a physician, I am perfectly well aware that it is brazen to announce a "cure" for any disease and that people would be highly skeptical, but on the other hand, I strongly believe that ketone ester will be a true cure, capable of reversing disease for those in the earliest stages. It may even result in some improvement for those in the more advanced stages, bringing back to life neurons that are faltering but not yet dead.

Over the next several weeks, I fine-tuned the article, adding a few more details and references, until I arrived at the version I planned to produce in quantity for the ICAD. With no response to my first letter, I sent a second letter to Justice O'Connor, this time with a copy of my article. I contacted the ASG requesting the status of the investigation, noting that some weeks had passed and I had not received a response.

NOW WHAT?

In early July, just two weeks before the ICAD conference, Dr. Veech approached me with the idea of obtaining levels of the ketones, beta-hydroxybutyrate and acetoacetate (the two types of ketones converted into cellular fuel), on Steve before and at intervals after ingesting coconut oil. We worked it out with the lab director at my hospital to have his personnel draw and prepare the samples for mailing, placing them in an extremely low-temperature freezer, according to a procedure provided by Todd King, who routinely runs this assay in Dr. Veech's lab. My job was to take the samples for overnight delivery to Dr. Veech's lab.

Ketone Levels and Coconut Oil

On July 11, we went to the hospital at about 7 A.M. for the first sample before breakfast. We then went to breakfast nearby, and I gave Steve 35 milliliter (ml), the equivalent of seven teaspoons, of coconut oil, noting the exact time. We returned to the hospital and additional blood samples were drawn at timed intervals thereafter up to three hours. Dr. Veech called me and suggested that we repeat the process with the dinner meal. Steve was up for it and so we did, taking samples before and at intervals up to three hours after receiving another 35 ml of the oil with dinner. On that particular day, he did not receive any other coconut products to avoid confounding the results. The next day, I delivered the samples in a special cooler for express shipping, and the day after we received the results from Dr. Veech. Steve's acetoacetate levels were higher than his beta-hydroxybutyrate levels (Figure 6.1).

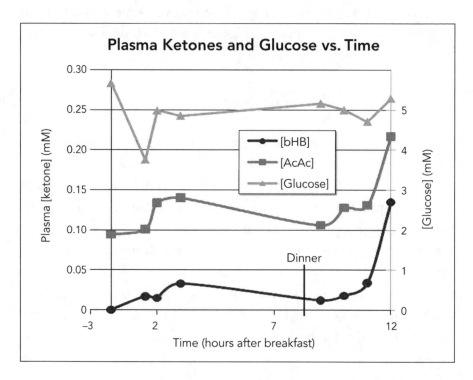

Figure 6.1. Measurements of glucose, acetoacetate (AcAc), and beta-hydroxybutyrate (bHB) at timed intervals up to three hours after Steve consumed coconut oil. The ketone levels were relatively low, but peaked at about three hours following the breakfast dose, and were close to baseline before dinner. The levels were still rising and considerably higher three hours after the dinner dose. (Diagram courtesy of Richard L. Veech, NIH.)

Dr. Veech was concerned that the ketone levels were quite low, with the exception that three hours following dinner, the levels were on the rise but had not yet peaked, so we didn't know how high they might have gotten before falling again. He was also concerned that the acetoacetate levels were higher than the beta-hydroxybutyrate levels. In the Accera trials, only beta-hydroxybutyrate levels were reported. He conjectured that during Steve's activity in the daytime, his muscles might have used up some of the ketones. In the evening, in a more sedentary state, there might be less use of the ketones by other tissues, and therefore more ketone was available to the brain during sleep, a time when the body is known to repair.

Prior to this small study, Steve received measured amounts of coconut oil for breakfast and dinner, but not for lunch. He sometimes received another coconut product if I happened to make a smoothie. As a result of the test, it was apparent that Steve should receive a measured dose of coconut oil for lunch as well.

Ketone Levels and Medium-Chain Triglyceride Oil

Two weeks later, just before the ICAD conference, Dr. Veech suggested that another set of ketone levels be performed, but this time after consuming MCT oil instead of coconut oil. He wanted to run the levels on a second individual as a control. It just so happened that my associate F had started using MCT oil shortly after I told him about Steve and his response to coconut oil. He has type 2 diabetes, lost his father to vascular dementia, and was very concerned about his own future health. He was more than happy to participate, and levels were drawn on him and Steve both before and after consuming 20 grams (21 mL or about 4 teaspoons) of MCT oil (see Figure 6.2 on the following page). This time, Steve's beta-hydroxybutyrate levels were higher than his acetoacetate levels.

Comparing the two studies showed that ketone levels from coconut oil were lower and peaked later than that from MCT oil, but were still present considerably longer than with MCT oil. The levels with MCT oil were higher and peaked at about ninety minutes for Steve, but were minimal by three hours. Also, the levels of

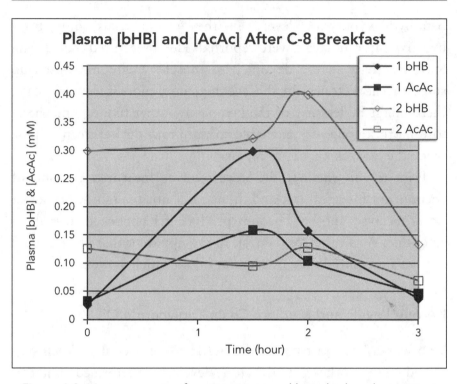

Figure 6.2. Measurements of acetoacetate and beta-hydroxybutyrate at timed intervals after consuming MCT oil. Steve (◆ ■) and my associate F (◇ □) were each given 20 grams of MCT oil with breakfast. AcAc and bHB levels were measured at intervals up to three hours after that. Steve's levels peaked at about ninety minutes, and F's levels peaked at two hours and were essentially back to baseline or below at three hours. (Diagram courtesy of Richard L. Veech, NIH.)

beta-hydroxybutyrate were more elevated than acetoacetate levels after taking MCT oil, whereas the opposite was true after taking coconut oil. F's dieting and losing a substantial amount of weight weekly at the time of the study may explain why his ketone levels were already elevated before taking MCT oil at breakfast.

Dr. Veech strongly advised me to include MCT oil in Steve's diet, pushing the quantity a little at a time until he vomited and had diarrhea, so, with Steve's approval, I did. However, it made sense to me that, since he had responded initially to coconut oil, there might be something else in it that was not present in the more refined MCT oil that could be helping Steve. So we continued to use coconut oil as well.

I began to experiment with a mixture of coconut and MCT oil, keeping a minimum of one tablespoon of coconut oil with each dose and increasing the amount of MCT oil gradually until we found Steve's limits of tolerance; then I backed off slightly. My rationale was that we would take advantage of the higher levels from MCT oil and the longer duration of the levels from the coconut oil. By mixing them, Steve should have ketone available to his brain around the clock. Is this necessary? Does the brain take up a volume of ketone and then store it, or is the ketone taken up, immediately processed, and used up? The answers are unknown at this time. To this day, I continue to base the way we are mixing the oils and dosing Steve three times a day on the assumption that it is wise to try to maintain a constant blood level of ketones.

Once we found Steve's limits of tolerance, we settled on a dose of four teaspoons (20 mL) of MCT oil and three teaspoons (15 mL) of coconut oil. For many months, if I tried to increase the amount of MCT oil beyond 20 mL, Steve had diarrhea. However, after a year, he was able to handle an increase in the mixture from 35 mL (seven teaspoons) per dose to 40 mL (eight teaspoons) and then 45 mL (nine teaspoons) several months later. As of 2011, this is the dose we have settled on three times a day with meals.

Two Days When We Missed Coconut Oil

There were two occasions when Steve missed getting his dose of coconut oil in the morning. The first was when he needed to fast for blood work, and the lab was so busy that it was nearly noon before he had a bite to eat. We decided to go to a restaurant, and by the time the food arrived, he was very tremorous and had considerable difficulty finding and using utensils. It soon occurred to me that the lack of coconut oil was the cause of this setback, and I pulled out one of the tiny bottles I carried with his premeasured dose. About twenty to thirty minutes after taking the oil, Steve smiled again and the shaking stopped.

The second occasion occurred in October 2008 during a vacation in California, a three-hour difference in time zones from our home in Florida. We slept in the morning after we arrived, and by the time we got to the restaurant to eat breakfast, it was about noon our time. We were sitting in a C-shaped booth with a front-row view of the ocean, and not many other people were there at that point. When the food arrived, once again Steve was very shaky and confused. He had a great deal of difficulty deciding which utensil to use and also had trouble keeping the food on his fork. He said he felt as if he were in a little box, the food was coming in at him, and he had to get out of the booth. I set up a chair for him at a table outside the booth. After he ate and had his oil, once again about twenty to thirty minutes later, he began to smile and joke, and the tremor disappeared. He said when the event was in progress he felt very claustrophobic and *he couldn't taste the food.*

The sense of smell is often blunted in the early stages of Alzheimer's, and some doctors use a test with common odors everyone should recognize in their diagnostic process. After Steve's experience in California, it occurred to me that perhaps the reason people with Alzheimer's disease lose interest in eating is that, at some point, not only do they have trouble smelling food but they can no longer taste the food as well, as the neurons that supply the taste buds are no longer functional. Perhaps the neurons involved in hunger and fullness go by the wayside as well.

ATTEMPTS TO INCREASE AWARENESS
AT THE MEDICAL CONFERENCE

Since first hearing about the International Conference on Alzheimer's Disease, I learned that about 5,000 researchers and physicians would be there from all over the world. Beside being the perfect opportunity to get out information about ketones and medium-chain fatty acids to an enormous number of people, I also saw it as an opportunity to learn as much as I could about the disease and the status of various treatments that seemed to be just over the horizon.

Plan A: Exhibit Space

Medical conferences usually have an exhibit hall where there are displays by pharmaceutical companies, equipment and supply manufacturers and distributors, hospitals trying to recruit nurses, and medical textbook publishers. This conference was no exception.

I contacted the person in charge of the exhibit hall, whom I will call ST, to advise her of what I wanted to do and learn the logistics of the process. I asked her whether there was any possibility of disseminating an article I had written at the conference, to which she responded in the negative. She said I would have to get a booth for $3,300, and she directed me to an exhibit hall chart on the company's website so I could pick out a location.

For a day or two, after mulling over the personal cost of the trip to Chicago, the exhibit, and the materials to distribute, I decided it was a small price to pay to get the information out to so many people. I talked with my sister Angela about the logistics of taking Steve with me, and she said that she and her husband John would help us in any way they could, either by staying with Steve at our home or by meeting us in Chicago. Angie researched flights while I looked into hotels.

I decided on the location of a booth and e-mailed ST with my confirmation. That same day I received the following response:

July 16, 2008
Hi Mary,
   Glad you found everything. I am copying DB, our exhibit manager, to reserve your space. The conference starts a week from Saturday, so you should make a commitment ASAP. We welcome your participation at ICAD.
Best regards, ST

As I read through the registration information, I learned that, in addition to the $3,300 booths, tables were available for $1,600. This seemed like a more reasonable alternative, given that I was just planning to distribute articles and not have a very fancy exhibit. I wondered why ST did not tell me about the tables and called her back to find out if there were still tables available. She sounded a bit miffed, but advised me that, yes, there were tables available, and she would reserve one for me. I completed the necessary reservation forms, including the payment information. A perk of having an exhibit was one free conference registration. And I could have up to three people assigned to the booth to help me, and Angie and John were more than willing.

Later that day I e-mailed ST again to confirm and pay for the table in the exhibit hall.

The next day she confirmed receipt:

July 17, 2008
   Thank you, Mary. I sent it to our exhibit manager at X Exhibitions. They will be in touch. ST

Our daughter Joanna had recently completed her bachelor's degree in graphic design and happened to be working part-time for a small local graphic design company. Her boss, Dave, who had read the article with interest, was willing to help, even given the relatively short time I had to get an exhibit together. He agreed to let Joanna format the article and then arranged to have 500 color copies made. I also arranged with a copier near our hotel in Chicago to print out 1,500 more copies that we could pick up before the conference started.

After a long weekend of working at the hospital and preparing for the conference exhibit, I received the following e-mail from ST:

July 21, 2008
Dear Mary,

I am very sorry to have to tell you that we have to deny your application and cancel your exhibit space in the exhibit hall for ICAD. The exhibit hall is intended for companies with products and services related to Alzheimer's disease and dementia. Any funds that you have paid will be refunded. As we previously discussed, we would welcome you to submit an abstract for our next research conference, or consider applying for a research grant. If you have not already done so, go to the website at www.alz.org/icad and enter your name to receive e-mail updates and announcements. Again, I am sorry you cannot exhibit and for your inconvenience.

Best regards, ST

After reading this, I was stunned and immediately called ST to try to convince her otherwise. I suggested that perhaps I could register the table under the name of my company, Spring Hill Neonatology, Inc. She said she would run it by the folks in charge. But next day, unfortunately, she informed me otherwise.

July 22, 2008
Dear Mary,

After additional discussion with our conference leadership, I regret to inform you that we indeed cannot approve your application for exhibit space. All applications for space are approved by the conference leadership to ensure that the exhibit hall space is the proper forum for the applicant according to the Association's policies. In your case it has been determined that it is not. You are still welcome to come to the conference as an attendee and attend all of the sessions, but you cannot display your material in any way. You may submit your material as a proposal for the next ICAD, or apply for a research grant if you wish. If you have registered for the conference and decide not to attend, I can see that your registration fee is refunded. Let me know if you want to do that.

Again, I am sorry this has not worked out as you wished.

Best regards, ST

I wrote yet another e-mail to her explaining in detail the many reasons why it was so very important for this information to get out as soon as possible to the Alzheimer's research community as well as the public. I pointed out that Accera, the makers of AC-1202 which had performed the MCT oil clinical trials, were approved for a booth and that the foundation of the dietary intervention discussed in the article I intended to distribute was based on their research. The millions of people with Alzheimer's should not have to wait for their product to come to market when it was available on the shelf now.

Later that day, ST wrote back.

Hi Mary,

There is no way that you can distribute your material at this conference. It does not qualify for the exhibit hall or any other form of display. Any presentations, either oral or poster, have to be submitted and reviewed by the Scientific Program Committee. You will have to find another way to distribute your material.

Best regards, ST

Still not ready to give up, I pointed out to ST that other groups were approved for exhibits that had no connection with Alzheimer's, such as a company selling bibles and a tourism company. I also suggested that she take my article to the medical director of the Alzheimer's Association for review, rather than relying on a nonscientist administrator to make this kind of decision.

July 24, 2008
Dear Mary,
   As you have requested, I have passed your comments on to our medical science department. As mentioned in previous e-mails to you, the exhibitors in the exhibit hall represent companies that are promoting products and services, not specific research findings—those are inappropriate for the exhibit hall. The proper forum for research findings at an Alzheimer's Association conference is through oral and poster presentations selected through the abstract submission process.
   We are glad you can attend the conference sessions and visit the exhibit hall as an attendee, but let us be perfectly clear that you cannot distribute your attachment any place at ICAD.
Best regards, ST

   I made another attempt to convey to ST that it would be obvious to any reader that my article was simply a case presentation that would support Accera's AC-1202 research, which the conference had already reviewed and approved, but I made no headway.

July 24, 2008
Mary,
   Your document was reviewed by our Medical Science Department and the approval of your application for an exhibit space at ICAD was denied. ST

   Obviously, I am not one to give up. I was actually quite taken aback that the people who manage the Alzheimer's Association would react to this particular information by going out of their way to suppress rather than, at the very least, investigate the concepts involved. Couldn't they consider the possibility that something in the diet could benefit people with the disease they had charged themselves to find a cure for?

Plan B: Taking to the Streets

Discouraged, but not ready to give up, I contacted the city government to find out if there were any laws against passing out information on public streets. My Plan B was to hand out copies of the article to people attending the conference as they entered and exited the convention center. I learned this was allowed, but we could not set up a table or stand of any kind, so plans for a poster exhibit were abandoned.

On the evening of July 26, Angie and John met us at the airport in Chicago, and we checked into the hotel. The next morning, we arrived early at the convention center to allow time to distribute copies of the article. To my surprise and dismay, the convention center and the grounds around it are so vast that most people coming and going were already on the private grounds before exiting vehicles. Many others were staying at a hotel with a direct indoor link to the center. Passing out copies to people on public streets was not going to be quite as easy as I had pictured.

We proceeded to the registration area where I checked in and learned that it would not be possible for anyone without a conference badge to sit in on any part of the conference or even enter the exhibit hall. We decided to split up at that point. John and Steve would do some sightseeing; Angie would scout out the area to see if there was a good place just off the grounds to pass out articles; and I would attend lectures. Unfortunately, we followed that plan through much of the four-day conference.

Plan C: Talking with Presenters and Attendees

I proceeded to the first plenary session. A plenary session includes all the participants in one room. In this case, the room was massive, far and away the largest hall I have ever seen at a medical conference. The speaker was at the front, and at various intervals there were very large screens, much like you would see at a rock concert, on which the speaker's audiovisuals were projected. I fully expected that the first plenary sessions would be devoted to an overview of what was known about Alzheimer's disease, so that attendees would start off the conference on the same page. This is customary at medical conferences. Instead, there were three talks back to back, each lasting forty minutes: the first was about mouse models of Alzheimer's disease; the second was about imaging, distinguishing diseases, and measuring progress; and the third was about biomarkers.

After a half-hour break, participants were divided into four groups in separate halls with sessions covering different areas of research. Twenty minutes were allotted per talk for two hours. There was a two-and-a-half-hour break in the middle of the day during which lunch was available. The afternoon was structured so there were six groups, with each talk lasting fifteen minutes for two more hours. On each of the four days of the conference, about 500 different poster presentations were set up in the exhibit hall, covering every conceivable niche of Alzheimer's disease except the topic of ketones that was most important to me and, in my estimation, the most promising one. That added up to an average of seventy-five oral presentations taking place in multiple rooms simultaneously several times a day over four days. During the final afternoon of the conference there was no wrap-up, no summary of what we'd learned, just a continuation of the same fifteen-minute talks in seven rooms over two hours.

My Plan C was to talk with as many attendees as I could about ketones to try to increase awareness and hopefully stimulate some of them to explore this area further. I stopped to talk with anyone presenting on such subjects as insulin, glucose, and nutrition-related research, among many others. I discovered that many of the attendees were physicians involved in treating patients and/or clinical research (testing on people rather than animals), and many more were Ph.D. researchers involved with laboratory and animal research.

With more than 2,300 presentations in four days, only one topic, a promising drug called Rember, made the news. So many tiny niches of research were represented that I could not help but think of them as small pieces of a very large puzzle: in this case, the answer to Alzheimer's disease, the cause and the cure. With more than 2,000 pieces to this puzzle, someone had taken the box, shaken it, and tossed the pieces in the air so they landed randomly on the floor, scattered in all directions and not even in the same room. I knew that some of the most important pieces of the puzzle were missing.

And who is putting the pieces of this puzzle together? In an ideal world, a group such as the National Institutes of Health or the Alzheimer's Association, with their vast monetary resources, would create a center, bringing together the top clinical and research physicians and scientists in every related discipline. These experts would not be owned by drug companies and would put aside their personal biases toward their own research to carefully and objectively sift through the pieces to work out this puzzle together. This would be a collaboration, not a competition. They would look beyond the research funded by the Alzheimer's Association and the drugs companies and beyond the U.S. borders to every part of the world. They would consider every chemical, nutrient, and microorganism that might play a role in the disease process for better or worse. They would use computers to compile and organize the information. A smaller group would oversee and orchestrate the process and keep it moving until all the pieces are put together. After all, this is urgent business for those of us who are losing our loved ones now. There is plenty of precedence for this type of activity to solve a problem. The Human Genome Project is one example in which the human sequence of DNA was completely worked out through collaboration.

A Surprise, an Experience, and Some Observations

One surprising event occurred the first day of the conference. While Angela was scouting out the conference center, she found the pressroom. At the next break, I inquired about leaving copies of my article for members of the press. I was told that only materials that had been previously approved by the Alzheimer's Association would be accepted for that purpose. In the hallway outside the pressroom, Athena Rebapis, a young reporter for www.intimetv .com, stopped to speak with us. I explained what had happened with Steve, and she asked if I wanted to be interviewed. I said, "Most definitely!" and we set up a time for the taping later that morning. Her director/producer, Troy Ferguson, was extremely interested and taped pictures of Steve's clocks, which were included in the presentation. An eight-minute segment with this interview appears in their program "Journey through Alzheimer's" along with other interviews from the Chicago conference, which can be viewed through a link on my website www.coconutketones.com.

Another interesting experience involved an individual who was almost certainly a security guard working for the Alzheimer's Association. He was a tall man with an Alzheimer's Association logo pin on the lapel of his navy suit, who seemed to spend an inordinate amount of time very close by. We first noticed him when we met in the lunch area near the exhibit hall on the first day of the conference. He actually sat down at the table without food where the four of us were eating and seemed to be eavesdropping. Thereafter, on several occasions he seemed a little too close when I was in the exhibit hall, particularly when I was speaking with poster presenters. Angie also noticed him when she was hanging out while I attended sessions. Considering how many people were attending the conference, his presence just seemed a little too much of a coincidence.

On my first visit to the exhibit hall, I found what I believed at that time was the reason why my exhibit was denied. I knew that Accera was scheduled to have an exhibit, and as you might expect, I decided to look for that booth right away. It was located directly across the aisle from the table exhibits where I would have been distributing my article. I stopped by the booth several times, hoping to catch their vice president, Dr. Lauren Costantini, an author of their research papers, but we were never in the same place at the same time. Accera had a poster presentation, but no one seemed to be available for discussion during the scheduled time. None of the written materials at their booth mentioned that the active ingredient in AC-1202, by then called Axona, is a medium-chain triglyceride. Instead, the product was presented as a "novel therapy" that increases ketones. I questioned a couple of their sales representatives at the booth, asking what the novel therapy was. For the most part, they either feigned ignorance or provided an evasive answer, such as, "It is a powder." When pushed, one of the reps finally told me that it was tricaprylic acid, one of the medium-chain triglycerides. I can only speculate why they would not divulge this information at this type of conference. I suspect part of the answer is that, in a conference attended by physicians and scientists, some astute people will know that the active ingredient in their product, MCT oil, is available over the counter. On the other hand, physicians are not likely to prescribe something new for their patients without some basic idea of what the product is.

The exhibit hall was quite a revelation. There were massive booths for the makers of the major Alzheimer's medications. One passed out expensive-looking engraved pens, and another, a four-port USB hub inscribed with the name of the products. The lines were long at these booths, and by contrast, there was very little activity at the Accera booth. Yet I knew that learning about ketones at their booth was perhaps the single most important piece of information that any attendee could acquire at this conference.

We hoped to distribute copies of my article to 5,000 conference attendees, but at most we were able to leave 300 in the city of Chicago; many of those were distributed at natural food stores and to passersby between Grant Park and the convention hall. Angie, John, and Steve also visited some of the local media and left copies. Overall, with the exception of a brief Internet TV interview, we were quite disappointed with the results of our attempts to get the message out.

THE GRASSROOTS APPROACH

We carried more than 1,500 copies of the article back home with us. I thought that since the attempts at getting this information out to the public at large by way of high-profile people, the media, and the Chicago conference were going nowhere, it was time to take a grassroots approach. I kept a box full of the flyers in our car, and we began to make a weekly circuit of the natural food stores in and around Spring Hill, leaving copies of the article for shoppers. We were invited to speak at a natural foods store in Spring Hill after the owner read the article. He posted a notice in his store, but only four people attended this first lecture. Shortly after, I received an invitation from the owners of another natural foods store to give lectures and to be interviewed for a health segment on a local radio program. The lectures were very well publicized, and the radio interview was aired a number of times. The attendance at the lectures increased to capacity, and several more were scheduled for people on the waiting list. There were eighty to ninety people at each talk.

People began sending the article out to other people. I regularly sat down with a list and e-mailed the article to as many on the list as I could during moments of free time, often very late in the evening and early in the morning. After e-mailing a copy to Bruce Fife, N.D., who has written many excellent books about coconut oil, an article appeared in his *Healthy Ways* newsletter summarizing what had happened with Steve, and he included my entire article in his next newsletter. I was contacted by a magazine distributed in natural food stores called *Energy Times,* and they likewise ran a story and created a link from which people could download the article.

The biggest break in getting the message out (before publication of this book) occurred several months later on October 28, when the *St. Petersburg Times* ran a story titled "Sketches in Progress" by Eve Hosley-Moore. The reporter spent considerable time interviewing Steve and me and attending one of my lectures. She also interviewed Dr. Veech and Dr. VanItallie. She eloquently conveyed the story of Steve's decline and his dramatic improvement after taking coconut oil, along with information about how ketones can provide an alternative fuel to the brain for people with Alzheimer's and those with certain other diseases. Steve's clocks were included with the story (Figures 4.1, 5.1, 5.2), and I believe this had more impact than anything else on what happened after the story ran. The article was also published online and can be viewed at www.tampabay.com/news/aging/article879333.ece.

Eve told me a few weeks later that it broke a record for "most e-mailed article," and it very soon "went viral" on the Internet. I began to receive regular requests to speak, to include my article or summaries of our story in newsletters, and to give radio interviews. Steve comes to all the talks with me and does not hesitate to answer questions and otherwise chime in.

I began to hear regularly from caregivers who were also seeing a positive response in their loved ones and occasionally from people who tried coconut oil and saw no response whatsoever. In Chapter 13, I share some of the many encouraging messages I have received.

There were very many days when I felt excessively stressed by the overload of full-time work, caring for Steve, and spending hours nearly every day trying to get the message out when I should have been relaxing and even sleeping. Then I would receive a phone call or an e-mail telling me about someone who had improved and how grateful the person was that I had written the article, and I knew my efforts were not in vain. This is often the impetus I need to keep going.

7

Steve: The First Year After Starting Coconut Oil

During the first two months, Steve primarily received coconut oil and occasionally small amounts of medium-chain triglyceride oil. He always received a minimum of two and a half tablespoons of coconut oil at breakfast and other unmeasured quantities of coconut oil and/or coconut milk later in the day. Steve's improvements over the first two months after starting coconut oil were:

- An increase in his Mini-Mental Status Exam score from 14 to 18 from the day before to several hours after starting coconut oil on May 20, 2008. He had additional MMSE testing at the local research centers and scored 17 on July 2 and 20 on July 23. Figure 7.1 on the following page charts the differences in Steve's MMSE scores before and after starting the oil.

- Improved clock drawing at fourteen and thirty-seven days after starting coconut oil. About two months after, when asked to draw a clock, he folded the paper in half, and then in half again, he said to try to center the clock in the middle of the paper. Then he became frustrated as he worked on the drawing because he "was not given a compass nor a ruler," which he wrote down on the paper before crumpling it up. A long-lost part of my "missing penny-finding" perfectionist accountant husband was surfacing again.

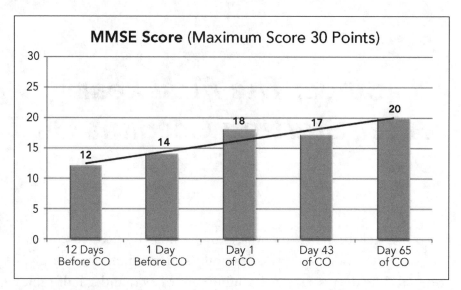

Figure 7.1. Steve's Mini-Mental Status Scores before and after starting coconut oil. Diagram by Joanna Newport.

- An increase in alertness, interaction, and ability to make conversation most noticeable in the morning.

- A return of certain aspects of his personality and sense of humor.

- An increase in animation in his facial expressions.

- Less distractibility, which allowed him to effectively resume certain activities, such as gardening and cutting the lawn, vacuuming, and helping with the laundry and dishes.

- Absence of tremor in his face and minimal hand tremor on occasion.

- Better listening comprehension.

- Increased recognition of family members.

- Increased libido.

- Improved ability to initiate and continue a course of conversation.

- Increased interest in exercise and desire to relearn.

- Keeping his pairs of shoes together and shoes and socks on both feet.

- Steve has said repeatedly that the "light switch came back on" and "the fog lifted" the day he started coconut oil, and he has often said that he has gotten his life back and has a future. His depression lifted.

After Steve's ketone levels were measured by Dr. Veech, he began to receive measured amounts of oil for breakfast, lunch, and dinner, plus additional coconut milk or oil used in cooking. We did this to maximize the amount of ketones he had available and provide him with a continuous stream of ketones around the clock.

IMPROVEMENTS AT THREE TO FOUR MONTHS

By three to four months after starting coconut oil, we were mixing MCT oil with coconut oil, and Steve was receiving a considerable amount of the mixture with each meal. We continued to see gradual improvements over this timeframe, including:

- Normalization of his gait and ability to run again.

- Disappearance of a visual disturbance that prevented him from reading. He explained at this point that during the prior one and a half years, when he would try to read, the words would go into "little boxes" sort of like "pixels" and would erratically jump around on the page, making it impossible to read even a single line. This problem disappeared and has not returned now nearly three years later.

- No longer showing any signs of depression.

- Relearning how to start the computer and use the mouse, but would become too frustrated to make progress in learning to type again.

Participation in a Clinical Trial

At the end of July, Steve entered into a clinical trial for an oral medication from Eli Lilly called semagacestat, a gamma-secretase inhibitor. This medication is expected to decrease the amount of beta amyloid building up in the brain, but it does not necessarily remove the beta amyloid from the plaques already present in the brain. As you may recall, beta amyloid is a protein normally made in the body whose function is not completely understood; when it accumulates in excess in brain tissue, it forms dense plaques, a hallmark of Alzheimer's disease. These plaques appear to be toxic to nearby brain cells and to interfere with communication between brain cells.

We had the option of entering an alternative trial with a vaccination that would remove beta amyloid plaques. However, one of the risks is a problem called "vasogenic edema" that could have severe consequences. The doctor explained that this would be more likely to occur in people like Steve who have the ApoE4 gene. They are more likely to have beta amyloid buildup in the walls of the blood vessels. Beta amyloid is removed fairly rapidly after the vaccine is administered, but when it leaves the blood vessel walls, they may weaken and allow fluid to leak into the surrounding brain tissue.

The oral medication has potential side effects as well, such as rashes, diarrhea, and a mysterious change in hair color, but none of them was as serious as vasogenic edema, which might cause actual damage to the brain. And so we decided to go with the oral gamma-secretase inhibitor. In this clinical trial, 60 percent of the participants would be placed on the drug and 40 percent on a placebo, but after twelve to fourteen months, those on the placebo would be switched to the actual drug. During screening for this trial, I told the physician and research assistant about what had happened with Steve with the coconut oil and MCT oil and gave them copies of my article. The company decided that, since Steve had been on this dietary intervention for at least two months, they would allow him to participate in the study.

Since we don't know with absolute certainty whether Steve was on the drug or placebo after July 23, we cannot be sure whether his improvements thereafter were purely a result of the coconut oil and MCT oil or the drug, or a combination of them. But the improvements prior to that were clearly related to coconut oil.

IMPROVEMENTS AT SIX MONTHS

By six months after starting coconut oil, now late fall of 2008, Steve was beginning to have improvements in his short-term and recent memory, but still had difficulty learning new cognitive skills. Here are two journal entries from those months:

December 11
"Steve seems to be holding on to his improvements, although after completing a month of OT [occupational therapy], his therapist Allison felt he was not able to make progress with the kind of cognitive studies she was trying—matching numbers or suits of cards, matching colored pegs, and so on. She said with some of these skills he functions at less than kindergarten level. The recent improvements I have noticed are better memory of things that happened the day before; he will bring something up himself and has his facts straight. He also complains of being bored and seems to need to do something more constructive. I take this as an improvement, since before he was perfectly content to shuffle things around in the garden or garage, basically without accomplishing anything. We attended several parties for the holidays that involved dancing, and he slow danced and even spent some time fast dancing with me. He had a big smile on his face, didn't get the steps down at all, loved to twirl me around, and seemed to enjoy himself. Last year I couldn't get him on the dance floor."

January 2, 2009

"Steve seems to be doing well. Recently, I have noticed that he will bring up events and conversations from one or more days ago and recall correctly the details. Last week, while I was working, he decided the doors were getting squeaky, found a small oil can, and oiled the hinges to all the various doors in the house. He was working at this when I came home. He also continues to complete jobs such as vacuuming with little or no prompting. He is in good spirits most of the time. He seems to be getting more and more bored lately. I believe he needs a purpose, so we will have to work on finding one for him. I take boredom as a good sign: before he was content to be aimless."

February 10

"Steve began his new job as a volunteer at Spring Hill Regional Hospital in the warehouse, working two days a week for three to four hours, helping to move the heavy boxes and put stickers on supplies, and working with one of the warehouse employees to make deliveries around the hospital. Around that time I wrote: 'On the days he is working, when I tell him today is the day, he jumps up out of bed to get ready and can't wait to get there. He is usually quite tired at the end of his shift but leaves with a smile on his face. I know all too well that he needs supervision, and I cannot thank the folks who work with him enough for everything they do to make this happen for Steve. It means so much to both of us.'"

April 2

"Two days ago Steve stayed in the waiting room while I went in to my doctor appointment. A couple of hours after, while we were eating, he told me about two articles he read in *Scientific American,* one about how Einstein may have been wrong and the other about neurons. This evening he started reading *The 36-Hour Day* (2001) by Nancy Mace and Peter Rabins, M.D., and announced that he was able to read the way he did years ago. He can actually comprehend. He took the book to the bedroom and came out laughing. He told me 'on page 113' they had written a section on hunting and Alzheimer's, and he thought it was hilarious that anyone would even consider going hunting with someone who had Alzheimer's disease."

SOME OBJECTIVE DATA AFTER A YEAR

Near the end of the first year after Steve began taking coconut oil, he received cognitive testing as part of the Eli Lilly semagacestat study. Remarkably, on May 5, 2009, his ADAS-Cog score had had improved by 6 points on a 75-point scale from when he started the study on July 23, 2008. Likewise his Activities of Daily Living score improved by 14 points on a 78-point scale during that same interval. Obviously, these results were very encouraging and gave us great hope.

8

Washington, D.C., and Dr. Veech

The week before President Barack Obama's inauguration in January 2009, Steve and I visited the Brooksville, Florida, office of U.S. Representative Ginny Brown-Waite. During the couple of days before the meeting, I spoke with Dr. Richard Veech and Dr. Theodore VanItallie to get their input on the important points to put together in a concise presentation. While we waited for Rep. Brown-Waite to arrive, Shirley, a liaison in her office, spent time with us, hearing about the events that had brought us there. She mentioned that she had a friend, now fifty-eight years old, with Alzheimer's disease, whom she saw over the holidays at a party and whom she did not expect to survive the year.

Representative Brown-Waite, a down-to-earth, straightforward individual, spent an hour and a half with us, listening intently to Steve's story and the basic science of ketones. She read with us some of the e-mails I received from people whose loved ones had improved. She promised to speak with Drs. Veech and VanItallie and investigate why the National Institutes of Health had not funded the continuation of this research. We left satisfied with the discussion and the belief that she would move this forward.

The following week, Steve and I took a road trip to Gasparilla Island, in southwest Florida, to share information with Dr. VanItallie and devise some strategy of how to push this issue. Dr. VanItallie was schooled at Harvard and Columbia University in the 1940s. After he completed a medical residency and then a fellowship in nutrition, he collaborated in the formation of the Institute of Human Nutrition at Columbia, where he served as director of the Obesity Research Center. He has received many awards for his nutrition research. At the time of our visit, Dr. VanItallie was eighty-nine, in excellent physical condition, and actively engaged in the pursuit of science twenty-four years after most people retire to a couch.

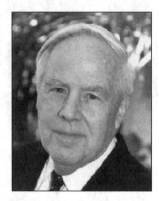

Theodore B.
VanItallie, M.D.

After lunch and a tour around the island, Dr. VanItallie, Steve, and I spent time trading research articles and other information. Dr. VanItallie's idea was to have a scientific meeting and invite ketone researchers to make presentations, as well as representatives of foundations that might provide funding for the research. He envisioned the proceedings of the meeting would be published in a prominent journal. We thoroughly enjoyed our visit and drove home that evening.

AN UNEXPECTED TRIP TO WASHINGTON

Then a fortuitous event took place. Shirley, from Rep. Brown-Waite's office, called me about two weeks after our visit to inform me that the husband of her friend with Alzheimer's disease reported that his wife had a response to coconut oil that was "unreal." She was now speaking in sentences again. I asked Shirley if she would share this information with the Representative and she said most definitely yes. She e-mailed me a copy of his message, which I then forwarded to Drs. Veech and VanItallie.

I decided to strike while the iron was hot and arranged a meeting during my next group of days off with Rep. Brown-Waite at her office in Washington, D.C., to include Dr. Veech. He, in turn, extended the meeting to include Dr. George Cahill, the physician who discovered that the brain could use ketones as fuel in

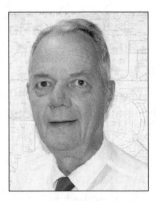

Richard L.
Veech, M.D.

the 1960s. Dr. Veech and Dr. Cahill are both Harvard-trained physicians and biochemists. Dr. Veech earned his Ph.D. at Oxford in England and trained with the quintessential biochemist George Krebs of Krebs cycle fame, and he later pursued a career in research with the NIH. Dr. Cahill served as director of metabolism at the Peter Bent Brigham and Deaconess Hospitals and later of the Howard Hughes Foundation, and he is a world-renowned expert in diabetes.

My sister Angela, my greatest support in all of this, came to our home with her husband a few days before the big meeting in Washington, D.C., to stay with Steve. With the meeting scheduled for 11:30 A.M. on Feb. 25, I took an early flight the day before in order to visit with Dr. Veech at his lab at the NIH in nearby Rockville, Maryland.

Meeting Dr. Veech

It was most exciting to finally meet Dr. Veech face to face. He is a tall, thin man, seventy-four at that time, personable, and genuine. He tells it like it is and faults himself for being less than diplomatic by nature. He made a point of taking me to the various labs to introduce me one by one to the members of his staff, several of whom are physicians. He had each of them explain their role in ketone research and share their most recent results. Two of the physicians, one an internist from Ghana, Dr. Osei-Hyeman, the other a neurologist from Japan, Dr. Kashiwaya ("Kashi"), spent time with me discussing Steve and his symptoms before and after starting the coconut oil/MCT oil regimen. Dr. Veech pulled out a small container of his ketone ester in crystalline form flavored with licorice and offered each of us a taste.

Later that night, Dr. Veech, Dr. Kashi, and I had dinner with Dr. Cahill. Like his colleague, Dr. Cahill is also tall and quite handsome, with more than a passing resemblance to the elder former President George Bush. We discussed the meeting planned for the following day, and I enjoyed listening to them reminisce about the many important scientists they have all known over the last half century or so.

The following morning, we met for breakfast and spent a couple of hours planning our strategy; then we took a taxi to Capitol Hill. We went through security to enter the Cannon Building, where Rep. Ginny Brown-Waite has her office. The security line came to a grinding halt when Dr. Veech pulled out his little bottle of ketones laced with licorice, which had to be thoroughly inspected, though he reassured the guard it was not poisonous or otherwise dangerous.

When we arrived at her office, we were advised that Rep. Brown-Waite was in the Capitol Building voting for the proposed Obama stimulus plan. We followed her aide underground and waited in the hallway while she was paged to come speak with us. Shortly thereafter, Rep. Brown-Waite emerged from the House Chamber. She immediately came up to me, shook my hand, and gave me a hug. She asked if I'd heard from Shirley about her friend's amazing response to coconut oil and advised me that she herself had been sending out the article to everyone she could think of.

After introductions, Dr. Veech briefly presented his paper slides to the Representative and Dr. Cahill explained the importance of ketones in the evolution of humanity—without ketones, humans, with our large brains, could not have survived. Rep. Brown-Waite advised us that she considered Senator Bill Young of St. Petersburg,

Florida, her mentor, and she wanted to get him involved in the process, since she was on the Ways and Means Committee as well as the Health Subcommittee and he was on the Appropriations Committee. She recommended that we draft a concise two-page report on the subject addressed to Senator Young and to her. She was paged to reenter the House Chamber to vote, and Dr. Veech gave the materials supporting his presentation to her aide. We followed her to the exit and left.

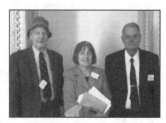

We were all extremely pleased with the success of the meeting, however brief. Dr. Cahill took a taxi to the airport, and Dr. Veech and I had another enjoyable meal, toasting our success, and then he drove me to the airport where I caught a flight back to Florida.

Left to right: George Cahill, Mary Newport, and Richard Veech in the Capitol Building, Washington, D.C., on Feb. 25, 2009.

This brief trip to Washington ranks very high among the most exciting days of my life.

ANOTHER TRIP TO WASHINGTON

A few weeks later, on March 20, Steve and I traveled to Washington to attend the Alzheimer's Public Policy Forums, a two-and-a-half-day conference sponsored by the Alzheimer's Association for the purpose of encouraging Congress to increase funding for disease research.

In preparation for the week in D.C., I arranged meetings with as many legislators as possible in order to enlist their help in getting funding for production of Dr. Veech's ketone ester and make them aware of the potential for MCT oil and coconut oil to improve lives now.

PM, from the regional Alzheimer's Association office in Florida, suggested that I contact someone in the Public Policy Office regarding coconut oil/MCT oil information. Believing this was a government office, I spoke with MS there, explained briefly the purpose of my call, and quickly sensed that he already knew about this. It did not take long, however, for me to realize this was a division of the Alzheimer's Association, and I had a sinking feeling that I should not have made the call. I e-mailed the article and a number of related research papers anyway, hoping that MS would read them and perhaps grasp, and even embrace, the information. A few days later, I learned how wrong I was on all counts.

I also learned that Maria Shriver, the wife of then Governor Arnold Schwarzenegger, would be testifying at the annual U.S. Senate Special Committee on Aging hearing for Alzheimer's disease, which we planned to attend as part of the Public Policy Forums conference. I called her office and faxed a cover letter and as much information to her as I could about ketones, stressing that this could be beneficial to her family members with Alzheimer's (her father Sargent Shriver) and her uncle Senator Ted Kennedy, who was suffering from a brain tumor. (Both of them are now deceased.)

A Conference at the NIH

The District of Columbia, with temperatures in the thirties and forties, was still quite cold in mid-March for people from Florida. We left our bags at the hotel and took the Metro subway to Rockville. I led and Steve followed, not always pleased about the activity and confusion around us. Getting on and off trains was particularly distressing to him, since little time is allowed to muddle through the people and pass through the doors before they close. I learned that the best way to navigate was to hold hands, to give Steve more of a feeling of security. The push-and-shove, "hurry-up" method only seemed to increase his confusion.

When we arrived at the conference room at the NIH, Steve met Dr. Veech for the first time, as well as Dr. Kashi and Dr. Osei-Hyeman.

They were very interested in Steve's condition and asked him many questions. Several others also attended from inside and outside the lab, many of whose faces were already familiar to me.

Dr. Veech had set up the conference beginning with me, so I gave a twenty-minute presentation about the progression of Steve symptoms and how I happened upon the information about medium-chain fatty acids and ketones, as well as Steve's response to the oils. Dr. Veech and the others each gave short presentations, complete with slides, of the various aspects of ketone research they were engaged in and the results. One of the many new things I learned that afternoon was that, in addition to ketones, medium-chain fatty acids also appear to enter the brain circulation and may also be used as fuel by brain cells.

Meeting with Senators and Opening Day of Forum

The next morning, Steve's right big toe, which had bothered him the day before, was now extremely swollen and tender, poor timing since were planning on sightseeing. Nevertheless, we took the bus tour of D.C., and then I spent several hours in the evening preparing for meetings with various members of Congress scheduled over the next few days. Dr. Veech had given me packets of information for each of the legislators, including a number of the important research papers related to the subject of ketones.

Steve and I had two meetings scheduled for Monday morning, March 23. The first was with Glen Schlesinger in the office of Florida Senator Bill Nelson; the second was with Taylor Booth on behalf of Florida Senator Mel Martinez, co-chair of the Special Committee on Aging. At each meeting, as succinctly as possible, I told the story of Steve, his history of early onset Alzheimer's disease, and how we came upon MCTs and their end-product ketones as a potential treatment for Alzheimer's and many other diseases with the problem of glucose uptake.

I told them about how Dr. Veech was making the ketone ester in his lab; how he did not have a facility large enough, much less the funding for such a facility, to produce the ester in enough quantity to do human testing; and how he could achieve levels with the ester many times higher than is possible with coconut oil or MCT oil. I noted that bankrupt ethanol plants could easily be converted to ketone ester production. I mentioned how medium-chain fatty acids are very concentrated in human breast milk and added to all infant formulas, and how ketones are important to the growth and development of the newborn brain and may also provide protection for the adult brain. I stressed that many of our fighting soldiers sustain traumatic brain injuries and die or are left with severe disabilities that might be alleviated if they could only receive an intravenous form of this ketone ester immediately after sustaining the injury. I added that many people here at home who suffer these types of injuries would also benefit.

Steve told them how he had come out of the fog since talking the mixture of coconut oil/MCT oil and how life was so much better since we had made this "discovery." I told them about my quest to make this information available to as many people as possible so they would have the opportunity to try it. I noted that we would appreciate any help they could give us with disseminating this information to the public and with obtaining or encouraging funding for Dr. Veech.

Taylor Booth from Senator Martinez' office advised that we should try to get a meeting with Senator Herb Kohl, the majority co-chairman of the Special Committee on Aging, particularly since they were holding annual hearings on Alzheimer's disease on Wednesday. We found the office for this Special Committee on the ground floor of the Dirksen Senate Building and spoke with MS about all of this. We learned that Joyce Ward, an aide in Senator Kohl's office, would be the best person to talk with, but she was extremely busy preparing for the hearings and therefore unavailable. I asked if it was possible to testify at the hearing and was advised that the agenda was set. However, MS noted that I could submit written testimony. We left some of the information with her and e-mailed more to her later, along with a letter to Senator Kohl.

Monday afternoon, we took the subway to the Omni Shoreham Hotel, where the Public Policy Forums conference sponsored by the Alzheimer's Association was taking place. The conference began with a Summit for Early Onset Alzheimer's Disease, followed by a roll call of advocates by state and an orientation. Shortly after we sat down, a man sat down at our table whom I recognized from Chicago. He was even wearing the same suit and had the gold Alzheimer's Association logo pin on his lapel. At that time, I suspected that his presence was security-related. This was just too much of a coincidence.

There were 500 people attending this conference, and most of them had a loved one with Alzheimer's disease. Many of the others worked for the Alzheimer's Association at its regional offices. This was an opportunity to get my message to 500 more people and whomever else they would pass it on to. I passed out as many copies of my article as I could during the breaks. As I handed it to them, I told people it was a case study about my husband with early onset Alzheimer's disease.

Steve hobbled along with his aching toe, and I could tell he was hurting more as the day went on. We took every opportunity to reduce walking, but Steve didn't complain and encouraged me to keep plugging away because all of this was so important and he "would live." The pain and swelling gradually subsided over the next twenty-four hours despite the walking.

Meeting More Senators and Second Day of Forum

We repeated this same process on Tuesday, March 24 (our thirty-seventh anniversary!), in the office of Senator Edward Kennedy, providing his aide, Craig Martinez, with a copy of additional information of the ability of ketones to shrink the type of tumors the Senator had. The meeting was rushed and had to be even more concise than usual to cover the most important details. Martinez seemed mostly unimpressed, but he took notice when I talked about traumatic brain injury and the troops.

We rushed from the Senate building to the Omni for the second day of the conference, arriving in time for the tail end of the research update, followed by a question and answer period. MS of the Public Policy Office had advised me that this would be the time to bring up the MCT oil/ketones. I was holding the microphone, preparing to ask my question, when the moderator, William Thies, Ph.D., the medical and scientific director of the Alzheimer's Association, decided there were to be no more questions. Coincidence? I was disappointed that I did not get to ask my question publicly, but I did take the opportunity to meet the speaker who gave the research update and ask if she received my information by e-mail the prior week. She did not recall seeing it, so I gave her copies of some of the information.

I then approached Dr. Thies, who seemed to know who I was, to see if he had received the packet of information I sent awhile back and to discuss the issue of why the Alzheimer's Association was so opposed to letting people know about the possibility that MCT or coconut oil could help. He told me that the idea needed extensive clinical testing before they would be willing to do that. I asked how he thought that could be accomplished, since it was unlikely a pharmaceutical company would undertake this. He suggested I contact the Alzheimer's Disease Cooperative Study at University of California in San Diego. I thanked him for the information.

Steve and I then proceeded to the ballroom for a luncheon. Ironically, as a result of my discussion with Dr. Thies, the only two seats I could find together were in the center in the second row. I say ironically because, after we settled into our seats, I realized that my chair was back to back with that of Maria Shriver, who was a speaker for this event and would also be testifying in Congress the following day. We would learn that her father, Sargent Shriver, ninety-three at the time, no longer knew who she was and no longer remembered what the Peace Corps was, even though he had worked so very hard to develop this program many years earlier.

I decided there was nothing to lose by approaching her. Packet of information in hand, I told her that I was a physician from Florida, caring for sick and premature newborns, and my fifty-nine-year-old husband, Steve, had the early onset disease. A nice looking man with salt and pepper hair and glasses peered over my shoulder as I presented the information. I asked if she was aware of the concept of "brain starvation" or "diabetes of the brain." The man replied that this topic was discussed in the upcoming HBO documentary, *The Alzheimer Project*. I told them about ketones and medium-chain triglycerides. I advised her that her husband might be familiar with MCT oil since bodybuilders use it to increase lean body mass. She listened very intently and circled items on the article I gave her.

Shortly thereafter, Maria Shriver gave her presentation about her father, and the man who peered over my shoulder was introduced as the producer of *The Alzheimer Project*. An eight-minute segment of the documentary was presented. As soon as there was an opportunity, I gave the producer a packet of information as well.

The afternoon session was all about strategy for the meetings we were to have as advocates on Capitol Hill the following day. A young lady presented the three points we were to make in these meetings on behalf of the Alzheimer's Association. Specifically, to reduce the two-year wait for Medicare to go into effect for those under age sixty-five who qualify for disability, to increase funding for Alzheimer's disease by $250 million over several years, and to create an Alzheimer's Center to study the disease and find the cure.

At that point, they wanted us to discuss these strategies with our neighbor to prepare us for the following day with legislators. I decided this would be a good time to distribute more of my articles. I simply told people, "This is a case study about my husband," and asked if they had received a copy yet. After distributing about forty to fifty of them, a young man walked up to the mike and announced there was someone distributing information about coconut oil and this was distracting people from the real message they were to take to Capitol Hill. MS of the Public Policy Office, who was seated on the stage, announced that they wanted everyone in the room to know that this was not from the Alzheimer's Association, they did not support it, and this was not to be taken to Capitol Hill. In retrospect, perhaps it was not the best time to distribute this information. However, it would be my last opportunity to get this information to a group of people who needed it. Of the 500 people attending, perhaps half had gotten a copy of the article. After that session, a few people came up to me, told me they had read it, and that they appreciated receiving the information.

We then broke down into groups by state to go over the meetings that were scheduled for the following day. MS went group to group to answer questions. When he arrived in our area of the room and finished his spiel, I told him that I would like to speak with him for a few minutes. Steve came with me, and we retreated to the hallway. I advised him that it was never my intention to have people take this as "the message" to Capitol Hill. My only intention was to get this information to 500 more people caring for loved ones with Alzheimer's. He told me that he thought it was irresponsible to push this kind of information based on one case. I told him that I had heard from many others whose loved ones have also improved and that all he needed to do was to look at the message boards for the Alzheimer's Association to see many accounts of this. In addition, Steve's case was just further confirmation of the studies performed by Accera. He reminded me that Dr. Thies had directed me earlier that day to the group in San Diego. I advised MS that, by the time someone applies for a grant and completes extensive clinical trials, years could pass and everyone in the room with Alzheimer's and the loved ones of the others would have seriously deteriorated or died. Shouldn't they at least have the opportunity to know about this and decide for themselves if they would like to try this dietary intervention?

A Full Day on the Hill

On Wednesday at 9 A.M., we attended a meet-and-greet with Senator Bill Nelson and left shortly after he did to speak with Melissa Bruce on behalf of Senator Daniel Inouye of Hawaii, then eighty-five years old. People over age eighty-five carry a 50 percent risk of Alzheimer's. Senator Inouye was chairman of the Senate Appropriations Committee and on the Health Subcommittee. In addition to the usual discussion, I pointed out that coconut is the starting point of ketones, and the economy of Hawaii could benefit from use of coconut oil, medium-chain triglycerides, and production of the ketone ester. Bruce seemed to get it and assured us that she would pass this information on to the senator.

We then walked posthaste to the Dirksen Building to attend the annual hearing of the Special Committee on Aging. We listened intently to testimony by Justice Sandra Day O'Connor, former House Speaker Newt Gingrich, Maria Shriver, and others. They encouraged the Senate committee to embrace the concept of the Alzheimer's Project Center, pointing out the Genome Project had been so successful. Gingrich testified that, with such a center, a means of prevention for Alzheimer's disease could be discovered by the year 2020. I could not help but think that prevention could be possible within the next year, along with stabilization and treatment of the disease a few years later, if the ketone ester was funded. I decided that I would take the suggestion of the young lady in Senator Kohl's office to submit written testimony. The members of the Special Committee on Aging at least would then be exposed to this information when reviewing the transcript of their hearing. We watched the press conference afterward and then beat a path to the offices of the U.S. Representatives on the other side of Capitol Hill.

We had a meeting with Anna Heaton in the office of our friend, U.S. Representative Ginny Brown-Waite, along with Peggy M, another advocate from our district who worked in the local Alzheimer's Association office. We wore our purple sashes and spouted out the information we were to convey. After lunch with Peggy, we met again with Anna and also with Justin, who was involved in appropriations, on the subject of ketones. Justin was already familiar with the topic, and the Representative herself came into the office to say hello and assure us that she was working on this issue. I advised her that we were able to get a meeting in the office of her mentor, Representative C. William "Bill" Young, shortly thereafter.

When we arrived at Representative Young's office, we were advised that he had been called away to an emergency meeting, and we would be meeting with his chief of staff, Harry Glenn. While waiting, we noticed a photo of Michael J. Fox shaking hands with the Representative. We had the pleasure of meeting with Glenn, who spent considerable time with us and listened with great interest. I emphasized the potential of ketones as a treatment for Parkinson's and added that I'd tried to get this information to Michael J. Fox through his foundation without apparent success. Glenn handed me contact information for a group in Sarasota, Florida, that studies traumatic brain injury. He also gave me some homework. He advised us that Fox had been a good friend of Representative Young's for many years and urged me to write a letter to him and send a package of information, stressing Parkinson's disease. Glenn offered to personally see that this was delivered directly to Fox. I told him that I would most definitely follow through on what he suggested.

We later joined Dr. Veech and a colleague from his lab at the hotel. We discussed the various meetings over the past few days, and we were all very pleased with the course of events. Dr. Veech encouraged me to write this book—the sooner the better. After a leisurely breakfast the following morning we returned to Spring Hill and reality.

STEVE ON THE ALZHEIMER'S ASSOCIATION AND CONFERENCE:
"[The conference] was a big show; that's all it was. . . . It was like when I worked for the mental health centers; they were always getting money from the government, but nothing was getting done, year after year. There is so little you can do, and they make a big party out of it. It's about people, and people hurting, and the hurting just doesn't ever stop. They keep fighting over and over for the money, and nothing changes. . . . And then there was the brouhaha about you [Mary] and your article . . . but I am glad you put the stuff out there. You had the cure in your hand and they ignored you."

9

The St. Petersburg Times *Runs Another Story*

In July 2009 I was contacted by a reporter for the *St. Petersburg Times,* Stephen Nohlgren, who had questions about ketones. He had seen a press release for Axona, a prescription medical food for people with Alzheimer's, and discovered that his paper had run the story about Steve and coconut oil the previous fall. We talked for some time—I filled him in on much of what had happened—and he decided to write a follow-up story.

LOCAL COVERAGE

As you remember, Steve had begun volunteering at Spring Hill Regional Hospital in the winter, putting stickers on supplies and helping to unload boxes of deliveries. Nohlgren and others from the paper met us at the hospital for interviews and videotaping. The online version of the story included a video showing Steve at work in the hospital warehouse and later at home, taking his lunchtime dose of medium-chain triglyceride/coconut oil in kefir and working around the house.

In conjunction with the article (next page), we were contacted by BayNews 9, a local cable channel, and they also interviewed and filmed us for a news story that appeared every half-hour over twenty-four hours. This video showed Steve backing his tractor out of the garage and cutting the grass.

TWIST ON ALZHEIMER'S FIGHT

BY STEPHEN NOHLGREN, *TIMES* STAFF WRITER
PUBLISHED SUNDAY, AUGUST 2, 2009

THEY ARE BRAIN BOOSTERS from caveman days that allow humans to survive on nothing but water. They nurture newborns right out of the womb. Now ketones—a kind of superfuel for brain cells—are drawing interest as possible treatment for Alzheimer's disease.

In March, a Colorado company began touting Axona, the first FDA-approved "medical food" for people with Alzheimer's. The key ingredient is a saturated fat that the liver converts into ketones. Meanwhile, a federal scientist is examining whether ketones might help soldiers think and fight better. He hopes to expand his work to people with Parkinson's disease and Alzheimer's.

Then there is Spring Hill resident Steve Newport. His wife retrieved him from an Alzheimer's funk fourteen months ago by loading him up with saturated fats found in coconut oil.

He says he feels "alive again." This does not mean the Promised Land is around the corner. Coconut and other ketone-producing oils can cause diarrhea and cramping. Cardiologists say they will clog arteries. Still, the science behind ketone bodies is intriguing and caregiver bulletin boards are sprinkled with hopeful anecdotes. An eighty-three-year-old woman in Connecticut is dressing herself again. A sixty-two-year-old man in California is cracking off-color puns. And in Spring Hill, Steve Newport mows the lawn without disassembling the John Deere.

The human body gets most of its energy from sugar, which comes from carbohydrates. But take away carbs, and the liver will start producing ketones—small fragments of carbon that can serve as a substitute fuel. Humans can survive about two months on nothing but water because the liver madly pumps out ketones. "Ketones are evolution's survival mechanism for starvation," says Theodore VanItallie, professor emeritus of medicine at Columbia University. A few years ago, VanItallie and colleagues treated five patients with Parkinson's disease with an extreme low-carb, low-protein diet that approximated starvation for twenty-eight days. Tremors decreased by 43 percent. One early hallmark of Alzheimer's is that nerve cells stop processing sugar and die. Maybe ketones can plug that fuel gap and keep those brain cells alive.

In March, a company in Broomfield, Colorado, called Accera, started marketing Axona. It produces ketones without starving the patient. The key ingredient is a saturated fat called caprylic acid. The liver converts a portion of it into ketones, regardless of what else a person eats. The Food and Drug Administration has not determined that Axona works, only that it is safe to eat and targets an identified nutritional deficiency.

Company literature says daily Axona servings improved cognition scores in people with mild to moderate Alzheimer's.

"It's conceptually very interesting. It seems to have a reasonable scientific basis," says Neil Buckholtz, head of dementias for the National Institute on Aging. "My major concern is that their clinical trials have never been published in peer-reviewed literature."

Accera chief executive officer Steve Orndorff says clinical trial data will be published in a few weeks. Axona costs about $72 a month and requires a prescription. It works in conjunction with traditional medicines for Alzheimer's. "This offers physicians for the first time in fifteen years a new therapy that works through a different mechanism," Orndorff says. "If we can show that Axona, coconut oil and other molecules work, we are going to open up a whole new area of research."

Mary Newport, a pediatrician who runs Spring Hill's neonatalogy clinic, scrounges for any Alzheimer's information she can find. Her husband is an accountant who began struggling with numbers in his mid-fifties.

Last year, she ran across a report of Axona's clinical trials, well before it hit the market. Not wanting to wait, she began feeding her husband large doses of virgin, nonhydrogenated coconut oil. . . . Coconut oil contains a mixture of saturated fats. The liver converts some into ketones. Others float around in the bloodstream, which is why cardiologists usually discourage its use. The effect on Steve Newport was immediate. "He said it was like someone had turned on a lightbulb," Mary Newport says. "He was alert, smiling, joking. He was Steve again. He was back."

One standard test for dementia is having a person draw a clock face. Before the coconut oil, Newport could manage only amorphous blobs. After the oil, his clocks looked like clocks. A story last November about the Newports appeared in some editions of the *St. Petersburg Times* and on tampabay.com.

Since then, Newport has continued to improve, his wife says. He still speaks in halting sentences, but he is reading again, volunteering at his wife's hospital and mowing the lawn. Before coconut oil, he would dismantle the mower, pour oil in the gas tank and forget about the lawn. Mary Newport acknowledges that she cannot pinpoint the source of her husband's continued improvement. About two months after she started the coconut oil, she also entered him into a clinical trial for a new Alzheimer's drug. She also began mixing in MCT oil, a supplement favored by bodybuilders. MCT oil also contains fatty acids that produce ketones.

In all, Steve Newport takes six to seven tablespoons of fatty oil a day, mixed into his food. Any more than that gives him diarrhea. To counteract artery clogging, his wife has reduced other fats in his diet. His cholesterol scores have not risen, she says.

Dr. Richard Veech, a metabolic specialist at the National

Institutes of Health, is working on the Holy Grail of ketone therapy: the ketones themselves. The Defense Department is paying to see if including ketones in field rations might give soldiers more stamina. Veech does not starve his subjects, nor feed them fatty oils. He manufactures ketones in the laboratory, then feeds them to his subjects. That raises their ketone levels twenty times higher than coconut oil or Axona does. The results in rats have been promising, Veech says, and tests on humans will begin soon at Oxford University, using rowing crews as surrogate soldiers. If he can figure out how to mass produce ketones, Veech says, he hopes to expand his work to Parkinson's and Alzheimer's.

After Mary Newport's posts on the Internet, other caregivers began spooning coconut and MCT oils into coffee and oatmeal. Not everyone showed improvement, but in Sandy Hook, Conn., eighty-three-year-old Mary Hurst started dressing herself again. Before the oil, she would never leave her nightgown and robe. She would sit in a chair all day, incommunicative "like a vegetable," says her daughter Diane Standish. Recently, Hurst walked into the kitchen and opened the refrigerator, something she hadn't done in years, Standish says. Asked what she was doing, Hurst retorted: Getting myself a piece of cake, do you mind? "She remembered that I had brought her a cake the day before," Standish says. "Miraculous."

Robert Condap of San Leandro, California, talks more after taking in coconut and MCT oils. When his wife, Gwen, was blow-drying his hair recently, he even cracked an off-color joke. "I was excited," she says. "That was an old part of him coming back." Jokes and clothes are small victories, maybe unmeasurable in scientific studies. But Gwen Yee Condap doesn't care. "This is not a cure. This is about improving quality of life," she says. "And we'll take any minimal improvement there is."

(Excerpted by permission from Stephen Nohlgren, *St. Petersburg Times.*)

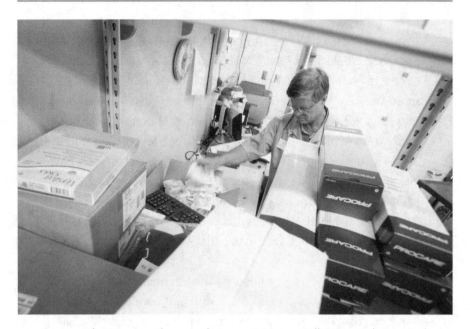

Steve volunteers in the warehouse at Spring Hill Regional Hospital
in July 2009.
(Reproduced by permission from the *St. Petersburg Times*.)

NATIONAL COVERAGE

Another major break in getting the message out came in October
2009 with publication of a report called "A Breakthrough in Alzheimer's Disease" in the *Health and Healing* newsletter of Julian
Whitaker, M.D., director of the Whitaker Wellness Institute in
Newport Beach, California. The article, several pages long, sum-
marized our story, discussed how ketones provide alternative fuel
for the brain, and outlined recommendations for incorporating
MCTs into the diet. This newsletter reaches about a quarter million people and is also available online by subscription. The number of hits to our website jumped substantially after the newsletter
went out, as did the number of people contacting me for more
information.

10

Steve: The Second Year After Starting Coconut Oil

A year after starting coconut oil, Steve still seemed to be heading in the right direction with continued gradual improvements, especially in his short-term and recent memory. He found work that was quite meaningful to him as a volunteer two days a week in the warehouse at Spring Hill Regional Hospital.

We were, however, about to enter a period of ups and downs.

SETBACK AND RECOVERY

Just when everything was going very well, I came down with bronchitis in June 2009, and, as hard as I tried not to pass it on, Steve caught it from me. Neither of us had had any significant cold or flu for several years up to that point, which I attributed to our healthy diet.

Steve was sick with constant coughing for several weeks. He took a product to suppress it that was a concentrated form of dextromethorphan, one of the active ingredients in many over-the-counter cold and cough medicines. Normally, I give him all his medications, but one day when I was working, he filled a 2-ounce cup, normally used for Nyquil, with this other product, instead of the two-teaspoon recommended dose. It was hours later before I knew he had taken it and discovered it when I noticed that a newly opened bottle was more than half gone. He then told me what he had done, but he seemed fine, so I didn't worry too much about it. I did tell him that he better not give himself any medication, but he should leave that up to me or our daughter.

A few weeks after the bronchitis, Steve had an outbreak of fever blisters on his lip that took more than a month to disappear, in spite of all the coconut oil he was consuming. In the previous year, he'd had a tiny blister for a few days just twice, a major improvement from the nearly constant battle he'd had for many years before starting coconut oil. On the day the blister showed up, he said he'd felt a sharp, stabbing pain on the scalp over the right side of his head.

During his illness, Steve told me at one point that he felt like he had "lost something," but couldn't explain what. He got up more often at night and became confused about where the bathroom was. He started putting some of his clothes on backwards, a problem that he didn't have before. We went to a Fourth of July dance, and he couldn't remember what to do with his arms and hands when we tried to dance. He started wearing just one shoe or sock again.

On the other hand, Steve was still able to do volunteer work and use the tractor to cut the grass, and his short-term memory still seemed improved over a year earlier. But needless to say, his negative changes worried me a great deal. I wondered if he was going to be able to recover from this setback. It was a very slow process, but he did recover almost completely.

In December 2009, Steve was able to dance at holiday parties, the shoes stayed on both feet, and his conversation flowed considerably better once again. He remained physically strong, with no hint of the tremor, visual disturbance, or slow gait that he'd had two years ago. In some ways, by January 2010, he seemed even better than before the illness. Here are some journal entries from that time:

January 13

"Steve is doing much better, is happy again and seems very much like Steve ten years ago with regard to his personality and interaction with me, although he still has a problem with 'doing things.' He surprised me last evening when we saw a classic film clip featuring Meg Ryan and Billy Crystal in a deli; he filled in the next line spoken by a lady at a nearby table, 'I'll have what she's having!'"

February 26

"On Joanna's birthday we ate at a Japanese restaurant and, much to our surprise, Steve picked up chopsticks and ate perfectly with them. Most people can't do this at all. Today, when we went to the hair salon, he said hello to our hairdresser Jackie by name and asked how her little boy was doing. Also, when Joanna told us she was going to see *Avatar,* he told her how wonderful it was and how the movie is 'in your face' [3-D]."

February 8 (Steve's Sixtieth Birthday)

"Steve is no longer depressed and usually bright and cheerful. He continues to volunteer in the hospital warehouse twice a week and wants to do more. It has been a long time since he has inexplicably taken something apart or lost his keys in the garage or done anything 'stupid,' as he says. He takes care of the yard and vacuums on his own.

"Steve recently told me that he feels like his accounting skills are still there, but can't access them. He can't use a calculator and can't even perform simple math. He can read short snippets, but can't stay with a novel. He has trouble keeping track of the day and the date. He doesn't drive and we seriously doubt that he ever will again. He needs reminders of how to do some very simple things and still needs a lot of help in that respect. It took many years for these skills to erode, and if those pathways in his brain have died, he will never get them back, unless he can learn these simple things from the beginning once again. His MRI in spring of 2008 showed considerable atrophy (shrinkage) of the brain, so there will be major limits on how much recovery we can expect, even if he is fortunate enough to take Dr. Veech's ketone ester at some point in the future.

"But, in spite of these persisting problems, the best part of his recovery is that 'Steve' is back. The personality and sense of humor that make Steve 'Steve' resurfaced in May 2008. My husband came back to me and he has not left. These aspects of Steve are stronger than they have been for many years. There are hours on any given day when everything is normal in our connection and interaction with each other. Not only are we husband and wife, but also we are good friends. This makes it easier for both of us to deal with the problems that persist. Steve has always been very aware of his memory issues and his limitations, and this makes it possible for us to talk openly about these problems. This goes a long way toward helping both of us cope with the nightmare that is Alzheimer's."

Eli Lilly Study

By the end of January 2010, Steve had been enrolled in the Eli Lilly semagacestat study for eighteen months. This was a crossover study, meaning that any time after twelve to fourteen months people who were on the placebo would be switched to the study medication. The drug is known to cause certain side effects, and a peculiar one is hair color change. But Steve did not develop the mysterious change until the beginning of February 2010, when we began to notice that his hair was coming in white at the roots.

Steve also developed several other possible side effects. He had an abrasion on his shin at the beginning of February that had not healed by March 1. When he nicked himself while shaving, the spots would open up and bleed while he was sleeping for up to five days. He had a strange episode where he nearly fainted and had an elevated CPK (creatine phosphokinase), an enzyme that increases as a result of damage to skeletal muscle, heart muscle, or brain. Since the drug is known to cause possible cardiac effects, this was of great concern. Fortunately, a repeat test at our local emergency room showed the elevation was related to skeletal muscle, but why this enzyme increased to very abnormal levels was a mystery.

We were scheduled to attend the Alzheimer's Disease International (ADI) Conference in Thessaloniki, Greece, March 10–13 (discussed in Chapter 11), and I had to decide whether to continue the study and risk possibly more serious side effects or discontinue the study. Considering that we might not have access to the kind of medical care we are accustomed to, we decided to withdraw Steve from the study. The apparent side effects disappeared, and he had a half-inch white band of white hair slowly work its way out as normal color hair began to grow in at the roots once again. Even though we could not be completely certain Steve was on the placebo for the first part of the study, all signs pointed in that direction.

Depression Revisited

Just a few weeks after Steve dropped out of the Eli Lilly study, his eighty-seven-year-old father lost his battle with diabetes and heart disease on March 23. Understandably, this triggered a new bout of depression that has not completely subsided more than a year later, as Steve deals on a daily basis with the many feelings and memories stirred up by the loss of a parent. A visit to Cincinnati to visit his mother a couple weeks after his father's passing found Steve more withdrawn and confused than usual. He called his mother "Grandma" and thought at times that his brothers had also died.

Steve began spending time talking to himself in the mirror as if he was talking to, and about, his father, and even named the image in the mirror "Paul," his father's name. These conversations were usually pleasant. On the other hand, he began seeing "Paul" in darkened windows in the evening and was often quite upset and confused by these images. I did not attempt to cover the bathroom mirrors, since I believed this was a therapeutic process for him, but I did hang curtains on the doors and windows that faced the courtyard to make the evenings more pleasant for him. Talking to oneself in the mirror is a common symptom as Alzheimer's disease progresses, so this was a disturbing setback for Steve. At the very beginning he told me that the image in the mirror looked like Steve from the neck down but like his father from the neck up (Steve looks more and more like his father as he ages). He also tells me at times that I look older than he expects when we look in the mirror together.

Steve also began having trouble finding certain rooms right around bedtime, and for a while I even had trouble convincing him to come to bed, since he seemed unsure that this was his bedroom.

Several weeks after we returned from Cincinnati, the pendulum seemed to swing back in a more positive direction. On April 25, I wrote, "[Steve] is better than he has been for a couple of months. He got the John Deere [tractor] out and cut the grass. He remembered how to operate it right away. He still does a good job vacuuming and worked in the warehouse [at the hospital] without a hitch. We saw in the news that there was a volcanic eruption in Iceland that stopped air traffic in Europe. A few days later he pointed up to our sky at sunset and said he thought the effects in our sky might be from the volcano."

But by the same token, Steve sometimes told me that he was going to go up the road to visit his mother and brothers, though they lived about 700 miles away in Cincinnati. A reminder of this was enough to keep him from wandering away. But fearful that he would follow through, our daughter Joanna made it her job to stay home with him whenever I was working. Caregiving has become part of her life as well—sad for one as young as she. She often said she believed she was doing this for a reason, and I cannot thank her enough for helping us this way.

A Stable MRI

On April 28, Steve had an MRI at the same facility at the University of South Florida where the previous MRI was performed in June 2008. We patiently waited for the written report to arrive at his physician's office. About ten days later, we received some amazing news. The bottom line of the report read: "Stable MRI brain in comparison to prior examination dated 6/16/2008." I called the radiologist who read the MRI, and he confirmed that he was sticking by this assessment.

Considering that Steve's MRI had deteriorated so much from normal to marked atrophy (shrinkage) between 2004 and 2008, this was quite surprising. It is much more likely that the atrophy would have continued to progress over the next two years. This appears to be further confirmation that medium-chain fatty acids and ketones are keeping his brain alive.

The first year after Steve started coconut oil and MCT oil was a year of substantial improvement. The disease process seemed to reverse a couple of years in some areas and even more in others. Overall, most of the second year was one of relative stability, even though there were ups and downs.

11

Two Overseas Trips: Greece and Scotland

In September 2009 I submitted two abstracts to the Alzheimer's Disease International (ADI) Conference in Thessaloniki, Greece, to be held March 10–13, 2010. Just after Thanksgiving, I learned that the case presentation about Steve had been accepted for an oral presentation (eight minutes to talk and two minutes for questions); the other abstract was accepted as a poster presentation. This second abstract was about other caregiver reports of forty-seven people with dementia and their responses to oils containing medium-chain fatty acids (discussed in Chapter 13). After considerable contemplation and discussion weighing the pros and cons with Steve, my sister Angie, Dad, Dr. Veech, and Dr. VanItallie, I decided to go. The opportunity to give an oral presentation, even though brief, to scientists and physicians from all over the world seemed important in my quest to get the message out.

OFF TO GREECE

The next question was whether to take Steve or not. Ultimately, the decision was his. He said he preferred to come with me rather than to stay with relatives. So Steve and our daughter Joanna came so she could help me with Steve. I thought it would be best for Steve, given his condition, to break up the trip, instead of traveling seventeen or more hours overnight from Tampa. The loss of a night's sleep could affect him for the entire trip. So we flew one day from Tampa to New York City, took a morning flight to London, just under seven hours, the next day, and the third day flew from London to Thessaloniki, nearly four hours more. We did manage to get five to six hours of sleep each night, but the 48-hour-plus journey left all of us fairly exhausted.

One of my major concerns in preparing for the trip was whether bottles of medium-chain triglyceride oil and jars of coconut oil would make it through security in our checked luggage. I mentioned this in an e-mail to Beth, a dietician at The Charlie Foundation (mentioned in Chapter 17), who happened to have an associate, Dr. Evangeliou, a pediatrician and professor living in Thessaloniki. Amazingly, he agreed not only to purchase the oils for us, but also to pick us up at the airport. He very kindly took us to our hotel and showed us some of the beautiful Byzantine churches along the way. It turned out that Dr. Evangeliou had been involved in ketone and ketogenic diet research.

When we arrived at the conference center the next morning, I checked in with my CD/PowerPoint presentation and was very pleased that the computer accepted it without a hitch. I am not usually that lucky. We attended a few talks together, but Steve and Joanna mostly hung out in the hotel lobby while I went to talks. They also attended a forum for people with dementia and their caregivers, where they bonded with Helga, a lovely person from Munich.

My Talk

The list of talks scheduled for the first afternoon session included a presentation by Samuel Henderson, Ph.D., from Accera, the inventor of Axona. His talk, also eight minutes, was titled "Ketone Bodies as a Therapeutic for Alzheimer's Disease." Steve and Joanna attended with me, and we listened to him discuss Accera's clinical trials with AC-1202 (an MCT known as tricaprylic acid) and the rationale for using an oil that produced ketones. To my surprise, he mentioned that I would be speaking on the same subject in the next group of talks, should people want more information about ketones.

During a short break, Joanna and I placed a handout on the seats of my slides with references, as well as a copy of the article I wrote in July 2008, "What If There Was a Cure for Alzheimer's Disease and No One Knew?" The presentation went very fast but very well. I talked about the problem of diabetes in the brain and the potential for ketones to bypass the problem as a sort of metabolic trick. I related what happened with Steve, showed pictures of his clocks, and displayed a chart of his Mini-Mental Status Exam scores and ketone levels. I discussed the even greater potential for Dr. Veech's synthetic ketone ester. There were a few easy questions at the end: "Can you cook with coconut oil?" "What other foods contain medium-chain fatty acids?" "Have other people responded to this?" The last question gave me the opportunity to mention my poster with responses of forty-seven people with dementia that was to be presented the next day.

All but a few of the 100 handouts were gone from the seats. A man from the Alzheimer Working Group (AWG) of Scotland spoke with me after the session and requested a copy of my presentation. Another physician from Mexico advised me that he was planning to make a presentation about this at their national conference later in the year. A physician from Japan asked me to take a picture of her with Steve. I was very pleased with the reaction and can only hope that the people who listened and understood will pass it on. Perhaps some of them will have the interest and resources to conduct a clinical trial.

The Poster Presentation

I left Steve and Joanna, who wasn't feeling well, behind the next day and went to get ready for the poster session. The poster exhibition was in the basement and had little traffic. When I arrived in the hall, Dr. Henderson was having a cup of coffee. When my poster was set up, I walked up to him and said, "At last we meet!" and we shook hands. He told me that he attended my talk. He said, "You know, I am just trying to get the message out too." He further told me that the Alzheimer's Association would no longer allow him to have a booth at their International Conference for Alzheimer's Disease. Also, they had put out a formal statement denouncing medical foods. I told him about my attempts to get a poster table at the 2008 Chicago ICAD and how I thought it was because of Accera's exhibit that the Alzheimer's Association had ultimately turned me down. He was surprised. He advised me that at least one other medical food company was no longer able to exhibit, but one of the bigger companies, a larger donor to the Alzheimer's Association, was still permitted to have a booth. We talked a lot about ketones, and I asked him questions about the science. We talked for at least an hour before we were asked to leave by the staff, who were removing all the tables in preparation for the next event.

That evening we attended a gala dinner, and Helga, Steve's new friend who also has dementia, sat with us. She talked about the possibility that we might come to Munich to talk about the ketone issue. There were presentations and awards, followed by a display of traditional Greek dance, then a medley of mostly American party dance music. The room turned festive as everyone flocked to the dance floor, and even Steve danced with me for a while. Joanna went to the balcony above the dance floor and took pictures and videos of the people dancing below as she moved to the music! We left when Steve began to look droopy. Not long after we settled in bed, it was Steve's night to have intestinal problems, which meant that I lost sleep as well, since things like that don't happen without my involvement.

The following morning, I picked up my poster and then, sure that Steve was past the worst of it, we walked along the waterfront for several hours in Thessaloniki. We were on to Athens the next morning. This part of the trip was for me. I had studied Greek literature for four years in college and thought that, if we were traveling all the way to Greece, we had to visit the Acropolis. The view of Athens from there is spectacular.

Heading Home via Athens, London, and New York

After that we moved on to London for two days before heading back to New York City. How did Steve do through all of this? Well, the trip was part dream and part nightmare! A lot of public transportation was involved, starting with airports and including taxis, subway systems, and buses. I took Steve by the hand whenever possible, and Joanna kept an eagle eye on him as well. On steps and escalators, I told him to follow Joanna while I brought up the rear. We must have uttered the phrases, "Come on, Steve!" and "Come on, Dad!" hundreds of times. I don't think Steve knew exactly what city we were in much of the time, so I reminded him a lot. At one point in Athens, looking at the signs in Greek, he remarked that we must be in Russia!

In London, Steve particularly enjoyed Madame Tussauds, and he was especially good that day, laughing and happy, in contrast to his mood the evening before. Just as I was beginning to enjoy the amazing view from the London Eye, a giant 443-foot ferris wheel, in the dark, he became uncooperative and tried to walk away from us several times. We had to reassure him that he was all right. Later at the hotel, I cried as I remembered what it was like to travel with the old Steve, before Alzheimer's disease. I missed his happy, smiling face, and I wondered, as I do every time, if I will see it again, and if this is the beginning of the end. When he woke up the next morning, smiling and talking like his normal pleasant self,

I was quite relieved to have my husband back once again. Perhaps with all the walking around, his muscles had used up most of the ketones from the oils and did not leave not enough for his brain, or maybe he was just tired. I was clearly expecting too much of someone with his condition to enjoy running around Thessaloniki, Athens, and London the way I wanted to experience it. So Joanna and I made a pact that we would end the tour of London when the sun started to go down. We had a much better day. After flying seven hours to New York the next day, sight-seeing there with our niece Anna, all three of us cheered when we started up the driveway to our home in Spring Hill the next day.

I decided that if we were to attempt such a trip again, we would fly directly to and from our destination and forget the whirlwind sightseeing. The stress far outweighed the benefit. And so we live and learn. Six months later, I would have the chance for a do-over.

OFF TO SCOTLAND

Early in the the summer of 2010, I learned that the Ketogenic Diets 2nd Biannual Conference was to be held that October in Edinburgh, Scotland. It was being organized as part of the International Symposium on Dietary Interventions for Epilepsy and Other Neurologic Disorders, and I soon learned that the organizers would consider the topic of MCTs to produce ketosis as a treatment for Alzheimer's. Ketosis, as you may remember, is the process that occurs when the body breaks down fats for energy instead of glucose. By that time, I had enough information from caregivers of sixty persons with dementia to submit an abstract, so I submitted the data from the caregiver reports and Steve's case study for consideration.

The conference's scientific committee accepted both abstracts for poster presentations, so then I had a new set of dilemmas: to go or not to go, and if I went, whether to take Steve or leave him with another caretaker. For a short time, I believed it would be impossible for me to attend this conference; however, I was encouraged by several colleagues to find a way to go. Dominic D'Agostino, Ph.D., an assistant professor at the University of South Florida (USF) who planned to attend, was one of them. Dr. D'Agostino helped a man from the United Kingdom with severe treatment-resistant seizures completely eliminate his seizures using a ketogenic diet. This evolved into research about the use of a ketogenic diet for navy divers as a possible means of preventing seizures, which they are prone to during deep dives. He has a very interesting lab with small hyperbaric chambers for use in animal studies and access to some amazing technology to carry out his work. Recently, D'Agostino and his colleagues at USF began studying caloric restriction, ketogenic diets, and the ketone ester for Alzheimer's mice. In addition, he was performing animal studies using ketone esters for epilepsy, oxygen toxicity, cancer, radiation, and traumatic brain injury. Should these animal studies have positive results, funding will be more likely for human clinical trials.

After deciding that I would attend the conference, I struggled with whether or not to take Steve. After investigating various options, I decided that both he and I would have more anxiety if he stayed at home than if I took him with me, and Joanna was more than willing to come along to help out.

Keeping It Simple

We left for Scotland on October 3 by way of Atlanta on an overnight flight to Amsterdam and then on to Edinburgh the next morning. All the flights to the United Kingdom originating in Tampa are overnight. The flight was packed and noisy, and we didn't sleep at all. I brought an e-book reader to keep us occupied, loaded with reading material for me and music for Steve to listen to through ear buds. In spite of the lack of sleep, Steve did amazingly well overall. There was the usual confusion going through security, including explanations of Steve's condition to security personnel.

After the sixteen-hour trip, we checked into our hotel in Edinburgh, two blocks from the conference hotel. We had a two-bedroom apartment with a full kitchen, dining area, and living room. The kitchen was stocked with a basket of breakfast goodies, and milk and juice were in the fridge. An organic grocery store was just around the corner, so we were able to relax and economize by having breakfast and lunch in our room. We tried to take a nap after we arrived, but there was too much noise on the street, so we took a walk to see the city, had an early dinner, and then crashed for fourteen straight hours. Steve had some interesting nightmares at the beginning of the night, involving scary breathing and big snakes, no doubt set off by the missing night of sleep, but thereafter he settled down. He had another bout of confusion involving images in darkened windows at a restaurant when we dined with other conference attendees late one evening. Otherwise, he handled our time in Edinburgh quite well.

While I attended the three-day conference, Joanna and Steve spent several hours each day exploring the beautiful city with a magnificent castle at its center. The conference was a six-minute walk from the hotel, and I sprinted back and forth each day to check on Steve during lunch breaks. In the evening, we continued the exploration process together and found unique restaurants on the Royal Mile where we experienced Scottish cuisine.

Making Contacts

I had a list of ketone and ketogenic diet researchers whom I hoped to meet at the conference, most of whom were speakers. I brought copies of a paper I prepared on ketone research ideas for treating newborns and shared them with several pediatric neurologists from Johns Hopkins School of Medicine who study the ketogenic diet for pediatric epilepsy: Eric Kossoff, M.D., Eileen Vinings, M.D., and Adam Hartman, M.D.

I took copious notes during the presentations and learned a great deal during the conference. In addition to the classic ketogenic diet, which is very high in fat and very low in carbohydrate and protein, some patients with severe epilepsy have complete relief from, or great reduction in, seizures with less restrictive ketogenic diets, including the modified MCT oil ketogenic diet, the modified Atkins diet, and the low-glycemic-index diet. These modified ketogenic diets generally result in lower ketone levels than the classic ketogenic diet. This means that some people are responsive to even relatively low levels of ketones in the range of those achieved with medium-chain fatty acids. If severe epilepsy can respond to mild ketosis, is it possible that other neurologic conditions, such as Alzheimer's, Parkinson's and traumatic brain injury, could likewise respond to this simple dietary intervention?

Thomas Seyfried, Ph.D., the premier researcher of ketogenic diets for brain cancer and a professor of biology at the University of Illinois, Urbana-Champaign, gave an amazing presentation. Dr. Seyfried has found that certain cancers, such as the brain tumor glioblastoma that affected Senator Ted Kennedy, can shrink by as much as 80 percent after a relatively short time on this type of diet. Potentially then, the tumor could be removed surgically without collateral damage to the brain caused by radiation, the current treatment of choice. Seyfried explained that most cancers can only use glucose as a fuel and cannot use ketones. Therefore, if you minimize carbohydrate and protein intake (protein can be used by the body to make glucose), the tumor will shrink due to lack of energy to keep the tumor cells alive. The brain and other organs in the body are spared because they can use ketones for fuel. Seyfried and his colleagues have published a case report involving a sixty-five-year-old whose tumor was no longer detectable on positron emission tomography (PET) or MRI scans after two months on such a diet (Zuccoli, 2010). During and after the poster presentation, I had a chance to talk for quite some time with Dr. Seyfried, and he encouraged me to submit Steve's case presentation to a scientific journal for publication.

The afternoon following the conference, we embarked on the journey home. This time we had a thirteen-hour overnight layover in Amsterdam, which we spent at an airport hotel, before taking the long flight home. I was pleased that we made the trip.

12

Steve: The Third Year
After Starting Coconut Oil

Steve: The Third Year
After Starting Coconut Oil

t the beginning of year three in the spring of 2010, I wrote,
"We can only hope that our persistence and strict adherence
to a diet that includes medium-chain fatty acids to keep ketones
available to Steve's brain will help him sustain this miraculous
reprieve from the nightmare. How long will this last? I don't know
the answer to this question, but believe that the clock has been set
back at least two to three years, and in some respects, even longer.
God willing, we will have many more good years together. As I
have often thought to myself, a lament I have heard from so many
others, if we can stay where we are now, it will mean everything in
this battle with Alzheimer's disease. While awaiting the availability
of Dr. Richard Veech's ketone ester, the next best strategy we can
employ is to stay on track with our healthy diet that includes
coconut oil and MCT oil, in order to provide with brain the
ketones as an alternative fuel. This will help provide Steve with the
best quality of life he can have while living with this disease."

SETBACKS AND RECOVERIES CONTINUE

The development of Steve's new symptoms at the end of the second
year was a tough reminder that we don't yet know what causes
Alzheimer's disease, much less how to treat it, and that the process
apparently marches on. Due to the setback that occurred after his

father died, we made the difficult decision for Steve to discontinue volunteer work.

In June, I found a study showing that music therapy is beneficial to people with Alzheimer's. We rediscovered how much Steve enjoys music after I loaded my computer with many of Steve's favorite albums by Barry Manilow, Neil Diamond, some Beethoven and the Beatles, as well as the soundtracks from some musicals he enjoys like *Fiddler on the Roof, South Pacific,* and *Phantom of the Opera.* Amazingly, he whistles along with an obvious recollection of the melodies. If I ask him if he would like to hear, for example, *South Pacific,* he will begin to whistle "Bali Ha'i," a song from the movie.

In July, I met a speech therapist, Andrea, who had considerable experience with Alzheimer's and stroke patients, and she began to work with Steve. On July 14, I wrote in my journal, "Andrea said they got off to a rocky start, but then he began doing pretty well. He could name sixteen of the twenty animal pictures immediately. He had trouble with four of the names because he was trying to come up with the subspecies, such as a 'capuchin' instead of a generic 'monkey.' He was overthinking it!"

Eli Lilly Drug Trial Fails

On August 17, I received a call from the research nurse for the Eli Lilly semagacestat drug trial. After reviewing the first eighteen months of data, the company learned that not only was there an increase in skin cancer, but that the people who received the drug had experienced *"accelerated worsening of the disease"* compared to the people on the placebo as evidenced by the ADAS-Cog and Activities of Daily Living Tests. This could explain some of Steve's new symptoms in late winter and early spring of 2010, when I believed he had crossed over to taking the drug. Steve's first reaction was to ask if they were going to give him a million dollars, a nice reminder that his unique sense of humor was still intact. My first reaction was relief that we had withdrawn him from the study at the beginning of March.

It is ironic that medium-chain fatty acids helped him improve so much that he qualified for a clinical trial with a drug that may have made him worse.

Gout and Prednisone: Another Setback

Steve was quite stable through the remainder of the summer and fall of 2010, with at least no obvious new symptoms. However, along with the holidays came another setback for Steve.

Just before Christmas, we had a stretch of very cold weather that was quite unusual for Florida. We went to a party at the home of longtime friends that involved caroling around their neighborhood. Steve merrily whistled along as we went door to door and we had a wonderful evening. The next morning, the big toe of his right foot was quite tender—indicating a flare-up of gout. Gout occurs in people who have high uric acid levels, and this substance will sometimes crystallize in certain joints, particularly in the large toes, which tend to be the coolest part of the body. Cold weather can trigger such a flare-up. I took him right away to see his doctor, and he prescribed prednisone, which usually reduces the pain and swelling within a few days. I was nervous about giving Steve prednisone because of the many side effects that can occur, including those involving the immune system, but I did not remotely anticipate what would happen next.

About four days after starting this medication, which is usually tapered off slowly over a few weeks, the pain and swelling in Steve's foot was gone, but he began pacing relentlessly through the house, agitated and suspicious of everything I tried to help him with. He refused to take a shower and change his clothes. He wouldn't come to bed. He began to constantly obsess about his father. The toilet became a mystery that had to be explained at times before he would use it, particularly in the late evening. I wrote in my journal on January 1, 2011: "It feels like Steve has fallen off a cliff and that is pretty much what I want to do right now. I don't know how I am going to get through this. Is this just a glimpse of the future, or is this our permanent situation?" My sweet Steve had turned into someone I barely recognized.

Since the pain and swelling were gone, we tapered the prednisone off more quickly than originally planned. By the middle of January, my question was answered as Steve gradually stopped the constant pacing and obsessing, and his pleasant demeanor and sense of humor returned. Even though he seems to recover after each setback, a little bit of something is lost each time, and we are left with one or more new problems to deal with. We won't be using prednisone again.

By early April, we took a trip to Cincinnati to see our families and stayed with my father and his wife as usual. At home, we have a king-size bed that is actually two twins side by side. At their home, we share a smaller double bed, which is normally not a problem. However, on this occasion I had great difficulty convincing Steve to come to bed. Finally, he told me he was worried. "About what?" I asked. He said, "I don't want to have any more children." He was worried that I would get pregnant if he slept with me! There wasn't anything I could say to convince him that it was safe to sleep with me. Fortunately, my father had an inflatable bed. When I suggested to Steve that I sleep on the inflatable bed and he could have the double bed, he said that would be fine, and he lay down and went right to sleep.

When we got home, once again he balked at coming to bed with me. I pulled our beds about six inches apart, and the problem was solved. Whenever a new behavior appears that doesn't make sense, there is no doubt a somewhat logical explanation for it.

It has been more than thirty-two months since Steve improved after he began taking coconut oil in May 2008. A lot has happened since then, and there have been some setbacks and recoveries, but overall Steve has retained most of the improvements we saw during the first months. There has been a big improvement in quality of life for both of us, and I believe we have gained at least two to three more relatively good years.

HOW STEVE IS DOING NOW

People often ask how Steve is doing now compared to when I wrote my first article in July 2008. Here is a comparison between the improvements reported on my website in the September 2009 update and Steve's status as of April 2011:

THEN (SEPTEMBER 2009)	NOW (APRIL 2011)
His gait has become normal.	Steve's gait is still normal.
He was unable to run for more than a year and can run again.	Steve can still run; he enjoys taking twenty-minute fast walks with me.
He had a visual disturbance that prevented him from reading. He describes it as the words moving around erratically on the page. This stopped after three to four months on the oils.	This problem has not returned. Steve does not spend much time reading; however, he can read accurately out loud, even complex words.
He has a mild tremor that only appears if he is late getting his oil.	The same.
He no longer feels depressed and believes that he has a future. He says he feels like he "got his life back." His libido also returned shortly after he started the oil.	Steve's father passed away in spring 2010, which set off some depression; however, his mood is much improved in the past few months.
He is much less distractible and able to stay with a specific task, such as yard work or vacuuming.	He is still able to do vacuuming, operate his rider mower, and will spend an hour or longer shredding old records for me.

Family members who talk to or see Steve every couple of months report that his conversational skills have improved each time they have contact with him.	Steve has retained his ability to carry on a conversation pertinent to the ongoing discussion.
His shoes used to get separated and he would very often wear only one shoe or sock. We used to have piles of the same-sided shoes and no match by the doors and in his closet! He would remove one shoe in his garage, and they would accumulate there. He is no longer having this problem.	Steve still keeps his shoes on and keeps them together.
Within the past six to eight weeks his memory for recent events is improving. He often brings up events that happened days to weeks earlier and relays telephone conversations with accurate detail.	This is about the same. He still remembers major events, such as our European trips.
He used to spend many hours rearranging his garage, but recently became "bored" and wanted to do something more. He now volunteers twice a week at the hospital where I work, helping in the warehouse with boxes and stickers and working with someone to deliver supplies around the hospital.	He volunteered for about a year at the hospital, but became a bit obsessed with wanting to have a paying job. He currently attends a four-hour social program for people with dementia twice a week, sponsored by Catholic Charities. He is a client, but does some shredding and vacuuming for them while he is there. He still doesn't get a paycheck!
Certain features of Steve's personality became more evident shortly after he started taking coconut oil.	Steve's sense of humor is still very much present and quite unique. He often teases me and also puts two and two together to come up with something unexpected. On April 6, we were in a restaurant and the server asked Steve if the "first bites" were good. Steve's response was, "Yes, and the second bites were good, too!"

Steve continues to take the half-and-half mixture of coconut oil and MCT oil. He receives three tablespoons at each meal and two tablespoons at bedtime. He eats a low-carbohydrate whole-food diet, with organic foods whenever possible, and receives about one tablespoon per day of cod liver oil and fish oil, as well as vitamins and other supplements. In spite of so many calories as oil, he currently weighs about ten pounds less than he did when he started taking the oils. His triglyceride levels have been 70 or less, and his HDL (good) cholesterol has increased from about 35 milligrams per deciliter (mg/dl) before starting the oils to 105 mg/dl.

As you know, "the light switch came back" on the day Steve started taking coconut oil. In spite of some setbacks, particularly this past year, this dietary intervention has brought about a significant improvement in his quality of life. We will continue to include coconut oil and MCT oil in our diet to provide ketones as an alternative fuel for the brain as a major component of our strategy to fight Alzheimer's disease.

13

Caregiver Reports

Since writing my article "What If There Was a Cure for Alzheimer's Disease and No One Knew?" in July 2008, I have received thousands of letters and e-mails from people who have loved ones with Alzheimer's disease, rarer and progressive dementias such as fronto-temporal dementia, posterior cortical atrophy, and Lewy body dementia, as well as a variety of other problems such as Parkinson's disease, Huntington's disease, multiple sclerosis, bipolar disease, and even glaucoma and macular degeneration. Improvement of eye problems may at first seem unexpected until one considers that the eye is an extension of the brain and specialized neurons are affected in these diseases. The involvement of nerve cells is the common thread that links all of these diverse conditions.

EXCERPTS FROM LETTERS AND E-MAILS

The following is just a sample of the numerous e-mails and letters I have received mostly from caregivers (though three people care for themselves) since 2008 reporting improvements and reflecting a range of ages and neurodegenerative disease conditions. Many of the people used coconut oil only, many others a mixture of coconut oil and MCT oil, and a few only MCT oil, MCT Fuel (a liquid energy formula made by TwinLab that contains MCTs), or Axona (the prescription medical food made by Accera).

Seventy-Eight-Year-Old Man with Fronto-Temporal Dementia

• December 2, 2008: "I read your article on the use of coconut oil; I also read that the Food and Drug Administration approved the drug Axona . . . and would like to try him on the drug. . . . He has improved significantly with the coconut oil." [I suggested she purchase MCT oil while waiting for Axona to be available, and I asked her for more information and to keep in touch about her husband's progress. Over the next months, she experimented with giving her husband the oils individually or in combination and eventually increased dosing from once to three times a day.]

• December 23, 2008: "My husband's memory has improved and his ability to speak and recall words is better. He has been taking MCT oil now for about a month, three tablespoons in the morning. What hasn't improved is his ability to make good decisions."

• February 1, 2009: "I decided to try just MCT oil, three tablespoons in the morning, but then I noticed that in the late afternoon he started to fade out on me. So I started giving him one tablespoon in the afternoon and he was better. I think he did much better on the coconut oil so I have switched him back to the coconut oil. I am still using some MCT oil."

• May 19, 2009: "Taking the oil three times a day in the proportion you suggested [four teaspoons of MCT oil plus three teaspoons of coconut oil]. I started him on the oil [five months ago] because of bizarre behavior, such as giving away thousands of dollars, melting a Netflix video in the toaster oven (because he needed to dry it), and putting a dishtowel in the microwave and causing a fire. Since I started him on the oil he has not exhibited this bizarre behavior. He still has problems but not as severe. . . . Since I started him on the oil, and especially now that he is taking it three times a day, he has improved dramatically. . . . I am assuming the oil works just as well with fronto-temporal dementia, since his behavior has improved."

• July 12, 2009: "He is not perfect, but he is very independent. . . ."

Seventy-Seven-Year-Old Man with Alzheimer's Disease

• November 13, 2008: "[My husband] has only been taking the coconut oil for two weeks but I can see a big difference already. The best thing that has happened so far is that my home has been peaceful for ten straight days. . . . It's hard for me to believe the wonderful change is from something as simple as coconut oil. To me, his improvement is a miracle. With my help this week he has fed the animals; fixed his tray (as a pilot he likes to eat off a tray since he did it for thirty years) with silverware, napkin, and plate; and this morning he got his own cereal. He has not done any of this since his hospitalization in June."

Eighty-Three-Year-Old Woman with Dementia

• January 1, 2009: [Seven weeks after beginning coconut oil.] "[My mother used to] sit in her chair all day like a vegetable. Some days she didn't remember who I was. . . . She would look at my father and ask who *he* was. . . . She did not have tremors, but was dizzy a lot, and could not walk very well. . . . Her day consisted of going from the bed to a chair in the living room. . . . She had no appetite and couldn't taste her food while on Aricept. . . . The transformation is truly a miracle. We noticed that she started slowly getting more coherent and the dead look behind her eyes was clearing. . . . We noticed that she slowly recognized people easier and remembered them more often. The repetition of questions stopped slowly . . . [and she now] gets around pretty well, I must say. Just this past week there were very important and profound changes. She has been sitting at the table, [and] actually eating her meals. . . . She decides to read the newspaper. Dad almost fell on the floor. . . . [She] now has all of her meals at the kitchen table with Dad and eats a decent amount of food. . . . She would get angry that someone was going to give her a shower. Now she goes willingly, enjoys her shower, and recognizes her home-health aid Sylvia when she comes. Both of [my parents] are diabetic and on medication, and their readings are always around 85–90. That made Dad nervous for a while. He never saw such low numbers, he thought that was bad."

• June 30, 2009: "Right now Mom is sitting by my kitchen table knitting. Something she wasn't able to do six months ago, because she couldn't remember what the needles were for."

• January 1, 2010: "Happy New Year! I wanted to give you a quick update on how my mother is doing since [my parents] moved in with me. I have a better handle on their whole situation and I can control how mom gets all her supplements. She is presently handling very well five tablespoons of oil a day. This is a combination of coconut oil and MCT. I mix them equally and put them in her tea, hot cereal, and protein shake in the morning, to which I add all her other supplements because she won't swallow the pills. . . . When I see mom sitting with pop having an actual conversation, playing with their great-granddaughter and being alert enough to enjoy her, I think of you and the great work you are doing. I remember the days when she fought us, soiled herself, refused to eat and didn't recognize anyone . . . ever!"

Fifty-Six-Year-Old Man with Dementia

• June 3, 2009: [Started on coconut oil and shortly after changed to MCT/coconut oil in a 4:3 ratio—one to one and a half table-spoons three times a day.] "There have been times in the last few weeks [when] I forget [my husband] has any problem at all. It is really amazing. I hate to think where he would be now if I had never come across your article. He is improving every single day. I am just so thankful for you!"

• June 3, 2009: "We just got his lab results. His total cholesterol went down from 140 to 120; triglycerides from 100 to 58; HDL from 53 to 54; LDL from 70 to 54. I am so pleased, as well is [he]. He has only been on the oil for two months! He does take Altoprev, Zetia, and Niaspan, but these are the best results we have seen in the past four years."

• August 20, 2009: "Each month I see improvements. He is participating in conversations, doing more things around the house to completion (i.e., laundry folding and putting away). Recently, we had family visiting us, and Fred actually went out and built a fire, helped with grilling . . . he was participating in life again. He is talking more, remembering to tell me things that happen during the day at home, remembering if someone calls and leaves a message for me. Recently, he asked me to take him to the camera store. He actually was able to tell the salesperson exactly what he wanted and how he wanted to use the camera. I was totally shocked. . . . If Dr. Veech needs test patients, we would certainly be interested."

Ninety-Year-Old Woman with Dementia

• June 26, 2009: "She scored 18 out of 30 on her mental exam and was really miserable. . . . For the past month, I've been visiting [my mother] almost every day, giving her chocolates made with coconut oil and MCT, and giving her the rest of the coconut oil pills I bought. She has infinitely more energy; she's coherent and genuinely happier. Last week they tested her again, and she scored a 26 out of 30. . . . She's attending exercise classes, church services, pizza parties—things she's been avoiding like the plague for over a decade, which is probably when she started having trouble, but no one knew it."

Eighty-Year-Old Woman with Dementia

• December 29, 2008: "After I read your article, I shared it with my siblings. We started my mom on coconut oil the day after Thanksgiving. We have seen a marked improvement in her cognition and functioning since it began. Her doctors seem skeptical but freely admit that there could be a connection."

Eighty-Four-Year-Old Man with Memory Loss

• August 13, 2009: "[My husband] seems to be more alive. He always was easygoing and it is nice to hear him have fun. He is outgoing in conversation, where before he just sat and listened, which was not like him. In the morning he makes the bed on his own and puts the throw pillows where they belong, and at meal-time clears the table and does the dishes and puts them away without my help. Before he did help with the chores but waited for me to start. Our nine-year-old granddaughter has him playing Wii. He can't see too well, but he jokes around with her and they laugh all the time. His short-term memory gives him a few problems at times but so does mine. On the whole I see quite an improvement since [he started] taking the coconut oil and I don't think it is just me hoping."

Woman with Alzheimer's Disease (Age Not Reported)

• July 2, 2009: "My mom is in the last stage. She pretty much has lost the ability to do anything for herself. Since [she] started the MCT Fuel and coconut oil . . . she actually has been slowly getting better. She is speaking actual words, if not whole sentences; she is stronger on her feet and legs, although she can't walk on her own; she is more alert to what is going on around her, rather than just sitting and staring off into space; and [she] is back to getting grumpy, which at this stage is acceptable. There are other small improvements as well. So which of all this is making the difference? I don't have a clue, but for my mom, she is better and that's all that matters to me."

Seventy-Seven-Year-Old Woman with Alzheimer's Disease

• January 14, 2009: "We have been doing this [adding one to two teaspoons of coconut oil to his wife's diet at each opportunity] since just before Christmas (about three-plus weeks) and she is definitely getting some results. Her cognitive signs are much brighter and she is exhibiting emotions that were not there before the last week."

• July 27, 2009: "Hilde was rather 'stoic' and paid little attention to things, paid little attention to surroundings, objected to being pushed or helped, would get up and walk and try to leave the 'dementia' assisted living facility to go home or find somebody or something, recognized family but immediately forgot that she had seen them or friends, etc. Today, Hilde is what several have called 'much brighter.' She is aware and curious about things going on around us. She recognizes more people, responds when spoken to, often questions something that she notices, is more cooperative with helpers. . . . During her stay in the hospital, Hilde forgot how to stand up and of course 'how to walk'—mostly [she] seems to be afraid. She had no physical therapy (PT) while there and now needs help in and out of bed, etc. She is currently receiving PT and in just four days shows some positive improvement."

Sixty-Eight-Year-Old Man with Peripheral Neuropathy

• September 19, 2008: "I started the coconut oil diet seventeen days ago. . . . Today is the fifth day in a row that I am pain free. All five nights I have slept through the night without waking up in pain. . . . I have found that I can actually go up and down the steps without a railing. I can go from room to room in my home without one hand on the wall for support."

Eighty-Three-Year-Old Man with Dementia

• July 16, 2009: "[My husband] tried the coconut oil, and like you, I found an immediate change. Since coming North different people have [talked] to me about his cholesterol with regards to taking the coconut oil. He stopped taking it and I found him going backwards. There was such a difference without the coconut oil that he has decided to start taking it again."

Twenty-Seven-Year-Old Woman in Coma After Car Accident

• January 2009: I had a conversation with the mother-in-law of a twenty-seven-year-old woman who suffered a traumatic brain injury as result of an auto accident in December 2008. She reported that her daughter-in-law was considered "vegetative" after about one month and had made no improvement whatsoever during that time. She was moved to a rehabilitation facility, where MCT oil was given to her three times a day. She woke up several days later, is now receiving physical therapy, and is expected to have a full recovery.

Seventy-Two-Year-Old Man with Parkinson's Disease

• June 20, 2009: "Now . . . the bigger news is that [he] is walking smoother, feels serene, looks good, is taking shorter naps, and with a momentary exception [is] sleeping well at night. He used to need to nap one to one and a half hours after a workout . . . now it is around thirty minutes. His Sinemet/Zandora [medication] used to be effective for about five hours and that was about a fifteen-to-thirty minute stretch. Even so, because he is spartan in nature, he would make it last five and one half hours at which time the tremor was obvious, he would be stiffer, and he would start to 'look bad' in the face. Now, with the oil, we have to be careful to watch the time instead of symptoms. Usually, I would notice the symptoms and ask if it weren't time for his L-dopa. Now he can go six hours without noticeable symptoms."

Sixty-Two-Year-Old Woman with Down Syndrome and Alzheimer's Disease

• August 26, 2009: "Condition before using coconut oil/MCT oil: 1. Would lean extremely far to her left side while eating (almost laying head on left arm on the table). Sitting (if sitting to her left, she would be laying on you) and walking with upper body leaning to the left and forward. Balance was poor. 2. Speech was at the point where only about 25 percent was understandable. The rest was garbled. 3. Almost complete loss of personal daily living skills. Had to be physically/verbally prompted. 4. Eyes were very foggy or glazed looking. 5. Had a cold almost monthly with outbreaks of cold sores. 6. Short-term memory gone and most of long-term memory gone. Could remember name and date of birth but not the year. Needed many verbal prompts to remember address and phone number. Needed verbal prompting to remember my name and family names. Unable to orient where she is as to where, why and when. 7. Episodes of dizziness, faintness, clammy, cold sweats. 8. Weight was 117 lbs. 9. Cholesterol was good.

"Condition after using coconut oil/MCT Oil: 1. Leaning syndrome is completely gone. Walks straight and with much better balance. 2. Speech is now . . almost 65 percent . . . understandable. Speech is garbled still when she is trying to tell me something that is not current with the conversation at the time. 3. Moderate improvement with personal daily living skills. Can perform some tasks independently and most tasks performed with just verbal prompting. 4. The first day she was given coconut oil, her eyes appeared clear and alert. Noticed that the glazed look returns when she is very tired or when not ingesting coconut oil/MCT Oil, or if she is ill, but not as bad as before starting the oils. 5. Since starting the coconut oil in February 2009, [she] has only had one cold and a cold sore. This occurred after lowering the amount of coconut oil in order to increase the MCT oil. 6. Short-term memory has slightly improved. [She] remembers her name and date of birth but not the year, needs only one or two verbal prompts at start to remember address and phone number. Has been able to remember other people's names more and to actually learn names of new people she sees on a regular basis. Remembers the days of the week Monday through Thursday and just more recently has started to say Saturday, which she couldn't say unless prompted to and then most times remembers Sunday after this. She keeps dropping Friday though. Very slight improvement in long-term memory such as remembering prior friends. 7. Only one episode of dizziness, faintness, clammy, cold sweats since starting the coconut oil /MCT oil. 8. Weight is now 134 lbs. with a gain of seventeen pounds since starting the oil. 9. Cholesterol numbers have slightly lowered five months after starting the oils."

Fifty-Five-Year-Old Man with Posterior Cortical Atrophy

• August 31, 2009: "Within an hour of taking his morning doses of caffeine and oils, [my husband's] speech clears up (ability to find words, to carry a thought through to conclusion, to refer to recent events). As time approaches for the next doses, the speech problems begin to reemerge but then resolve as the treatment kicks back in. I tend toward cynicism and have worried that I have been seeing effects only because I so desperately want to see them. But others have noticed it, too. Several weeks ago I had warned a friend who sees Steve only occasionally what he should expect, as Steve's decline since May had been severe. In the intervening weeks I had begun the therapy with Steve. . . . This friend pulled me aside yesterday and asked what I had been talking about. He said he did not detect anything unusual with Steve until near the end of the day (when it was time for his next doses). Each day the baseline of Steve's condition seems to move a bit higher. MMSE 18 of 30 on August 6, 2009. [He was] hospitalized in May 2009 for 'precipitous collapse of his cognitive abilities' (he could not spell simple words, [was] unable to complete sentences, lost [his] ability to comprehend what he was reading, had mixed up his meds, hit a stationary object with his car for the fifth time in the past several months). [He showed] 'mild diffuse cerebral volume loss' and 'mild biparietal lobe atrophy' on scans. He has recovered his dexterity with things such as fastening seatbelts and tying shoes. He is operating remote controls a bit more readily. He is asking me less frequently to help him with a word on a sign he cannot make out. There are still some lapses, though. We met with our lawyers last week to prepare our affairs . . . and the next day Steve could not remember the meeting had even occurred. But there is no question in my mind that the decline is on pause and that some capacity is actually returning."

• April 14, 2011: "He has at least maintained at a steady state over the past year. The skills he at least partially recovered (reading, using a computer, tying shoes, fastening seat belts) soon after beginning the coconut/MCT oils in 2009 have all remained intact. In fact, some of his motor skills have continued to improve. When I first met him over eight years ago, he shuffled his feet badly when walking. He now walks normally, and his legendary clumsiness is all but gone. We live in a gated community and he walks 5.5 miles a day by himself, having struck up acquaintances with quite a few other residents along the way. He now knows considerably more people than I do, and he often comes home with stories about events in the community and other news he picks up on these conversations. . . . Now he sets a pace that I can barely match on the few occasions I accompany him. On the other hand, he still clearly has memory impairment. But I find he frequently reminds me to follow up on something that I have forgotten. . . . He takes one packet of Axona in the morning, two tablespoons of coconut oil mid-morning, a 10 dram-vial [1 dram equals $1/8$ ounce] of MCT oil mid-afternoon and again mid-evening. He has not had a single cold sore since beginning the oils. That's the [principal] reason I leave coconut oil in the mix, despite his general practitioner's horror that he eats so much of it."

Eighty-Seven-Year-Old Man with Vascular Dementia

• August 11, 2009: "In a short period of five days my dad is getting up from bed [and] talking to people; he recognizes people and is coming back to his own self day after day with coconut oil. . . . Mom calls it a miracle." Before coconut oil she reports: "He was all day in bed and up with manic episodes at nights. Not talking and not being able to recognize even family members. . . . He was silent and mostly bed-bound. After five days he is talking and getting up from bed, walking around the house as if he recognizes everything and doing things he forgot to do for a while."

Ninety-One-Year-Old Woman with Alzheimer's Disease

• August 20, 2009: "I am convinced the [coconut oil just under two tablespoons] is helping [my mother] and here is why: She tries to write out a grocery list every week. The lists have become more and more illegible as time goes by. I was shocked last week when she gave me the list—it was *astoundingly* more readable, with fewer misspellings, items written along the lines of the paper and in handwriting that is much more recognizable as my mother's. . . . Usually, if she is forced to answer the phone, her voice is pained and she sounds gravely upset, until I am able to calm her down and get her out of her funk. Last week I called and she answered the phone. At first, her voice was tentative, but when I told her it was me she was pleasant and sounded content. . . . I had given up talking to her by phone because she began to have trouble holding it to her ear and hearing. . . . I called [my parents] today and my father asked if I wanted to talk to Mom. . . . He gave her the phone and she had no trouble immediately talking to me and hearing me. She was pleasant, seemed happy and asked me how 'everyone' was doing. As far as I know, there have not been any side effects and she has not complained about taking it."

Woman with Glaucoma (Age Not Reported)

• October 22, 2009: [Letter to physician, copied to Dr. Newport.]

"Dr. Robert: I am a glaucoma patient receiving care at [your facility]. In early September, a friend of mine sent me an account of Dr. Mary Newport's success with MCT (medium-chain triglycerides) and coconut oil for her husband's early onset Alzheimer's disease.... Recognizing that glaucoma is a neurodegenerative, age-related, genetic disease like Alzheimer's . . . and realizing that there is a direct link between neurons in the brain and retinal neurons . . . it just seemed logical to me to add some coconut oil to my diet to see if ketone bodies could enhance energy/oxygen uptake to my damaged retinal cells in order to maintain, and maybe even improve, my existing vision.

"My husband (his mother died of Alzheimer's) and I began taking the oil the first week in September. I started with a few tablespoons . . . one in the morning, another midday, and one more in the evening. The second night, as I was sitting at my computer, I suddenly realized that the screen seemed much clearer and easier to read, with enhanced contrast and clarity. This was very strange for me at that time of the night, when my tired eyes and blurry vision are usually telling me to go to bed. I also noticed that the tool bar at the top of the screen, which I always thought was gray-white, was suddenly pink. In fact, I was picking up light pink and light blue colors in several blocks in the screen that I had never seen before! I am in the computer business with a son and his wife, so my first thought was that my LCD display might by dying . . . but that wasn't the case this time. The next day, when the tool bar color was gray again, I decided to take a tablespoon of the oil right away, and in about thirty-five to forty minutes, the pink returned. This was repeated over and over again for the next several days. *There is no question re: cause and effect*! In fact, I began using my perception of pink color on my screen, and its intensity, as a gauge of ketone saturation in my body. If the pink fades out, it is time to take another tablespoon of the oil!

"I am currently taking about eight tablespoons total each day, which seems to be perfect, and incidentally, matches Dr. Newport's dosage experience and the speed of the oil's effects on her husband's condition. I am excited about the improvements in my vision, which are dramatic and continuing. Both rods and cones seem to be benefiting from the extra ketone energy they are getting. I am now able to drive at night and see better at dusk. My eyes accommodate faster from dark to light and light to dark. My depth perception is also better, and as a result, I am walking with less hesitancy. I think that these are all improvements in my central vision, not peripheral vision, which is hard to judge."

• July 12, 2010: "My glaucoma is stable, no further deterioration at this point."

Sixteen-Year-Old Boy with Seizures

• September 6, 2009: "Joe has been taking the coconut oil capsules, 2 caps 3 times a day, for about a week now, plus I added organic coconut oil chased with lemonade. A few days in, Joe started complaining about feeling seizures throughout the day, but he skipped a day without having his evening two- to three-minute grand mal. I'm convinced you're onto something, because even feeling those weird small seizures today, he actually wanted to read and finished a simple workbook that two days before he was unable to comprehend. Today, he's had two meals cooked in coconut oil, coconut ice cream, coconut juice plus two tablespoons oil, one in AM, one in PM, as well as the six capsules. He went out and played Frisbee in the heat—no seizure—and has cleared out the dishwasher twice today and as I'm writing this, collecting all the dirty cups around the house. He has not stopped talking all day and still no grand mal and less comments on small seizure activity.

My goal Tuesday is to pick up the MCT oil. I'll let you know how it goes."

• September 10, 2009: "We got three and a half days with no grand mal seizures until yesterday when he missed his morning dose of meds, oils, and aminos because of blood work."

Seventy-Two-Year-Old Man with Parkinson's for Ten Years

• March 25, 2010: "Glen has just retired this Christmas after being a practicing architect for 50 years. He works out four days a week, eats well, and [takes] supplements. We have read all that we could find on the dietary use of coconut products and have been on a supplementing program for three months. I use coconut milk in place of dairy milk in all my food prep and cook a lot of Thai food. He also takes two grams of coconut oil three times a day before meals in capsule form, making six grams plus food intake per day. While supplementing, Glen has experienced an appreciable reduction in tremor severity, a significant enhancement in bowel function, mental agility and recall. We particularly noted a rapid decline and deterioration in motor function and mental agility while temporarily out of product."

Man with Symptoms and Family History of Huntington's Disease (Age Not Reported)

• July 12, 2010: "My husband is at risk for Huntington's disease. He's doing very good on the combinations of oils [two tablespoons of MCT and coconut oil mixture in 4:3 ratio]. If I back off on it, I notice the unintentional movements start to come back and the unsteady gait. The stuff was back-ordered once so I had to cut way back for about a week and a half. It can be a challenge to get at least two tablespoons down him each meal. However, I do believe it takes that much to keep the symptoms at bay."

• September 9, 2010: "I just wanted to update you on my husband,

Stormy (showing symptoms of Huntington's disease [HD]). Unbeknownst to us, his sister (who has been tested and does not have the HD gene) and her husband who visited us a little over a year ago (about the time I noticed symptoms) also noticed symptoms in him. They did not mention it because we did not. They came back to visit about a few months later and still did not say anything. However, we just saw them again; six more months have gone by and my husband and I told them about it and what we were doing (it gets hard to hide the oil when you spend days with someone). She said that the last time they were here that they thought he was a lot better, but they couldn't imagine why that would be and that the coconut/MCT oil must be helping. So as it turns out I was not the only one noticing signs and not the only one noticing that they are abating."

Sixty-Two-Year-Old Man with Early Onset Alzheimer's Disease

• October 21, 2010: "My husband has been diagnosed with probable Alzheimer's disease. In June 2010 I happened to read a question about Alzheimer's disease and coconut oil on a discussion forum. I decided to Google it and came upon your blog about your husband. We decided to try the oils, and after about four months now, my husband has improved in many areas.

"From June 17 to July 28, 2010, [my husband began] taking a mixture of coconut oil and MCT oil, three to four teaspoons, three times a day. Results after 6 weeks: more awareness of time and place; better able to read and retain what was read; improvements in reading aloud; initiates conversation/better at following conversation, though often certain things still don't register/better at keeping up conversation. This is the most noticeable improvement, commented on by many: more interested and sociable; much less depressed; finds he can do work (rewriting lecture notes into book form) more easily; slight tremor improved.

"Between July 28 and October 21, 2010: I increased his dose to one tablespoon of coconut oil and two tablespoons of MCT oil, three times per day. No nausea or diarrhea at all. When I ran out of MCT oil for a few days, I substituted three tablespoons of coconut oil, three times per day—noticeably worse reading and short-term memory. By the end of September/beginning of October, short-term memory seems improved: less repeating questions, several times remembered names previously forgotten, remembered events in more detail than I would have expected, but this is of course all very subjective. He has written some e-mail messages for the first time in about a year; brought up himself that he wants some money in his wallet, so that he can pay for things himself. Before, he had never asked for that for several years. The very latest change, not more than a week ago, is the partial lifting of the anosognosia [lack of awareness of one's own disability] that has been strong from the very beginning."

Sixty-Two-Year-Old Man with Familial Amyotrophic Lateral Sclerosis (FALS)

• December 23, 2010: "I have been waiting for over a year to thank you for your videos. My reason for waiting is as follows. I inherited ALS from my mother, who died in 1986. Mine started in early 2007 and was officially diagnosed as FALS in September 2008. The first signs came in my right leg with major muscle loss starting in the gluteus maximus and other related muscles affecting running and the knee.

"In late 2009 I saw your videos on how coconut oil had helped your husband. So I then obtained a large container of it, and started taking four tablespoons each day in early November 2009. In December 2009, I took six tablespoons per day, and in January 2010 I started taking eight tablespoons per day. My logic said, 'If four tablespoons is for a normal person then I needed more!' It's been almost one year now with very possible results. Some of these are:

1. Stable weight. Staying around 68 to 70 kilograms [149 to 154 pounds].

2. More muscle mass in my upper right leg! Before I started taking the coconut oil if I reached up on the underneath of my leg I could feel the leg bones. Today I cannot do that! What I feel now is some muscles rather than bones.

3. The circumference of the leg has increase by about one-quarter inch, which is not much. But it's not gotten smaller so to me that's a positive. Also, my left leg has increased about the same amount. I credit this to the fact that I now use my left leg much, much more due to the weakness of my right knee.

4. The right leg feels completely different than it did before taking the coconut oil. It now feels more awake, and a part of me again. Before it felt asleep and non-responsive. It is still not right, but it's better. What I've realized is that the first muscles to go are the ones that have not responded yet, but I'm hopeful!

5. Some improvements in ankle and leg movement over 2009 and 2010.

"As for official documentation of these improvements, I only have my loosely kept journal. However, based on a recent blood test, my cholesterol, etc., are fine! Therefore, I plan to continue taking the eight tablespoons daily, and check my weight and leg measurements each month to see what happens."

Sixty-Three-Year-Old Man with Early Onset Alzheimer's Disease

• February 15, 2011: "We came across your story less than a month ago. My father, Mick, is sixty-three years old and suffering from early onset Alzheimer's disease for the last six years. He was just entering the phase where we were truly feeling we were beginning to lose him. He is at home with my mother, but we have been thinking more and more about very regular respite. An article about your experience came like a bolt from the blue when I was researching other means of home support, etc. Dad has been taking one tablespoon of coconut oil daily for the past three weeks, and the results are noticeable to us all. [He is] more focused, better able to converse, seems a bit sharper sometimes. It's amazing. We (and I mean my entire extended family and many friends) are now on coconut oil—I have been telling everyone. Maybe it's coincidence, but all of the health food shops seem to be sold out of the stuff these days! If it holds him at the stage he is at for a little longer, we will be so thankful. Our only regret is we didn't hear about you sooner. My Dad, even of late 2008, was a very different man."

Fifty-Seven-Year-Old Woman with Early Onset Alzheimer's Disease

• March 1, 2011: "Greetings from Ireland. My wife Elizabeth, now aged fifty-seven, showed signs of Alzheimer's as far back as summer 2007. . . . From September 2009 to March 2010, Elizabeth's condition deteriorated to the extent she had to leave work and was subsequently retired on health grounds. Early onset Alzheimer's was confirmed by Elizabeth's consultant in September 2010 and by her neurologist in October 2010. The neurologist told me there was no cure, and I should look about getting assistance. Two days after visiting the neurologist, I found your website and started Elizabeth on coconut oil on October 28, 2010. I initially gave her one tablespoon, three times daily, and over the following three to four weeks put her up to two tablespoons, three times daily. I also gave her a fish oil supplement. After about two weeks, I saw an improvement, and looking back I think she reversed back through the mood swings she encountered on the way down. Elizabeth continued to improve and put back on the weight she had lost by the end of December, and as I didn't want her to continue to gain weight I sourced MCT oil. I started Elizabeth on one tablespoon of MCT oil and one tablespoon of coconut oil, three times daily on January 7, 2011. Over the next two weeks, I progressed her to two tablespoons of MCT oil and one tablespoon of coconut oil, three times daily. Elizabeth continues to take the fish oil supplement, and we eat salmon two to three times weekly. She is now much improved and I continue to see improvement in little things she can now do that she had difficulty with a short time ago. I hope she will continue to improve."

[I asked the caregiver for more detail about his wife's improvements:]

• March 4, 2011: "I will give you an outline of how Elizabeth was and how she is now. Her personality completely changed, she would become aggressive for the smallest thing; now [she is] a completely different person to live with, [her] personality [is] back as if a switch had been flicked, and [she is] back to her old self. [She] had problems dressing, putting shoes on wrong feet, putting clothes on inside out, or having difficulty putting them on; now [she is] much improved at dressing. [She] was always a woman who took great care of her appearance and especially her hair; she stopped taking care of herself and stopped looking after her hair, she wouldn't even comb it; now [she] has returned to taking great care of her appearance. [She] stopped watching her favourite programs on television, I would put them on for her, she would sit staring at the wall and get up in the middle of them and go to bed; now [she is] back watching her programs and looks forward to seeing them. [She] had lost interest in her grandchildren, would say hello when she would meet them but then sit and withdraw into herself, not even being aware of what they were doing; now [she is] back enjoying their company, only yesterday we visited our daughter who has three boys under five and she spent two to three hours playing with them. [She] had difficulty knowing what time of day it was, unable to read clock; now [she is] aware of the time and able to tell me the time if I ask her. [She] would go to bed in the afternoon and I would have difficulty getting her to get up again; now [she] never goes to bed in afternoon. [She] had difficulty knowing where she was and basically looked lost especially out shopping; now [she is] comfortable in shops and knows where she is. Our children are all surprised at the improvement in their mother and they have all started using coconut oil as have a lot of their friends."

Thirteen-Year-Old Welsh Terrier with Cognitive Problems

• [Mrs. DG asked me if I thought coconut oil could help her thir-teen-year-old Welsh Terrier who was having cognitive problems. I told her about a study by researchers at Accera, the company that developed Axona, using MCT oil with elderly dogs, and there was a significant improvement in the dogs (Studzinski, 2008; Taha, 2009). I suggested she try one-quarter teaspoon of coconut oil for each ten pounds the dog weighed, two or three times a day. I received this e-mail several weeks later:]

"Dr. Newport, I am very encouraged with the use of the coconut oil for my Welsh Terrier. She is getting up in the morning for breakfast without my having to do anything physical to awaken her. In fact, this morning she wanted to go into the larger exercise area and knew exactly how to navigate the doors to reach the area she wanted to enter. . . ."

CHARTING RESPONSES FROM CAREGIVERS

As you can see from these e-mails and letters, some people respond rather quickly to medium-chain fatty acids, and others more gradually, with improvements occurring over months rather than days. Steve had immediate improvement in some aspects of the disease, but some of the other changes became more apparent after three to ten months, such as resolution of the visual disturbance that prevented him from reading and his improvement in recent memory.

As people began to contact me with questions, I asked them to please let me know how their loved one responded to incorporating medium-chain fatty acids into their diet, even if there was no response. I did not prompt them about what types of responses they might expect. I thought it would be more interesting and helpful to hear from people, in their own words, what they noticed about their loved ones' responses.

By May 2009, I had received reports from many others about the responses of their loved ones. At that time, Dr. Veech suggested that I put together a spread sheet documenting the reports I had received, which could help in the quest to fund research into the ketone ester. The vast majority reported positive responses, but some reported no improvement whatsoever. Not everyone reported improvements in memory and/or cognition, which can be relatively easily documented with testing. Many of the reported improvements were in other aspects of human life, such as increased social interaction, improved ability to make conversation, and resumption of activities that had fallen by the wayside.

When the spreadsheet was complete, I thought it would be interesting and helpful to make a chart showing whether there was a response or not and what types of responses were reported. I attempted to group the various types of responses into several different categories for charting purposes. Arguably, there may be some overlap among the groups, as some improvements related to conversation might be considered cognitive improvements, but I was trying to think of these from a practical point of view. Even though I heard from people with other types of neurodegenerative diseases, I limited the chart to the forty-seven people with dementia. This information was submitted and accepted for the poster presentation at the Alzheimer's Disease International Conference in Thessaloniki, Greece, in March 2010. By the time abstract submissions were due in July 2010 for the ketone symposium in Scotland (both events were described in Chapter 11), I was able to expand the chart to sixty people with dementia whose caregivers provided sufficient information. These are the types of responses that people reported:

Improved Memory/Cognition

- Higher scores on memory or cognitive test
- Improved clock drawing
- Better cognition
- More alert
- Brighter
- Improved awareness
- Less foggy
- Less hazy
- Recognizing people or places
- Less distractible
- Better sense of direction

Improved Social Interaction, Behavior, Mood

- More interaction with others
- Better sense of humor
- Less agitation
- Improved behavior
- Less hostile
- Less aggressive
- Happy
- Improved mood
- Less anxiety
- Less depression

Improved Speech, Conversation

- Speaking again
- Clearer speech
- Less repetitiveness
- Making sense
- More logical
- Improved conversation
- More talkative
- Improved verbal skills
- Better word recall

Resumption of Lost Activities

- Showering again without help
- Performing self-care again
- Doing things around the house

- Doing household chores again
- Preparing meals again
- Resumed a hobby
- Reading again

Improved Physical Symptoms

- Less tremor
- Getting out of bed without help
- Able to walk again
- Walking without assistance
- Improved strength
- More ambulatory
- More energy

- Less stiffness
- Improved balance
- Less dizziness
- Fewer episodes of faintness, clamminess, sweating
- Improved gait
- Fewer episodes of seizure/twitching

Improved Sleep

- Fewer nightmares
- Sleeping better

- No longer sleeping excessively

Improved Vision

- Visual disturbance gone

- Able to see more clearly

Improved Appetite

Table 13.1 presents the percentage of the sixty people who showed improvement within each of these categories after consuming medium-chain fatty acids. For a graphic depiction of these results, see Figure 13.1 on the following page.

TABLE 13.1. IMPROVEMENTS OBSERVED AFTER CONSUMING MEDIUM-CHAIN FATTY ACIDS

OVERALL RESPONSE	NUMBER AFFECTED	PERCENT AFFECTED
Improved	54/60	90
Improved memory/cognition	37/60	62
Did not improve	5/60	8
Stable over 6 months	1/60	2
SPECIFIC RESPONSES		
Improved social/behavior/mood	29/60	48
Improved speech/verbal skills	21/60	35
Resumption of lost activities	16/60	27
Improved physical symptoms	12/60	20
Improved sleep	4/60	7
Improvement, otherwise unspecified	4/60	7
Improved appetite	2/60	3
Improved vision	2/60	3

Measurable and Immeasurable Results

After putting this information together, it occurred to me that many of the positive responses to this dietary intervention with medium-chain fatty acids were not easily measurable. When clinical trials are carried out for Alzheimer's disease, the testing often focuses on improvements in memory and activities of daily living. Some of the improvements reported here by caregivers may be more difficult to quantify, such as social interaction, mood and behavior, and improved sleep and appetite. It is possible that certain areas of the brain are more sensitive to mild ketosis than others, and this could vary from person to person. Some people may not have improved memory, but at the same time may have responses that are very meaningful to them and their loved ones,

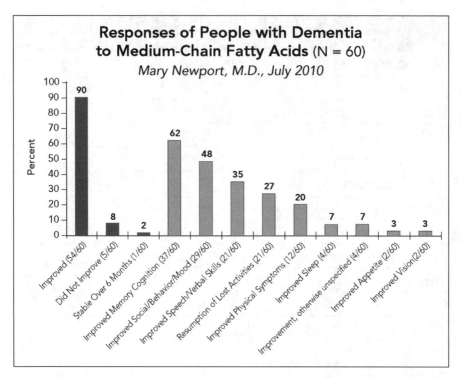

Figure 13.1. Responses of people with dementia to medium-chain fatty acids as reported by their caregivers. Reports were sent by e-mail or letter and were spontaneous, not prompted with regard to type of information. Specifics of the responses were then categorized to create this graph. Of the 60 individuals, 32 were males, 27 females, 1 unknown; 43 of 60 reported age with range of 50 to 94 years (average 76.3.); 36 used coconut oil only, 3 MCT oil only, and 21 a combination of coconut oil and MCT oil. Positive response is presumably due to metabolism of medium-chain fatty acids to ketone bodies for use by neurons as an alternative fuel in brain cells with decreased ability to transport glucose. Diagram by Joanna Newport.

improving their quality of life overall. These types of responses should not be overlooked when studying potential Alzheimer's treatments, including this dietary intervention. Ideally, a mechanism will be developed to document improvements in these other aspects of Alzheimer's disease for use in clinical trials.

PART TWO

Ketones, Medium-Chain Fatty Acids, and the Ketone Ester

Several of the chapters in this section, specifically those on ketones and their discovery and medical implications, may appear to some readers as too biochemical or technical. If you do not have a scientific or medical background, then you may want to revisit these chapters after you read Part Three of the book or you may choose to skip them entirely. This information is not essential to using this dietary intervention. The nature of the brain, Alzheimer's disease, ketones, fatty acids, and the like, although extraordinarily interesting, are indeed technical. For those readers who are eager to know the science behind the discovery, the information in Chapters 14–19 is a primer introducing you to ketones.

14

Type 3 Diabetes and Alzheimer's Disease

A basic understanding of how cells are constructed and how they operate will allow for an appreciation of ketones and for their importance in the body, but especially in the brain.

The individual cells that make up the many tissues of our body are extremely complicated structures, much more than the simple cell with a nucleus and cytoplasm that older generations learned about in grade school. Each cell of our body requires fuel to operate. This fuel must pass through the membrane of the cell and be carried to a specialized part of the cell, called the mitochondrion, where it is processed into energy. The cell then uses this energy, called ATP (adenosine triphosphate), to keep itself in working order and also to produce proteins and other substances, which are different for each type of cell.

An amazing amount of activity goes on within the cell membrane. The processes that take place there decide what can enter and what can leave the cell. The cell membrane is made up of fatty molecules that line up in such a way that the fluids outside of the cell are repelled, thereby keeping the environment out of the cell. At the same time, the fluids inside the cell are protected, keeping the contents of the cell inside. Receptors for various substances sit on the cell membrane and act like keyholes in this process. When the right substance (the key) comes along and attaches to the receptors (the keyhole), this unlocks the door into the cell for a particular substance to enter.

One important example of this transport process, relevant to our concern here, involves the transport of glucose, the simplest form of carbohydrate, into the cell. When you eat something that contains carbohydrate, or sugar, it is broken down into smaller glucose (blood sugar) molecules, and this event signals the pancreas to release insulin, a hormone. Insulin (the key) must attach to the insulin receptor (the keyhole) so that glucose can be allowed into the cell. A transport protein, named GLUT for glucose transporter, carries glucose through the cell membrane and releases the glucose inside of the cell. Different types of cells use different GLUTs. Once inside the cell, the molecules of glucose make their way to the mitochondria, the energy plants of the cell. This sets off a complex chain reaction involving many enzymes and other substances to make the final, important energy particle called ATP.

When everything is normal, every cell membrane has insulin receptors so all the cells can use glucose as fuel. But if insulin receptors are absent, there is no way for glucose to enter the cell and be turned into ATP. This in turn can lead to serious health problems such as diabetes mellitus.

DIABETES MELLITUS

Diabetes mellitus is a group of conditions that involves a problem with the way the body metabolizes glucose; specifically, the levels of glucose in the blood are abnormally high, although the reasons for this differ. Diabetes is one of the most common chronic conditions, affecting nearly 26 million people in the United States, or 8.3 percent of the population, according to the National Diabetes Fact Sheet 2011 from the Centers for Disease Control (CDC) and Prevention. In addition, an astounding 79 million people, or one in four, have prediabetes, meaning that levels of glucose are elevated but not quite to the levels of those seen in diabetes. People with prediabetes are at high risk of developing diabetes but can often avoid this by close attention to diet and exercise.

Diabetes becomes more common as we age, affecting about 3.7 percent of people between twenty and forty-four and gradually increasing to nearly 27 percent of people who are sixty-five or older. Also, about half the U.S. population sixty-five and older have prediabetes, therefore more than three-quarters of the people in this age group either have diabetes or are at high risk of developing diabetes.

People with diabetes mellitus often develop other chronic conditions: it is the leading cause of kidney failure, representing about 44 percent of cases, and is also the leading cause of new cases of blindness in people between the ages of twenty and seventy-four. In addition, people with diabetes are at greater-than-normal risk of developing high blood pressure, heart disease, and stroke, as well as damage to the nervous system, such as impaired sensation or pain in the extremities, skin breakdown, and difficulty with wound healing. The brain is affected as well—the diabetic is more likely to develop dementia than the nondiabetic (Akomolafe, 2006; Pasquier, 2006).

Type 1 Diabetes Mellitus

In type 1 diabetes mellitus, the pancreas fails to make insulin, and glucose builds up in the bloodstream, unable to get into cells. Without this basic fuel, the cells cannot continue to function, and when enough cells malfunction, the various organs of the body shut down. Type 1 diabetes can develop rather suddenly, and the person may become acutely ill, even slipping into a coma as the blood sugar rises and the blood becomes acidotic. In this instance, the fat cells begin to release extremely large quantities of fatty acids, which are then converted in the liver to ketones. The ketone levels become extraordinarily high—much higher than the levels proposed by Dr. Richard Veech for use in his ketone ester. This is called diabetic ketoacidosis, and the affected person will die unless insulin is administered.

Type 1 diabetes used to be called "juvenile-onset" diabetes, since most cases start during childhood and adolescence, in fact, about one in 400 children and adolescents have type 1 diabetes. More than 90 percent of cases of diabetes under age ten are type 1. Overall, nearly 3 million people in the United States have type 1 diabetes.

A person afflicted with type 1 diabetes must continue to receive insulin on at least a daily basis, sometimes two or three times daily, in order to survive. Blood sugar levels can vary significantly depending on the foods that are consumed and need to be monitored throughout the day. Blood sugar levels guide the diabetic about how much insulin to use for each injection. Some diabetics are so unstable, or "brittle," that they must use a pump that injects insulin at programmed intervals under the skin.

It is very important for the diabetic to adhere to a healthy diet and to keep the blood sugar within reasonable limits. The well-controlled diabetic can expect to live a longer and healthier life than the "poorly controlled" diabetic who ignores his or her doctor's and dietician's advice.

Type 2 Diabetes Mellitus

In type 2 diabetes mellitus, the pancreas is able to make insulin, but may have trouble making enough insulin to handle the amount of glucose in the circulation. In fact, insulin levels may be higher in some people with type 2 diabetes than in someone without the disease. In some cases, certain types of cells do not respond normally to insulin because some of the insulin receptors may be defective or may not be on the surface of the cell membrane where they belong. Other agents may also interfere with insulin receptors. As a result, glucose may not be able to get into the cell in sufficient amounts. This is called insulin resistance. Eventually, when the energy in the cell is depleted, the cell will die.

Type 2 diabetes was formerly known as "adult-onset" diabetes. About one in five people over age sixty-five in the United States have type 2 diabetes, and it is becoming much more common in younger people, representing about one-third of cases in ten- to nineteen-year-olds. Overall, there are about nine people with type 2 diabetes for each person with type 1 diabetes. Obesity that results from an excess of calories, so common in the United States today, is thought to play a major role in the rising rates of type 2 diabetes and related diseases. Modification of diet to reduce overall caloric intake, and paying close attention to the types of carbohydrates consumed, can play a very important role in preventing and controlling the disease.

Diabetics who experience one or more episodes of severe hypoglycemia (low blood sugar) are even more likely to have memory and other cognitive problems as they age. Episodes of low blood sugar happen most often when too much insulin is produced in relation to how much carbohydrate is eaten. This can be a very serious problem, particularly for people with type 1 diabetes who have difficulty controlling their blood sugar. Confusion and other problems related to cognitive functioning are common symptoms of low blood sugar. Consuming medium-chain triglyceride (MCT) oil appears to protect people with diabetes from experiencing these cognitive problems during hypoglycemic spells (Page, 2009). There will be more about this research study in Chapter 18.

The effects of insulin go well beyond simply letting glucose into cells. Insulin also reduces the use of fat as a source of energy, causes lipids to be stored in fat cells, and causes glucose to be stored in the form of glycogen in muscle and liver. Insulin affects the activity of numerous enzymes, causes the walls of arteries to relax, and increases cell growth and survival. These are just a few of the more important effects of insulin.

Type 3 Diabetes Mellitus

Until just a few years ago, it was commonly believed that insulin was made only in the pancreas, a gland located just behind the stomach. Then, in 2005, Suzanne M. de la Monte, M.D., Jack R. Wands, M.D., and their associates at Brown University and Rhode Island Hospital reported that insulin and some of the related insulin growth factors are, in fact, made in the brain (De la Monte, 2005).

I am going to repeat this because it is such a profound discovery: the brain can make its own insulin.

The earliest reference I have been able to find suggesting that a dementia such as Alzheimer's may involve a problem with glucose metabolism is in a 1970 German paper by Siegfried Hoyer, M.D., and others (Hoyer, 1970). The researchers found decreased levels of glucose and a lower cerebral metabolic rate (the speed at which energy is used) in the brains of some people with dementia. Building on further work by Hoyer and many other groups begun in the 1970s and exploding in the 2000s, de la Monte's group presented more evidence supporting the developing concept that insulin resistance and a deficiency of insulin in the brain are responsible for cognitive impairment and Alzheimer's disease. They coined a new term, "type 3 diabetes," to refer to Alzheimer's disease (Steen, 2005) and published another paper in 2008 with evidence that Alzheimer's disease is type 3 diabetes. In the summary of this article, they state: "Alzheimer's disease represents a form of diabetes that selectively involves the brain and has molecular and biochemical features that overlap with both type 1 diabetes mellitus and T2DM [type 2 diabetes mellitus]."

Dr. de la Monte and her associates have learned there is a gradual progression of insulin deficiency and insulin resistance in parts of the brain in people with Alzheimer's. This means the brain does not make enough insulin and some cells in the brain do not respond normally to insulin. The researchers also found that this process worsens gradually over time. In one of their studies, they looked at the brains of people who died with advanced Alzheimer's disease. They found that:

- Levels of insulin and factors related to making and using insulin are greatly reduced.

- All the signaling pathways involved in the use of energy are abnormal.

- The functioning of mitochondria is abnormal.

None of the people with advanced Alzheimer's they studied had either type 1 or type 2 diabetes. Thus, the concept of type 3 diabetes, or diabetes that affects only the brain, was born (Steen, 2005). Researchers have also learned that obesity and type 2 diabetes can increase the risk of developing Alzheimer's and hasten the progression of Alzheimer's, but do not appear to cause it. Given that diet can be modified to reduce weight and reverse type 2 diabetes, then changing to a healthier diet could delay or slow the progression of Alzheimer's disease. The primary goal with such a diet would be to increase the effectiveness of insulin by reducing how much carbohydrate we eat, especially simple sugar. Our bodies need carbohydrate, so eliminating it completely is not realistic or desirable. But most people in this country consume too much, which could spell big problems for us as we age. If we want to avoid dementia and a host of other problems, we need to eliminate as much carbohydrate as possible. (For more on what constitutes a healthy diet, see Chapter 22.)

Dr. de la Monte and her group then looked at the brains of

people who died at various stages of Alzheimer's disease. They found that the loss of insulin and neurons with insulin growth factor receptors begins early in the disease. (Neurons are highly specialized brain cells that are responsible for transmitting information throughout the body.) This worsens with each stage of the disease until it is very severe and occurs throughout the brain in the most severe cases of Alzheimer's.

In their reports, de la Monte and her group have suggested that some of the treatments for type 1 and 2 diabetes might also help people with type 3 diabetes. For example, insulin administered as a nasal spray can penetrate into the brain. Insulin given this way is showing some promise as a treatment and is currently in clinical trials.

The problem with insulin is not the whole story, as Dr. de la Monte acknowledges in her papers. What causes this defect in insulin production and use in the first place? Inflammation in the brain is a major factor in Alzheimer's disease. Is the problem with insulin a result of inflammation? And what about the "plaques and tangles" that are seen in the brains of people with Alzheimer's? Two avenues of research have been exploring these issues. Simply put, some researchers believe that the amyloid plaques cause the destruction of neurons that results in Alzheimer's disease, and some believe that the tangles cause Alzheimer's. For example, those in the beta-amyloid camp believe that a treatment that removes beta-amyloid from the brain will stop the worsening of the disease process and may even reverse it. Many groups of researchers throughout the world are working on every aspect of these issues.

A CHAIN REACTION OF CELL DESTRUCTION

After reading everything I can find, I believe we will learn that neither the plaques nor the tangles cause Alzheimer's disease. I believe these are byproducts of brain cells, specifically neuron cells, are dead and dying as they disintegrate, or that they are a response to the disease process that causes cell destruction and death.

To further explain the tangles of Alzheimer's, the neuron cell has thin extensions from it that allow it to connect with other cells (Figure 14.1). In general, the shorter dendrites receive signals from other cells and the axons transmit signals to other cells. The axons of one neuron can be very lengthy, up to several feet long. Inside of the body of the neuron and its axons and dendrites is a skeleton made of neatly arranged tubules that support the cell, much like our own skeleton. As the neuron deteriorates and dies, the tubules in this skeleton are chemically changed and become disorganized instead of neatly arranged. Eventually, the tubular structure pulls up out of the axons, wads up, and forms a tangle inside of the cell. Once this begins, it is unlikely anything can be done to bring this cell back to life.

I believe that the problem of glucose not getting into the cells is ultimately responsible for the malfunction and death of these cells. If adequate amounts of glucose cannot get into the neuron cell, and there is no other fuel to replace it, the whole chain of events

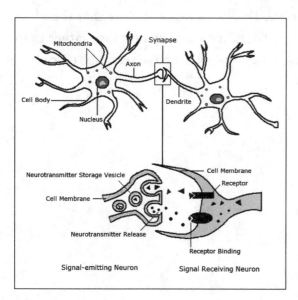

Figure 14.1: Neurons have a membrane that is designed to send information to other cells. The axons and dendrites are unique structures designed to transmit and receive information. The connections between cells are known as synapses. Neurons release chemicals known as neurotransmitters into these synapses to communicate with other neurons. Diagram by Joanna Newport.

that comes thereafter is affected. Without enough fuel, the mito-chondria cannot manufacture enough ATP. Without ATP, the cell cannot make the proteins it usually makes, may make defective proteins, and/or may not have enough energy to release their pro-teins and enough of the chemicals called neurotransmitters that it needs to communicate with other cells.

I believe that up to a certain point, this process may be revers-ible. If the cell can get some form of fuel, so that certain substances are replenished, the mitochondria can make more ATP again. Then there may be some recovery and reversal of the process, much like someone whose heart has stopped and is brought back to life by a defibrillator. But without enough ATP, proteins and other chemi-cals accumulate inside the cell; the cell membrane deteriorates, no longer able to fulfill its purpose of deciding what gets in and what gets out; the proteins leak out and accumulate outside the cell; and the skeleton of the brain cell collapses and begins to wad up, form-ing the tangle inside the cell.

While the process of how cells function is far more complicated than what I've discussed here, it is clear to me that if a cell cannot get enough energy and is in the process of dying, at some point reversal will not be possible. I want to make it clear that the ideas presented in these last two paragraphs are my opinion, rather than proven facts, and they are based on what I have read up to now.

15

What Causes Alzheimer's Disease?

What triggers the chain of events that ultimately results in the death of brain cells? Despite the very many millions of dollars spent on research into this question and the thousands of researchers all over the world working on it, there is no answer. At present, we do not know with certainty what causes Alzheimer's disease.

Heredity plays a major role in whether we will develop Alzheimer's or not, but environmental factors appear to influence how our genetic makeup will play out as we age. Any number of toxins or infectious agents could get the ball rolling, or at least contribute to the disease process. A history of traumatic brain injury is a well-known risk factor for the disease. The following are examples of research related to just a few of the suspects.

GENETICS

About 0.1 percent of people with Alzheimer's have the familial form of the disease, passed to them as a dominant mutated gene from their parent, and these unfortunate people usually develop the early onset form of the disease (before age sixty-five). The vast majority of people with Alzheimer's have the sporadic form of the disease, meaning that it is not the result of a specific genetic mutation. However, our genetic profile can place some of us at greater risk than others.

A number of different genes have been shown to either have a protective effect or carry a greater risk of developing Alzheimer's if they are in our DNA, but the best known of these is apolipoprotein E (ApoE). This is a substance that transports lipids in the plasma and central nervous system and plays a central role in maintaining and repairing neurons. There are three common forms of this gene known as ApoE2, ApoE3, and ApoE4. They are distinguished by substitution of a single amino acid on a critical part of the gene that determines how the gene folds and therefore how it functions, or potentially malfunctions (Zhong, 2009). For example, people with an ApoE4 gene are more likely to have recurrent fever blisters, with ramifications that will be discussed later in this chapter (see "Herpes Virus Infections").

We receive two of these ApoE genes, one from each parent, and the combination of the two genes determines our level of risk for Alzheimer's, although even the greatest level of risk does not guarantee that we will develop the disease at all. Possessing one ApoE4 gene increases the risk by three times, and if both genes are ApoE4, the risk is fifteen times greater. In addition, people with two ApoE4 genes, who represent about 2 percent of the population, are more likely to develop early onset Alzheimer's. People with ApoE3 genes, but no ApoE4 gene, carry average risk, and if you are lucky enough to possess two ApoE2 genes, you carry the lowest risk (Blennow, 2006).

EPIGENETICS

A relatively new field called epigenetics studies the effects of environmental factors, such as air pollution or chronic exposure to pesticides, and lifestyle choices such as diet and smoking, on how our genetic makeup plays out. Researchers have learned that these factors may turn on or turn off certain genes and can be passed on from one cell to its daughter cells after cell division occurs, and therefore stay with us for life. If the cell involved happens to be a sperm or egg, these effects can be passed on to the next generation. So not only are we affected by what our mothers ate while carrying us in the womb, we may be affected by what either of our parents ate before they even conceived us (NIH 2009 Progress Report on Alzheimer's Disease).

Toxic Metals and Chemicals

Abnormally high levels of metals, such as lead, mercury, aluminum, iron, and cadmium, or exposure to certain pesticides, fertilizers, or other chemicals in our food have been implicated as possible causes or contributing factors to developing Alzheimer's disease, since high levels of one or more of these have been found in some people with Alzheimer's. Accumulations of these metals could damage DNA and other structures within our cells. Any of these could produce oxidative damage (from oxygen free radicals), as well as inflammation in the brain, one of the hallmarks of the disease. As just one example, a well-known controversy involves whether mercury causes or contributes to Alzheimer's disease. Some people with Alzheimer's have high levels of mercury, possibly the result of the material and the process used for filling cavities in the past. There are experts who have come out in favor of, and others opposed to, removing these fillings to reduce the risk of continued exposure to mercury. The problem with removing the fillings is that mercury is released in the process, so special precautions need to be taken.

Diet

Dietary deficiencies, such as certain B vitamins, vitamin D, and docosahexanoic acid (DHA, an omega-3 essential fatty acid), have been considered as contributing to dementia, as have excesses of certain substances in our diet. In addition to providing evidence of Alzheimer's as diabetes type 3, Drs. Suzanne de la Monte and Jack Wands have looked at some potential substances in our diet that might cause or worsen this problem of insulin deficiency and resistance.

Alcohol

One of these substances is excessive intake of alcohol, which Drs. de la Monte and Wands say, "causes progressive toxicity and degeneration in the liver and brain due to insulin resistance" (De la Monte, 2009). As part of this process, damage to cells occurs from oxidation (attacks by oxygen free radicals), and mechanisms that produce inflammatory response are activated. The inflammation that results in the liver promotes the manufacture and accumulation of ceramides and other toxic lipids that cause insulin resistance. These toxic lipids cross the blood/brain barrier and damage brain cells as well. Much of the damage that occurs in the brain from toxic lipids appears to be related to insulin resistance (De la Monte, 2009).

Ceramides are a particular family of lipids that is highly concentrated in the cell membrane and one of the largest components of sphingomyelin, a major part of the lipid bilayer of the cell membrane. The lipid bilayer is the lineup of lipid molecules that repel watery fluid to keep the outside world out of the cell and the contents inside the cell. Ceramides also act as both positive and negative signaling molecules, substances that are involved in communication within the cell and cell membrane. One of their jobs is to signal a sequence that leads to the death of a cell, another is to signal the sequence to divide to make a new cell. Toxic ceramides have been implicated in a number of disease processes including cancer, diabetes, and neurodegeneration. Some of the very interesting things these researchers have learned in relation to alcohol and the brain are that:

- The cholesterol content of the cell membrane is reduced by exposure to alcohol (ethanol*).

- Depletion of cholesterol in the brain impairs the binding of insulin to its receptors, which also results in reduced glucose uptake into the cells that is stimulated by insulin.

- Replacing the cholesterol in the cell membrane partly (but not completely) restores the ability of the insulin to bind to the receptors and glucose to be transported into the cells.

* Note: Researchers believe that ethanol may remove other important lipids from the cell membrane.

Nitrosamines

Nitrosamines are another group of substances de la Monte and her group have studied that may play a role in the development of insulin resistance in the brain (De la Monte, 2009; Tong, 2009). Like excess alcohol, nitrosamines produce ceramides or toxic lipids that cross the blood/brain barrier and can cause insulin deficiency and insulin resistance in the brain, and therefore chronic exposure to nitrogen fertilizers, nitrates in water used to irrigate crops, and consumption in food and water could contribute to the process of neurodegeneration (De la Monte, three 2009 articles).

Found in tobacco and nitrogen fertilizers, nitrosamines are also commonly used as preservatives in processed foods, such as white flour and therefore anything that contains white flour; in processed cheeses; and in most bacon and luncheon meats. Even formulas and foods made for infants are not free of these compounds. Look for "nitrites" or "nitrates," or any words that contain "nitrite" or "nitrate," for example, thiamine mononitrate, on food labels. Certain vegetables naturally contain some nitrates, however, at much higher levels if grown in the conventional manner with nitrogen fertilizers; therefore, organically grown vegetables are a better choice. Many beers and some hard liquors are made with a process involving nitrosamines, and some contain high levels of these compounds. Thus, someone who chronically drinks certain brands of beer or scotch may have a greatly increased risk of damage from toxic ceramides due to the combination of alcohol and nitrosamines. Manufacturers of these beverages are not required to list nitrosamine content on the label.

It is very possible that a great many people in the United States consume foods with nitrosamines compounds at virtually every meal, and this may even begin in infancy. Our diet has evolved more and more in this direction over the past half century. Could this in part explain the simultaneous, growing epidemic of Alzheimer's and other diseases that involve insulin deficiency and/or insulin resistance?

INFECTIOUS AGENTS

Research published in March 2010 by Stephanie Soscia, a postdoctoral fellow at Massachusetts General Hospital, and others presents some findings that no doubt come as a shock to those in the beta-amyloid camp. The researchers found that beta-amyloid, the protein that forms the classic plaque deposits that accumulate and damage nearby brain cells, is actually antimicrobial. Beta-amyloid killed eight different bacteria that were exposed to it. This is a profound discovery, considering the millions (billions, more likely) of research dollars spent looking for substances that will reduce beta-amyloid in the brain. There are currently vaccines in clinical trials and oral medications that intend to do just that. Perhaps some of the supplements we take to try to reduce beta-amyloid (turmeric is one example) work by preventing or eliminating infection and therefore reducing the need for beta-amyloid to be made in response to infection.

When we develop an upper respiratory infection such as the

common cold, the cells overproduce mucus in reaction to it. When we cut ourselves, if the wound becomes infected with bacteria, the body reacts by producing white blood cells and other substances that accumulate as pus to fight the infection. Could it be that these abnormal collections of beta-amyloid plaque are part of the brain's immune response to repeated flare-ups of infection in the brain and not the cause of Alzheimer's disease? Alzheimer's appears to start in one part of the brain and then spreads until the entire brain is involved. This is compatible with how infections spread in other parts of the body.

Herpes Virus Infections

Researchers Ruth Itzhaki, Ph.D., and Mark Wozniak at the University of Manchester in England may have found the cause of Alzheimer's disease, at least in some people. They have learned in the course of their research, spanning at least thirteen years, that there is a strong association of a history of fever blisters, also called cold sores, in people who are ApoE4+. Herpes simplex type 1 (HSV1), the virus that causes fever blisters, is not usually found in younger brains but is found in nearly all elderly brains. They speculate that the immune system isn't as effective in fighting this virus as we reach old age. The researchers found evidence of HSV1 within 90 percent of the beta-amyloid plaques in the autopsied brains of six elderly ApoE4+ people who died with Alzheimer's disease. They also looked at four brains of similar aged people who were ApoE4- and did not have dementia as controls, and likewise found the virus within 80 percent of the plaques; however, there were many fewer plaques. Seventy-two percent of the viral DNA found in Alzheimer brains was associated with the amyloid plaques (Wozniak, 2009).

This is strong evidence that beta-amyloid is a response to infection in people who are ApoE4+. Perhaps people with this genetic profile are more susceptible to the disease and/or don't fight the virus as well. In the discussion of this study, the researchers conclude that "the infected cell, after suffering severe structural damage, dies and disintegrates, releasing amyloid aggregates which then develop into classic plaques after other components of dying cells are deposited on them. Presumably, in ApoE4 carriers, Alzheimer's disease develops either as a consequence of HSV1-induced plaque accumulation or as a direct consequence of virus induced cell death or inflammation" (Wozniak, 2004).

This group has also found that HSV1 infection produces a marked increase of beta-amyloid 1-40 and 1-42 (specific toxic types of beta-amyloid found in Alzheimer's) within cultured neurons and glial cells and also results in increased beta-amyloid 1-42 in mouse brains following infection with this virus (Wozniak, 2007). In addition, HSV1 increases Alzheimer's disease-like tau (protein that forms the classic tangles) within the infected cells (Wozniak, 2009).

HSV1 and certain other viruses live inside of nerves. Periodically, something triggers the virus to multiply, and an outbreak of infection occurs. This infection usually appears on or near the lips, but can appear elsewhere on the body. The nerves to the lips, called the trigeminal nerves, actually originate deep inside the brain. If an outbreak of the virus can appear on the lips, why not closer to the origin of the nerve deep inside the brain?

Some infections do not reoccur once we are exposed to and have overcome them. Those of us who have had measles or mumps developed a good immunity to the infection so that we would not expect to ever have this type of infection again. The herpes family of viruses, which also includes chickenpox, the virus that causes herpes zoster, commonly known as shingles, is different in that we develop only a partial immune response. The virus remains alive but dormant (asleep) within our nerves. As our antibody levels to these viruses drop, the infection can occur over and over. Some people are much more likely to experience repeated infections than others.

Steve is ApoE4+ and has had a lifelong history of fever blisters, often breaking out every few weeks and sometimes lasting a month or longer. When we were moving from Cincinnati to Charleston, he had an outbreak around one of his eyes. The optic nerves of the eyes connect with the occipital cortex, where vision originates in the brain. Perhaps this explains the visual disturbance that kept him from reading for nearly two years. It is well known that the eyes are a porthole to the brain.

It just so happens that the C:10 and C:12 medium-chain fatty acids in coconut oil dissolve the lipid capsules of HSV1 and other members of the herpes family of viruses, effectively killing them. This may be another good reason to add coconut oil to the diet. Certain medications that control the herpes virus, such as valacyclovir (Valtrex), could be effective and are being considered for clinical trials in this regard (Thormar, 1987; Kristmunsdottir, 1999; McGrath, 1997).

There is evidence in at least some cases that a viral illness triggers the onset of type 1 diabetes. Insulin is made in the islet cells of the pancreas. If these cells can be permanently altered by a virus in such a way that they no longer produce insulin, then why couldn't the same process happen in the cells that produce insulin in the brain?

MITOCHONDRIAL DYSFUNCTION

Alzheimer's and Parkinson's disease are just two of many diseases that involve dysfunction of mitochondria. The exact reasons for such dysfunction are not certain.

One of the interesting facts about our mitochondria is that, unlike the cells in our bodies, the DNA that controls these tiny organelles comes exclusively from our mothers. Jia Yao and others reported in the August 2009 issue of *Proceedings of the National Academy of Sciences* (*PNAS*) that, in a female mouse model of Alzheimer's disease, mitochondria in neurons in the embryo (early stage unborn mouse) were already producing less energy than controls. They found decreased levels of pyruvate dehydrogenase (PDH) enzymes and mitochondrial respiration as early as three months of age in these mice. This did not occur until the equivalent of menopause in the normal mice. As Alzheimer's disease progresses, certain enzymes that control energy production within the mitochondria decrease both in quantity and in their level of activity. As a result, less ATP is made. Without enough ATP, the cell malfunctions and eventually dies. As more and more cells die, the symptoms of the disease emerge.

Certain lifestyle choices may speed up or slow down the cumulative effects of mitochondrial damage and malfunction. Food choices may play a critical role in the outcome. It is possible that treatments will come along to slow down this process as well. The ketone ester may be one of them.

TRAUMATIC HEAD INJURY

A number of studies have been performed looking at whether there is a connection between head trauma and Alzheimer's. Two review studies that combined results of many smaller studies both concluded that head trauma severe enough to cause loss of consciousness increased the risk of Alzheimer's by a factor of 1.5 to 2 for men, but not for women (Mortimer, 1991; Fleminger, 2003). In addition, in 2009 the *New York Times* reported results of a study commissioned by the National Football League (NFL) showing that NFL players developed Alzheimer's or similar memory-related diseases nineteen times more often than the normal rate for men ages thirty through forty-nine (Schwarz, 2009).

CONNECTING THE DOTS

How do the aspects of Alzheimer's disease discussed above interconnect? Is there a single explanation that could link them together?

In researching a possible connection between nitrosamine compounds and viral infection, I happened upon an article detailing research that took place in the lab of George Cahill, Jr., M.D., the doctor who discovered that the brain can use ketones as fuel. The article was entitled "Studies of Streptozotocin-induced Insulitis and Diabetes" and published in the *PNAS* in June 1977 (Rossini). Previous studies with streptozotocin (STZ), a nitrosamine compound, used a single large injection known to cause diabetes within one or two days by destroying the beta cells in the pancreas that produce insulin. This substance has been used to provide animal models of diabetes for various studies. Single smaller doses of this substance do not produce this effect. This 1977 study built upon the researchers' previous study in which a small injection of STZ was given daily to mice for five days and found to induce diabetes within five to six days.

This time the researchers administered STZ alone or in combination with one of three other substances; two of the substances, nicotinamide and 3-O-methyl-D-glucose (3-OMG), were thought to reduce or delay the diabetogenic effect of STZ and were shown to do so in this study. The third substance, antilymphocyte serum, was used to determine if the damage to the cell is a result of the cell's own immune response to STZ, and they found this to be true. But an unexpected finding in this study was that a marked increase in the number of virus particles (a type C mouse virus) was found in the surviving beta-pancreatic cells within six days of the injections. They speculated that the virus might induce proteins within the cell that initiate the immune response and, further, that STZ may alter the function of the beta cell in such a way that it changes from an insulin-producing cell to a "cell primarily synthesizing virus."

If one connects the dots among the various reports in this section, the following hypothesis emerges as one possible mechanism for the development of Alzheimer's disease: nitrosamine compounds found in everyday foods produce toxic ceramides in the liver that cross the blood/brain barrier, destroying insulin-producing cells in the brain and altering other brain cells to produce insulin resistance. This process results in the inability of cells to take up glucose for fuel, leading to poor functioning, and eventually death, of the cells due to lack of energy. As the cell dies, the skeleton of the cell is damaged and retracts to form the tangles that are hallmarks of Alzheimer's. These toxic lipids also allow viruses already present within the brain to transform cells into virus-replicating factories. An increase in beta-amyloid occurs as part of the innate immune response to infection, and the characteristic plaques are formed to try to contain the virus. This immune response produces the inflammation typical of Alzheimer's, resulting in collateral damage to nearby cells.

This hypothesis is my attempt to connect the dots between the research findings presented in this chapter and has not been proven at this time. This or any number of other mechanisms could result in the clinical picture that we call Alzheimer's disease.

16

Ketones Basics

In the October 2003 issue of *Nutrition Reviews*, the lead review article "Ketones: Metabolism's Ugly Duckling" was written by Theodore B. VanItallie, M.D., and Thomas H. Nufert and included a comprehensive discussion of:

- The discovery of ketones

- The physiology and metabolism of ketones

- The role of ketones in starvation and carbohydrate restriction

- The recognition of ketones as a metabolic fuel

- How ketones are used now to treat disease, such as epilepsy and rare genetic defects

- The potential for treatment of other diseases with ketones

I highly recommend this article for anyone who wishes to read a more technical and detailed discussion of what is currently known about ketones than I'm providing here.

My goal is to provide information about ketones so that most people will be able to understand them. Much of what I discuss is based on that article, as well as information from other articles written by Richard Veech, M.D., George Cahill, Jr., M.D, Oliver Owen, M.D., Sami Hashim, M.D., and their many associates, and a number of others who have researched and written about ketones.

Information about the ketogenic diet largely comes from the book entitled *The Ketogenic Diet* (2007) by John M. Freeman, M.D.

THE CHEMISTRY OF KETONES

Organic chemistry is the study of compounds that contain hydrocarbons, various combinations of carbon and hydrogen that are the basis of living organisms. A number of other elements may be included in these compounds, such as nitrogen, oxygen, phosphorus, silicon, and sulfur. The various types of compounds are grouped and named according to the way the particular elements are arranged. Some examples of groups of organic compounds are esters, amides, aldehydes, fatty acids, and ketones, to name just a few.

The Chemical Structure of Ketones

For those who did not take chemistry, very simply, an atom is a single particle of an element, such as hydrogen or carbon, and a bond is a connection between atoms. A molecule is a group of two or more atoms. Each type of atom has a specific number of possible bonds it can make with other atoms. For example, hydrogen can make one possible bond and oxygen two bonds. A water molecule is one oxygen atom that attaches its two bonds to two hydrogen atoms, or H_2O (Figure 16.1).

The carbon atom can have four possible bonds

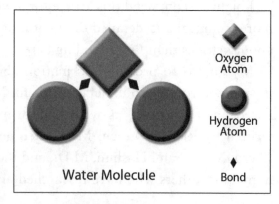

Figure 16.1: A water molecule. Diagram by Joanna Newport.

to other atoms. The defining feature of ketones is a single carbonyl group, which is an oxygen atom connected by two bonds to a carbon atom. Also attached to the carbon are two more carbon atoms, and each of these carbon atoms is attached to a variety of atoms or groups of atoms. In the simplest ketone, called acetone, the other two carbons use their three other bonds to attach to hydrogen atoms (Figure 16.2).

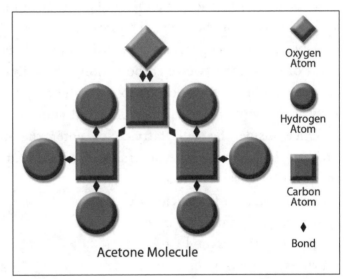

Figure 16.2: The ketone body acetone. Diagram by Joanna Newport.

Many different kind of ketones are found in nature, but in the human body there are three ketones, also called ketone bodies, that we will be talking about. These are acetone, acetoacetate, and beta-hydroxybutyrate. Acetone is the simplest ketone, while acetoacetate and beta-hydroxybutyrate are more complex molecules. You should know that acetone made in our bodies is the same acetone found in fingernail polish and paint thinner. Most people are familiar with the odor of acetone. When a person has an excess of ketones in the blood, some of this acetone will be exhaled, so the person's breath may smell like acetone. Also, some of the acetone is disposed of by the kidneys in the urine.

How Ketones Are Formed

The process of making ketones is called ketogenesis. This is a complex process (Figure 16.3), but I will attempt to explain it simply.

Ketones are produced when the glucose stored in the body is used up and fat is broken down to be used as energy. Triglycerides, the storage form of fat, are converted to fatty acids in the adipocytes (fat cells) or fat tissue by a process called lipolysis. Fatty acids can be used as a metabolic fuel by a number of tissues such as muscle or the heart. The fatty acids released from fat are transported to these tissues and cross the cell membrane. Fatty acids of more than twelve carbons (long-chain fatty acids) require special membrane transporters to enter the cell, but medium-chain fatty acids, with twelve carbons or less, do not.

Once inside the cell, fatty acids enter the mitochondria, a process that requires special transporters for fatty acids longer than twelve carbons. Inside the mitochondria, the fatty acids are split repeatedly into two carbon fragments called acetyl-CoA by a process known as beta-oxidation. An additional set of reactions occurs when fatty acids are transported to the liver. They are converted in the liver cell mitochondria first to acetyl-CoA as in other tissues, but then the acetyl-CoA is converted through several biochemical reactions to the ketone acetoacetate, which

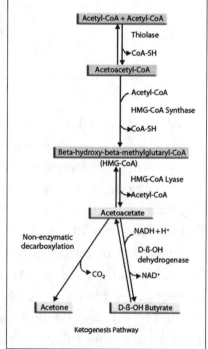

Figure 16.3. Ketogenesis pathway.
Diagram by Joanna Newport.

is then converted to the other two ketones, acetone and beta-hydroxybutyrate. So when fatty acids are converted in the liver to ketones, this entire process is called ketogenesis. The ketone bodies then leave the liver and are transported throughout the body, where they can be used as an energy source in the mitochondria of a number of tissues, including the brain.

WHY KETONES ARE SO IMPORTANT
IN THE HUMAN BRAIN

As you know, mitochondria are tiny structures inside of cells in which energy is manufactured. Certain cells, such as heart muscle, neurons, and liver cells, can have a thousand or more mitochondria inside of each cell. Amazing to think a cell that cannot be seen with the naked eye can have a thousand of anything so complex inside of it! When a fuel such as glucose (after being converted to pyruvate) or ketones enters the mitochondria, a chain of events takes place leading to the generation of the basic source of energy, ATP, that drives our cells. The way cells use ATP is much like how a car takes electricity from a battery in order to run. Ketones are a more efficient producer of ATP than pyruvate, improving the hydraulic efficiency of the working heart by over 30 percent (Kashiyawa, 1997).

Fatty acids made from stored fat can be used by the heart for fuel but are too large to cross the protective blood/brain barrier into the brain circulation. But ketones are able to pass into the brain on a special monocarboxylate transporter and can be used by the neurons and other brain cells for fuel.

The fact that our brains can use ketones is very important in our evolution as a species. Compared with other animals, the size of the human brain is very large relative to our total body weight. The considerably larger cerebral cortex, the part of the brain that provides us with higher intelligence, accounts for most of this difference.

Glucose as Fuel

The brain in an average adult weighs just over three pounds, just about 2 percent of the total body weight, but it has a very high-energy requirement. When we are at rest, the brain consumes about 20 percent of the calories needed to carry out basic bodily functions. This represents about 100 to 120 grams of glucose per twenty-four hours. In the infant and child, the brain is even larger relative to body weight, and the brain may consume as much as 40 to 50 percent of the basic calorie requirement. The pregnant mother has to provide enough energy for two large brains and may need 200 to 220 grams of glucose every day to provide enough energy for herself and the baby.

For many millennia, our ancestors, and even people in our world today, have endured periods of feast and famine. Our bodies are only able to store enough glucose in the liver (glycogen) to last about forty-eight hours, but then must tap into muscle to make new glucose. This is a very complex process, called gluconeogenesis. During starvation, about 60 percent of this process occurs in the liver and 40 percent in the kidneys. Very simply, protein from muscle is changed into specific amino acids and released into the bloodstream mostly as glutamine and alanine. The glutamine is mainly converted to glucose by the kidneys. The liver uses the alanine, some recycled lactate and pyruvate, which come from red cells and kidney cells, some glycerol from fat, and even some ketone body, to make glucose.

While glycogen stores in the liver are used up within a couple of days, gluconeogenesis can continue for at least forty days. But the calories that we can make from gluconeogenesis alone are not nearly enough to provide the basic calorie requirements of the body and brain for an extended period of time. If glucose were the only fuel our brains could use, a starving human would last only about two weeks before consuming so much muscle that survival would no longer be possible.

Fat as Fuel

When we have an abundance of food, we store extra calories in the form of fat. When our energy needs exceed our calorie intake, we begin to tap into these stores of fat, which are broken down into fatty acids. As we continue to starve, our muscles, including our heart muscle, switch over from using glucose to using primarily fatty acids as fuel. Medium-chain fatty acids can cross the blood/ brain barrier but are not made in the body in a form that can be released into circulation to fuel the brain. The only exception to this is that the lactating mother can manufacture medium-chain fatty acids in the breast that become part of the milk for the baby.

Since our brains require so much fuel to survive, when we have used up our stores of glucose, how does the brain survive starvation? As our bodies change over to using stores of fat as the main source of fuel, some of the fatty acids are converted into ketones in the liver. The presence of ketones in general circulation actually increases the blood flow to the brain by as much as 39 percent, at least initially (Hasselbalch, 1996). Ketones cross the blood/brain barrier and are taken up very rapidly by brain cells as fuel. Ketones also perform other important functions, which will be explained shortly.

Ketones as Fuel

Ketone bodies do not require insulin to enter the cell, but rather are transported into the cell by a much simpler mechanism than glucose. The ketone body bypasses some of this complex process and enters directly into the Krebs cycle, the chain of chemical reactions that produce acetyl-CoA and ultimately the basic energy molecule ATP. During starvation, about 60 percent of the energy requirement of the brain can be provided by ketones, thus sparing muscle from being broken down to provide energy. Since our brains can use ketones as fuel, we can potentially survive for two months or longer without food, instead of just two weeks. The more fat tissue available, the longer we can survive, since fatty acids can be used by muscle and ketones made from fatty acids can be used by the brain and other tissues.

The average adult will have a low level of ketones after fasting overnight, but these levels drop as soon as we eat our morning meal. We begin to see a significant increase in ketone levels after about two days without food. The levels of the ketone bodies acetone and acetoacetate rise and then begin to level off after about ten days in the 1 to 1.5 micromoles per liter (mmol/l) range, but the levels of beta-hydroxybutyrate continue to increase very dramatically for a time before leveling off in the 6 to 7 mmol/l range. As long as we have fat available, we continue to make ketones.

The infant, child, and pregnant or lactating woman is able to start making ketones considerably sooner than the average adult, reflecting their even greater need for brain fuel during starvation. The newborn uses ketones for as much as 25 percent of the energy requirement during the first days of life (Bourgneres, 1986). Most new mothers learn quickly there is not much breast milk available during the first days after the baby is born. Human babies are quite fat relative to other creatures, and ketones help them get through this period until their mother's milk is more available.

If our brains did not have the ability to use ketones as fuel, it is unlikely that we would even exist as a species today, or at least not as the very large-brained, intelligent species we are. Our ancient ancestors, and even many people today, have gone without food for extended periods and survived, thanks to the role fat and ketones play in providing fuel.

THE DISCOVERY THAT KETONES ARE AN ALTERNATE FUEL IN THE BRAIN

The fact that the brain can use another fuel was discovered and reported in 1967 in an article entitled "Brain Metabolism during Fasting" in the *Journal of Clinical Investigation* by Dr. George Cahill and his associates, who included Dr. Oliver E. Owen. In 1965, at about the same time that Dr. Cahill decided that it would be important to reinvestigate the effects of starvation in humans since better methods had become available to measure biologic fuels and hormones, Owen began a fellowship in Cahill's lab at Harvard. Owen detailed the history of this discovery in his article "Ketone Bodies as a Fuel for the Brain during Starvation" in *Biochemistry and Molecular Biology Education* (2005).

Early Studies Reveal Backup Fuel

The first subject was an obese nurse who was highly motivated to participate in the researchers' study of prolonged fasting. She was referred to their clinic for weight loss due to her concern about having a heart attack. As a nurse she was well aware of the procedures involved. After a few days on a balanced diet, the researchers began a starvation protocol in which she received only water, vitamins, and salt tablets for a period of forty-one days. They chose forty-one days because that was the period of time that Jesus fasted according to the Bible. They took blood samples from catheters placed in arteries and veins around her brain and liver to measure various metabolites. Much to their delight they found that her brain had survived this lengthy period of starvation by using ketones and greatly reducing the use of glucose. About two-thirds of the fuel used by her brain was provided by beta-hydroxybutyrate and acetoacetate.

Dr. Owen reported, "The fact that the brain could derive energy from substrates other than glucose was of monumental importance for understanding human survival during starvation. Our findings explained why normal size humans can survive sixty days or more without food; the brain obtained most of its energy requirements from ketone bodies, a fuel derived from fatty acids. This finding resulted in a total reappraisal of the hierarchy of fuels used by different tissues of humans" (see Figures 16.4 and 16.5).

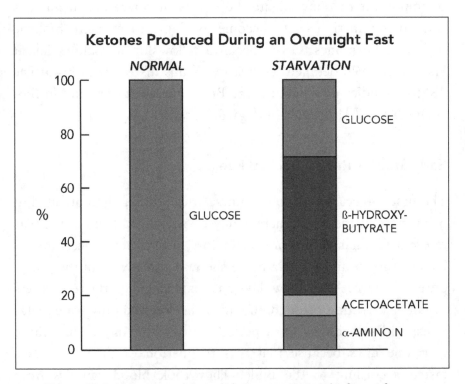

Figure 16.4. Ketones produced during an overnight fast. After an overnight fast in normal individuals, virtually 100 percent of the fuel used by the brain comes from glucose. During starvation, ketones supply two-thirds and glucose just one-third of the fuel for the brain. Data from Owens, 2005.

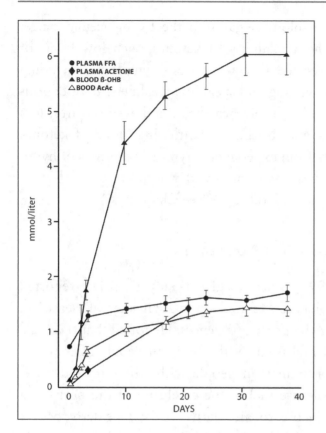

Figure 16.5. Levels of ketones are nearly zero when we eat regularly. While fasting, the levels begin to rise after one or two days, and beta-hydroxybutyrate in particular increases dramatically if starvation continues for more than five days. Data from Owens, 2005.

Dr. Cahill's group studied two more obese patients in the same manner and confirmed that "during prolonged starvation, the brain extracts significant quantities of acetoacetate and beta-hydroxybutyrate from the blood, thus sparing the metabolism of glucose. We grasped immediately that the metabolism of ketone bodies rather than glucose was the predominant source of energy, sparing muscle protein and ensuring survival during starvation." They also learned that during starvation, glucose levels drop and then level off after about three days, and this is paralleled by a similar drop in insulin levels.

An even bolder experiment followed (Cahill, 1980). Three obese college-age men were starved for several days until their beta-hydroxybutyrate levels increased. They were then given a dose of insulin to drive down blood sugar into the hypoglycemic range. Normally, without the availability of ketones, such low levels of glucose would be expected to cause serious symptoms, including confusion, difficulty thinking and speaking, weakness, poor coordination, paleness, sweating, rapid heartbeat, and even seizures, loss of consciousness or coma. In this study, the high level of ketones protected the subjects from experiencing typical symptoms of hypoglycemia. Other studies have confirmed this protective effect of ketones in the face of low blood sugar (see Chapter 18).

Later Studies Reveal a Fuel Preference

Fast forward to 1991, when Siegfried Hoyer, M.D., reported "Abnormalities of Glucose Metabolism in Alzheimer's Disease" in the *Annals of the NY Academy of Sciences*. He found that there is a shift in the types of fuel used by the brain in people as they age that is even more prominent in people with Alzheimer's disease. Young, normal people use fuel in the cerebrum of the brain in a ratio of 100:1 of glucose to alternative fuels; in elderly people without Alzheimer's, this ratio is 29:1; and in people in the early stages of Alzheimer's this ratio is 2:1. This means that someone in the beginning stages of Alzheimer's requires that about one-third of the fuel for brain cells comes from alternative fuels. Dr. Hoyer speculated that possible alternative fuels could be fatty acids and amino acids present in the brain, such as glutamate, that could be converted to glucose, but he did not specifically mention ketones in this article as a possible alternative fuel.

We know from the work of Drs. Cahill and Owen that ketones could also provide this alternative fuel. Since most of us do not have ketones circulating and readily available to the brain, it stands to reason that brain cells lacking this necessary fuel would malfunction and eventually die. Treatment with foods that contain medium-chain fatty acids, which are converted to ketones in the liver, or, even better, direct treatment with ketone bodies themselves, could provide the brain with this necessary fuel.

CONDITIONS THAT CAUSE THE BODY TO MAKE KETONES

The body makes ketones in response to a number of conditions, including fasting. As we fast overnight while sleeping, a relatively tiny amount of ketones are made, but as soon as we eat a typical breakfast, they disappear. If we continue to fast for a period of two or more days, the levels of ketones increase very significantly. As a modern-day example of the biochemical miracle of ketogenesis, one need only recall the images of people emerging from beneath the piles of concrete where they were trapped without food for as long as fourteen days after the disastrous 2010 earthquake in Haiti. Upon being pulled from the rubble, many of these people were alert, smiling, talking and even singing, their cognitive function apparently intact. With their stores of glucose gone in less than a day or two, ketones came to their rescue to preserve their brains and allow them to survive while awaiting release from their concrete prisons.

Helpful levels of ketones are produced by the body through exercise and diet. However, not all production of ketones is healthy. Life-threatening levels of ketones can also be produced in diabetics, called diabetic ketoacidosis (discussed later).

Diet and Ketosis

Most of us in the United States do not have to struggle with the problem of feast and famine. The standard American diet (sometimes called "SAD"!) is very high in carbohydrate, or sugar. As a result, there is not much ketone circulating in the bloodstream, since plenty of glucose fuel is available.

One way to produce ketones through diet is to consume an extremely high-fat, low-carbohydrate diet, called the "ketogenic diet." This diet is sometimes used to treat children, and occasionally adults, who have severe epilepsy. This diet is also relatively low in protein, allowing enough protein for the child to grow or for the adult to maintain lean body mass. The Atkins and South Beach diets are less restrictive forms of the ketogenic diet and result in a milder "ketosis" (more on these diets in Chapter 17).

There is yet another way that ketones can become available to brain cells through diet, and that is the basis of the dietary intervention discussed in Part Three in this book. When a person eats foods that contain medium-chain fatty acids, they are absorbed from the small intestine and transported directly to the liver, where they are partly converted to ketones. The ketones are then released into the blood circulation. Some of the medium-chain fatty acids are also released into the circulation and are used immediately as energy. Medium-chain fatty acids are known to be used directly as fuel by muscle mitochondria (Turner, 2009); are small enough to cross the blood/brain barrier; are not stored as fat but rather used immediately as fuel by tissues; and may be used as fuel by the mitochondria in the brain. Animal data shows that medium-chain fatty acids are used in the brain (Johnson, 1990). Further studies need to be done to determine what specific tissues, in addition to muscle, are able to use medium-chain fatty acids directly.

The most concentrated food sources of medium-chain fatty acids are coconut oil and palm kernel oil, which contain about 55 to 60 percent medium-chain fatty acids. These are saturated fats, but do not behave the same way in the body as long-chain saturated fats that doctors worry about (see Chapter 21). Oils normally consumed in this country, such as soybean, olive, canola, corn, peanut, safflower, and sesame, do not contain any medium-chain fatty acids. Some foods that do contain medium-chain fatty acids are goat's milk, whole cow's milk, butter, heavy cream, and goat and feta cheese, although not nearly in the concentrations found in coconut and palm kernel oils.

We can take advantage of the biochemical process that naturally occurs in our bodies when we consume fats with medium-chain fatty acids. The more medium-chain fatty acids we consume, the more ketones we produce. If you do not eat medium-chain fats on a given day, you are not likely to produce a significant amount of ketones, unless you are starving for a couple of days or longer or you are on a ketogenic diet.

Medium-chain fatty acids cross the blood/brain barrier, where they are used by brain cells for fuel. Considering the process that occurs in Alzheimer's and certain other neurodegenerative diseases, it is very conceivable that medium-chain fatty acids are an important source of fuel for the brain. They might even be considered essential fatty acids for some people: the brain needs medium-chain fatty acids, but we cannot make them; therefore, we need to consume them. So there appears to be a great advantage to including foods with medium-chain fatty acids in the diet on a daily basis. Not only will that provide the brain with ketones, but also with medium-chain fatty acids that can be used directly as fuel by certain brain cells.

More extensive research is needed to learn about the various functions of medium-chain fatty acids in the brain and other organs in addition to their function as fuel.

Exercise and Ketosis

We produce ketones when we exercise. This was first described in 1909 by G. Forssner, who noticed that the levels of ketones always increased in his urine after a brisk 4-kilometer walk lasting over thirty-six minutes. In 1911, L. Preti reported the same phenomenon in a patient who had a minor stomach complaint after climbing up and down stairs until exhausted. In 1936, F. C. Courtice and C. G. Douglas reported that following moderate early morning exercise after fasting overnight, ketones begin to rise upon completion of exercise and continue to rise for at least nine hours. They hypothesized that the muscles, which were glucose-deprived due to lack of food overnight, use the circulating ketones while the exercise occurs. When the exercise ceases, the liver continues to make ketones for a short period, which then accumulate in the circulation. This phenomenon was thereafter called the "Courtice-Douglas effect" and is also known as "post-exercise ketosis." In all three of these studies, the subjects were on some kind of a restricted diet, reported as either low carbohydrate or high protein, for a period of time before the experiments. Later researchers noted that if a high-carbohydrate meal was taken before the exercise, there was no increase in ketones.

While research on post-exercise ketosis continues to confirm early findings (Passmore, 1958; Johnson, 1974; Koeslag, 1979), let's now fast forward to the new millennium. A protein found in the brain has become a focus of interest in the fight against Alzheimer's and other neurodegenerative diseases. Brain-derived neurotrophic factor (BDNF) is undergoing intense study due to the role it plays in the areas of the brain that are especially susceptible to degeneration in Alzheimer's disease, the hippocampus and dentate gyrus, part of the hippocampus that helps form new memories. BDNF has widespread functions throughout the brain, such as promoting the growth and survival of neurons and strengthening of synapses (Blurton-Jones, 2009). Synapses, you may recall, are the connections between neurons in the brain that are so important to learning and the formation of memories. Therefore, BDNF is important to normal cognitive functioning. Levels of BDNF are reduced in the brains of people with Alzheimer's. When levels of BDNF are below normal, neurons are more susceptible to damage and degeneration.

Within just the past few years, researchers have learned that BDNF increases in the brain in response to learning and exercise. This increase in BDNF appears to be the mechanism by which learning and exercise improve cognitive function and stave off memory decline in the hippocampus (Vaynman, 2004; Yamada, 2002).

But what substance specifically stimulates the brain to make BDNF when we exercise? Is it possible that the increase in ketones related to exercise stimulates the brain to make BDNF? The answer to this question is not known for certain at this time.

Diabetic Ketoacidosis

When doctors worry about the possible dangers of raising ketone levels, they are thinking about diabetic ketoacidosis. When a person with type 1 diabetes does not have an adequate supply of insulin to allow sugar to enter the cells, and blood glucose levels become extremely high, the person may develop a condition called diabetic ketoacidosis and may even go into a coma. Among other metabolic events, large amounts of ketones are suddenly released into the circulation. The levels of ketones become dangerously high, as much as five to ten times higher than in the situation of starvation or on a classic ketogenic diet. If the person is not given insulin in short order, this condition may be fatal. Diabetic ketoacidosis is a common presentation for children and adults signaling the beginning of type 1 diabetes.

The levels of ketones from consuming very large amounts of medium-chain fatty acids would never remotely come close to reaching the levels of diabetic ketoacidosis. The levels of ketones are fifty times higher in diabetic ketoacidosis than after consuming a large quantity (20 grams) of MCT oil (see Table 16.1).

TABLE 16.1. COMPARISON OF BETA-HYDROXYBUTYRATE LEVELS UNDER VARIOUS CONDITIONS

CONDITION	BETA-HYDROXYBUTYRATE (MMOL/LITER)
Exercise[1]	0.25
Coconut oil and/or MCT oil[2]	0.25 to 0.5
Classic ketogenic diet[3]	2 to 5
Starvation[4]	2 to 7
Beta-OH Butyrate Ester[5]	2 to 7 (proposed levels)
Diabetic ketoacidosis[6]	25

Sources:

1. Levels of ketones after running for 90 minutes (Koeslag, 1979).

2. Levels of ketones based on Accera Studies (Henderson, 2009) and levels at NIH (Tables 6.1 and 6.2).

3. Levels of ketones on a classic ketogenic diet (Gilbert, 2000).

4. Levels increase between two and ten days' duration of starvation (Owens, 2005).

5. Proposed levels (Veech, 2001).

6. Levels can reach as high as 25 mmol/l (Veech, 2001).

17

The Discovery of Ketones and the Ketogenic Diet

One of the earliest scientific articles about ketones appeared in the German literature in 1865 by J. Gerhardt. This article discusses the discovery of ketones in the urine of people with diabetes. Thirty years later, another German article discussed the presence of an abundance of ketones in the urine of people who were in diabetic coma (Hirschfield, 1895). For many years thereafter, ketones were simply thought to be abnormal byproducts of disease, such as diabetes. Even today, many doctors think of diabetic ketoacidosis when they first hear about the discussion of ketones and Alzheimer's disease. They worry that their patients might become acidotic if they consume medium-chain fatty acids. This is simply not true (see section on Diabetic Ketoacidosis in Chapter 16).

ORIGIN OF THE KETOGENIC DIET

The story of the effect of ketones in treating disease actually begins much earlier. There are historical references to fasting as a successful treatment for epilepsy and seizures in the Bible and again in the literature of the Middle Ages. In 1921, a pediatrician, Rawle Geyelin, M.D., reported at an American Medical Association convention successful treatment of three patients with epilepsy by an osteopath, Hugh Conklin, D.O. One of these patients was a ten-year-old boy with severe epilepsy who endured two very long periods of fasting, after which he had no seizures for the next year. Dr. Geyelin also reported that eighteen of twenty-six patients he treated showed marked improvement, and two were seizure-free for more than a year. He found that a twenty-day fast appeared to have the best results. Drs. Geyelin and Conklin did not know at that point that starvation produces high levels of ketones, and that these high levels of ketones were almost certainly responsible for the reduction of seizures in their patients.

Use of Ketogenic Diet as a Treatment for Disease

Also in 1921, R. M. Wilder, M.D., reported in a brief article in the *Mayo Clinic Bulletin,* "The Effects of Ketonemia on the Course of Epilepsy," that the ketone bodies acetone, acetoacetate, and beta-hydroxybutyric acid appear not only in the urine of people in diabetic ketoacidosis, but also in the urine of normal people who are starving. Not only that, but ketones appear in the urine of people who consume "a diet that contains too low a proportion of carbohydrate and too high a proportion of fat." Thus, the classic "ketogenic diet" as a treatment for disease was born about ninety years ago.

In the classic ketogenic diet, about 80 percent of calories come from fat and the other 20 percent from protein and carbohydrate combined. Protein is limited because it can be converted in the liver to carbohydrate—when carbohydrate stores have been used up—by a process mentioned earlier called gluconeogenesis. At the same time, it is necessary to provide enough protein to prevent the breakdown of muscle and other tissues in the body, the so-called lean body mass. For children on a ketogenic diet to reduce epileptic seizures, protein is strictly calculated to allow for preservation of muscle and adequate growth. A ketogenic diet is not an easy one for most people to follow for the long haul, due to the small amount of carbohydrate allowed and the requirement to measure accurately every morsel of food eaten. But adhering to the classic ketogenic diet has a distinct advantage: it produces levels of ketone bodies considerably higher, in some cases ten times or more, than levels produced by ingesting oils with medium-chain fatty acids.

A review of the literature shows that, from the 1920s to 1960s, considerable research investigated the ketogenic diet and epilepsy. Other researchers studied the production of ketones during starvation in various groups of people and for various lengths of time. Better methods were developed for measuring ketones, and many of the details were worked out regarding how ketones are made and how they are broken down in the body. Lab animals were used in many cases to discover these details, and then these studies were duplicated in humans to confirm their findings. Some of the men who worked out these details in the 1960s are still actively involved in the study of ketones today: Drs. George Cahill, Sami Hashim, Oliver Owens, Theodore VanItallie, and Richard Veech. (There will be more about these physicians and their work in Chapter 19.)

The ketogenic diet as a treatment was largely put on the back burner for many years in the middle of the twentieth century, as various anti-seizure medications came into widespread use. The ketogenic diet was a topic of discussion during my own medical school and pediatric training and was used on occasion at that time for children with the most relentless forms of epilepsy. Little did I know at that time the role ketones would play in our own lives several decades later.

POPULARIZING THE KETOGENIC DIET

In the early 1990s, Jim Abrahams, a Hollywood director, came upon the ketogenic diet in the course of his own research as a potential treatment for his twenty-month-old son, who had severe epilepsy. Little Charlie endured as many as 100 seizures a day, in spite of treatment with strong anticonvulsants that resulted in heavy sedation. He did not even improve with brain surgery. The family decided to undertake the diet in spite of resistance from five pediatric neurologists Charlie had seen. Within days, the seizures stopped completely. Abrahams was angry that doctors had not made his family aware of the ketogenic diet. He soon learned that Charlie was just one of hundreds of thousands of children treated for epilepsy every year who did not have access to the ketogenic diet as a treatment due to lack of awareness of this option. He made it his mission to inform parents of other children with the disease and to educate doctors, hospitals, dieticians, and nurses, as well as promote research into the ketogenic diet.

In 1994, Abrahams founded The Charlie Foundation for this purpose (www.charliefoundation.org) and has had considerable success in achieving these goals. In 1992, he made a movie starring Meryl Streep, *First Do No Harm,* about a family dealing with severe epilepsy and their discovery of the ketogenic diet as a treatment for their son. In 2004, *Dateline NBC* aired two segments, and in 2008 a follow-up story about Charlie and the ketogenic diet greatly increased awareness and stimulated research. The first major international symposium covering the ketogenic diet took place in April 2008, and the related articles were published in a special edition of the medical journal *Epilepsia* in October 2008. The next symposium took place in October 2010 in Edinburgh, Scotland.

It is important to note that children with epilepsy who are on a strict ketogenic diet can greatly reduce the frequency of seizures and even become seizure-free over time, but it requires extremely rigid adherence to the diet. Very recently, the diet has been tried by older people, and some adults with epilepsy benefit significantly from the ketogenic diet as well. However, not everyone with epilepsy responds dramatically to the diet, but many have a considerable reduction in seizures, by half or more.

People with Alzheimer's disease, Parkinson's, and other neurodegenerative diseases who do not see improvement by consuming oils with medium-chain fatty acids should consider going all the way with the ketogenic diet. Conversely, modification of the ketogenic diet to include medium-chain fatty acids may allow for a slightly less-restrictive diet and assurance that some ketone production will go on, even if there is a slip-up in how much carbohydrate is consumed. Some research has shown that this type of modification might allow for more carbohydrate in the overall diet, which may be easier for some families (Huttenlocher, 1971).

Two Popular Forms of the Ketogenic Diet

The Atkins diet is one popular version of the ketogenic diet used for several decades. With Atkins, the primary focus is on reducing carbohydrates, but protein and fat can be eaten in unlimited quantity. There is a two-week induction period in which carbohydrates are limited to 20 grams per day; thereafter, carbohydrates are increased by 5 grams per week until weight loss stalls, then it is stepped back to the previous level. Considerable water is lost from muscle initially, which is very encouraging on the scale, but it does not represent true loss of fat, which is the desired goal. With restriction of carbohydrates, ketones are produced, since the body is forced to break down fat for fuel. With unlimited protein, however, it is conceivable that, for people who consume large quantities of it, not much ketosis may be going on, since the body can also convert protein to carbohydrate.

The South Beach diet is very similar to Atkins except there is more emphasis on eating "good" carbohydrates—foods with a low-glycemic index that do not cause the sudden spike in glucose followed by a spike in insulin levels that are characteristic of "bad" carbohydrates.

18

Medium-Chain Triglycerides and Ketones

The terms medium-chain fatty acids and medium-chain triglycerides are somewhat interchangeable. In fats and oils, such as coconut oil and medium-chain triglyceride oil, three molecules of a particular fatty acid join together with a glycerol molecule to form a triglyceride. Thus, medium-chain fatty acids join together with glycerol to form medium-chain triglycerides. Medium-chain triglyceride oil, also called MCT oil, is usually a combination of several different types of medium-chain triglycerides. The medium-chain triglycerides found in MCT oil are usually derived from coconut or palm kernel oil.

MEDIUM-CHAIN TRIGLYCERIDES AND KETONES

The fact that medium-chain triglycerides are metabolized to ketones in the liver is not new information. When I read this in the Accera patent application, I recalled learning this in my medical school biochemistry class in 1974.

In 1906, scientists G. Embden and F. Kalberlah reported that when caprylic acid, one of the medium-chain fatty acids, was pumped through the circulation of dog liver there was a prompt increase in the liver's output of acetoacetate, one of the ketone bodies. In 1959, H. Schön and others fed medium-chain triglycerides (C:8 through C:12) to a group of people and found an increase in blood and urine levels of ketones; they also found that this did not occur when they were given long-chain fatty acids.

In 1966, Dr. Theodore VanItallie and his associates, Dr. Sami Hashim and Dr. S. Bergen Jr., confirmed these findings and expanded upon this research. They gave 100 milliliters (more than 3 ounces!) of either MCT oil or corn oil, along with some casein (a milk protein) and dextrose (a sugar), to twenty patients, six of whom had diabetes. Some of the people received both types of oil at least two days apart. All the people had a significant rise in their ketone levels after consuming the MCT oil, the diabetics on average slightly higher than the nondiabetics. After consuming the corn oil, there was a relatively negligible increase in ketones. The increase in ketones occurred even though the people also received glucose and protein. These researchers published several other studies in which they reported that:

- Medium-chain triglycerides are absorbed directly from the intestine without the need for digestive enzymes, which are required for the longer-chain fatty acids.

- Medium-chain triglycerides are transported directly to the liver by way of the portal vein.

- Part of medium-chain triglycerides are converted to ketone bodies in the liver.

Dr. Hashim and his associates continued to study the use of medium-chain triglycerides in the pediatric population into the 1970s and beyond. They confirmed that medium-chain triglycerides are absorbed very easily, even in the premature newborn (Tantibhedhyangkul, 1971 and 1975). They studied the addition of various percentages of MCT oil to formulas, finding for example, that calcium was more readily absorbed from the intestine if the infant formula contained higher levels of MCT oil. Thus, by the time I began my pediatric residency in 1978, it was a new practice to add MCT oil to feedings of premature newborns to help them grow faster. Special formulas were developed for premature newborns that included MCT oil and coconut oil and/or palm kernel oil, which contain about 55 to 60 percent medium-chain fatty acids. Virtually every infant formula used in the United States today contains a large amount of MCT oil and coconut and/or palm kernel oil.

EARLY RESEARCH AND DEVELOPMENT WITH MCT OIL

The May 9, 2000, issue of *Proceedings of the National Academy of Sciences* included an article entitled "D-beta-hydroxybutyrate Protects Neurons in Models of Alzheimer's and Parkinson's Disease." This was the landmark report on ketone research from the National Institutes of Health laboratory of Dr. Richard Veech and his associates, Yoshiro Kashiyawa, Takao Takeshima, Nozomi Mori, Kenji Nakashima, and Kieran Clarke. (This report will be discussed in more detail later in this chapter.) One important statement in the opening summary of this paper is relevant to our current discussion: "The ability of ketones to protect neurons in culture suggests that defects in mitochondrial energy generation contribute to the pathophysiology of both brain diseases [Alzheimer's and Parkinson's]. These findings further suggest that ketone bodies may play a therapeutic role in these most common forms of human neurodegeneration." I don't know if this article led to what happened next or if the timing is just a pure coincidence.

On May 1, 2000, a U.S. patent application was filed by Samuel T. Henderson, Ph.D., of Broomfield, Colorado, entitled "Use of Medium-Chain Triglycerides for the Treatment and Prevention of Alzheimer's Disease and Other Diseases Resulting from Reduced Neuronal Metabolism" (discussed in Chapter 4). This application has been revised and continued since 2000. Dr. Henderson had the brilliant insight to consider the possibility that the relatively mild ketosis that occurs after consuming MCT oil would be sufficient to bring about improvement in people with Alzheimer's disease, as well as other neurodegenerative diseases. This is a profound discovery that had very important ramifications eleven years later for Steve, and now for many others as well.

Dr. Henderson put two and two together and acted on it. He personally experienced the nightmare that is Alzheimer's, losing a close family member to the disease, and he wanted to do something about it. He and his associates formed a company called Accera in 2001 where they developed a food product, initially called AC-1202, in which the active ingredient is the medium-chain triglyceride known as caprylic triglyceride, also called C:8. They determined a dose of C:8 that most people could tolerate and that would also be sufficient to increase ketone body levels significantly, aiming for a level of about 0.5 millimoles per liter (mmol/l) of beta-hydroxybutyrate.

First Study with MCT Oil in People with Mild to Moderate Alzheimer's

The Accera company decided to seek Food and Drug Administration approval for their product and conducted clinical trials. One of the trials tested for tolerance of different versions of the product in normal healthy people. Other studies evaluated the effectiveness of the product in people with mild cognitive impairment and Alzheimer's disease. Several research centers in our area of Florida were involved in these clinical trials. The product AC-1202 was given a name, initially Ketasyn, which was later changed to Axona.

The results of Accera's first study were published in 2004 in *Neurobiology of Aging* (Reger, 2004). The purpose of the study was to "explore whether hyperketonemia improves cognitive functioning in individuals with memory disorders." The researchers "tested the hypothesis that acute elevation of serum beta-hydroxy-butyrate levels through an oral dose of medium-chain triglycerides would improve memory and attention in individuals with AD or mild cognitive impairment." They included people who were considered to have mild to moderate impairment, with an average MMSE score of 22 out of a possible 30. They also looked at the differences between people with and without the ApoE4 gene; ApoE4+ is a known risk factor for Alzheimer's disease (discussed in Chapter 15). There appear to be some differences in how glucose is used by people based on whether they are positive or negative for this gene. Dr. Henderson and his group suggest that the ApoE4 gene may affect the way other substrates are handled in the body, including ketone bodies.

This first study included just twenty people, of whom nine were ApoE4+. Each person was studied on two different occasions, making it a crossover study in which the person serves as his or her own control. At one visit they received AC-1202, and for the other they did not. They were instructed not to eat from 8 P.M. the evening before the study. In the morning, blood was drawn and then they were given the mixture containing either MCT oil or the placebo. Ninety minutes later, blood was drawn again and they were given a series of four memory and attention tests over thirty minutes. They then had one more blood draw.

The results were quite impressive, at least for people who did not have the ApoE4 gene. The level of beta-hydroxybutyrate increased by an average of 7.7 times compared to the level before taking the MCT oil. The ApoE4- people had an average improvement of more than 6 points on the 78-point ADAS-COG memory test *on the day they received the MCT oil* compared to the placebo day. In another test called "paragraph recall," a trend showed that the ApoE- people with higher beta-hydroxybutyrate levels had the most improved scores. The two other tests showed no apparent effect of the treatment. As a group, the people who were ApoE4+ actually showed slight worsening on the ADAS-COG test.

In their conclusions, the researchers stated: "The rapid improvement in some areas of cognitive functioning suggests that ketones may function as an alternative fuel for cerebral neurons in MCI [mild cognitive impairment] or AD patients. . . . Future studies may also confirm the differential treatment effects for ApoE4+ and ApoE4- subjects in a larger sample with several MCT doses. Additionally, the cognitive effects of long-term elevation of beta-hydroxybutyrate levels may support the feasibility and efficacy of MCT administration as a novel therapeutic strategy."

There's an interesting sidelight about this study. In order to conduct a valid study, the people receiving the treatment and the people administering the tests must not know whether the subject is receiving the active ingredient or the placebo. So the active ingredient must be disguised in such a way that one cannot tell the difference between the two doses. In this study, the MCT oil was blended with about 5 ounces of heavy whipping cream. For the placebo, an additional amount of cream was added instead of MCT oil. There is some irony in their use of this cream to disguise the MCT oil. According to the U.S. Department of Agriculture (USDA) National Nutrient Database, the amount of heavy whipping cream added to the MCT oil provided an additional 6 grams of short- and medium-chain fatty acids, so in the placebo, the people actually received about 10 grams of these ketone-producing fatty acids. Their results might have been even more impressive had they used something other than cream to disguise the MCT oil!

One of the most significant take-home points from this study is that some people with memory impairment improve after just one sizable dose of medium-chain triglycerides. Steve improved the very first day he consumed 35 grams (seven teaspoons) of coconut oil. He said that "the lightswitch came back on" and "the fog lifted." Steve is positive for the ApoE4 gene. So why did he respond when the folks like him in Dr. Henderson's study did not? The primary difference between their study and what happened to Steve is the type of oil used. The Accera study used just one type of medium-chain triglyceride, caprylic triglyceride. Coconut oil contains all the medium-chain fatty acids, as well as long-chain fatty acids. Perhaps another fatty acid was responsible for his improvement. In addition, when Steve's ketone levels were measured after he consumed MCT oil, his beta-hydroxybutyrate levels were higher than acetoacetate levels, but the reverse was true after consuming coconut oil. Perhaps the ketone body acetoacetate plays a more important role for people who are ApoE4+. Certain types of brain cells may prefer acetoacetate to beta-hydroxybutyrate, and perhaps these cells are more affected in people who are ApoE4+ like Steve. It has been suggested based on studies that acetoacetate may play a greater role than beta-hydroxybutyrate in controlling seizures using the ketogenic diet (Hartman, 2007).

There is yet another possibility. Given that medium-chain fatty acids are not stored as fat and can cross the blood/brain barrier, perhaps one or more of the other medium-chain fatty acids in coconut oil are taken into the mitochondria of various types of brain cells to produce this improvement. Further study of specific medium-chain fatty acids needs to be undertaken to learn more about exactly what happens to the portion of these fatty acids that is not converted to ketones.

In 2004, when the first Accera study was published, Steve had an MMSE of 23 and had just been diagnosed with dementia. His MRI scan was read as "normal" at that point in time; four years later, his MRI showed considerable shrinkage in his brain, classified as severe in the areas affected by Alzheimer's disease. I have wondered so many times what our life would be like now if the results of this study had caught the attention of the media.

Second and Larger Study in People with
Mild to Moderate Alzheimer's

The results of a second, larger study by Accera were first reported at a neurology meeting in 2007 (Constantini, 2007), but they did not appear in a journal in detail until more than a year after Steve's dramatic improvement from coconut oil (Henderson, 2009). This study was also described in the patent application for AC-1202 that I found on the Internet in May 2008, but it was not made available for the scientific community until more than a year later. There were 152 participants in this study with mild to moderate Alzheimer's disease, of which eighty-six people received AC-1202 and sixty-six received the placebo. This time the treatment was continued for ninety days, and both the placebo and the MCT oil were in a powdered form that the subject could reconstitute in a liquid drink. This time the subjects were given 20 grams of MCT oil, a reduction from the 40 grams used in the first study. One hundred-forty people completed enough of the study to have their data included in the final results. This time, once again, the people taking AC-1202 who were ApoE4- showed improvement on the ADAS-COG test as a group over the ninety days; the ApoE4+ people as a group followed the same path as people on the placebo, declining over that period of time. Neither group showed an improvement in MMSE scores.

I have subsequently learned from one of the authors of the report that nearly half of the ApoE4+ people did, in fact, improve on the ADAS-COG. However, when they were looked at as a group, there was no statistical improvement. It would be helpful for this information to be available in their report, since some physicians may not believe it worthwhile treating someone who is ApoE4+ with Axona, when it may very well be beneficial.

Doctors know very well that many people have trouble remembering to take their medications, which can obviously have an impact on the effectiveness of the treatment. The researchers were able to keep track of how compliant the subjects were, and there was a greater than 2-point difference in improvement in the people who were compliant compared to those who were not. Also, many of the people in the study had to reduce how much AC-1202 they were taking due to adverse effects. About one fourth developed diarrhea. The people who were able to tolerate a larger dose of AC-1202 showed greater improvement in their scores. Another interesting point was that, on average, the people who had higher beta-hydroxybutyrate levels had more improvement.

At the end of the ninety days, there was a two-week "washout" period. The people were taken off AC-1202 and tested again. Compared to where they started out, the people who were ApoE4- showed some worsening in their ADAS-COG scores, but were not quite back to where they were at the start of the study. The sad news here is that they were taken off the treatment. I suppose this was deemed necessary to demonstrate that MCT oil had, in fact, brought about the improvement.

Third Study with MCT Oil in People with Mild Cognitive Impairment

The Accera group performed another study of 159 people, this time with mild cognitive impairment, which often leads to Alzheimer's disease (Costantini, 2009). Once again, the people receiving Axona showed improvement in response to the treatment, particularly those who were APOE4-.

Study with MCT Oil and Diabetes

In 2009, Kathleen Page, M.D., at Yale University School of Medicine and others published a study in which they administered MCT oil to people with "intensively treated" type 1 diabetes who were also prone to severe hypoglycemic (low blood sugar) attacks. Ten of the eleven people they studied were using a pump that continuously administers insulin under the skin; the eleventh person required multiple shots of insulin each day. Most of the people had between six and thirty episodes of hypoglycemia per month. The researchers deliberately caused hypoglycemic attacks in the subjects. Some of the people received MCT oil, the others placebo. Nine of the people were studied twice. On one day they received MCT oil (40 grams) and on another day the placebo, effectively serving as their own control.

The people who administered the battery of cognitive tests did not know whether the subjects received MCT oil or placebo. They also measured plasma, glucose, insulin, fatty acids, and ketone levels (beta-hydroxybutyrate). The ketone levels increased to an average of 0.35 mmol/l. When compared to the placebo, the researchers reported, "MCT prevented the decline in cognitive performance during hypoglycemia" in five of the seven tests administered. Their findings "suggest that MCT could be used as prophylactic [preventive] therapy for such patients with the goal of preserving brain function during hypoglycemic episodes. . . ."

In summary, studies have shown that consumption of MCT oils can bring about cognitive improvement in people with memory impairment and protect cognitive function in diabetic people who experience severe hypoglycemic episodes. Presumably, these effects occur because ketones and possibly medium-chain fatty acids are available to the brain as an alternative fuel to glucose.

A COLLECTION OF SUPPORTING EVIDENCE

In January 2011, Stephen Cunnane, Ph.D., and collaborators published a review in *Nutrition* entitled "Brain Fuel Metabolism, Aging, and Alzheimer's Disease," detailing what is currently known about the connection between the deterioration of the process of glucose metabolism in the brain and the development of Alzheimer's disease, as well as the role ketones could play in the prevention and treatment of Alzheimer's disease (Cunnane, 2011). This review cites 217 research articles to support the concepts they present. The scientists state that to the best of their knowledge: "Hypometabolism [decreased uptake of glucose] is currently the earliest measurable abnormality in the brain that is connected to Alzheimer's disease so its features and the reasons for it should shed light on the etiology of Alzheimer's." They point to PET scan studies showing small areas of lower brain glucose metabolism in people as young as thirty years old who are ApoE4+ and similar findings in the offspring of people with Alzheimer's decades before symptoms occur.

Cunnane and his colleagues say that ketone metabolism is an important feature of brain function, as evidenced by two observations: "(1) The amounts and activities of ketone-metabolizing enzymes in the brain are not changed by glucose status and always exceed the amount necessary to supply the brain's total energy needs; and (2) during infancy the brain appears to have an obligatory requirement for ketones." Therefore "the brain is always prepared to burn ketones." On the other hand, they explain why glucose is still essential for the brain and why ketones cannot completely replace glucose as a fuel. They discuss the Henderson and Page studies, demonstrating that mild elevation of ketone levels can maintain normal brain function even when blood glucose levels are low enough to cause deficits.

The researchers have learned from PET scans and other types of studies that use of ketones by the brain does not appear to be affected by aging or by Alzheimer's disease, but is lower in diabetes mellitus. They have also discovered that the plasma concentration of ketones is directly proportional to the percent of energy supplied by ketones to the brain. Thus a ketone level of 0.4 to 0.5 mmol/l, which can be achieved by taking medium-chain fatty acids, can provide 5 to 10 percent of the brain's energy needs. This is equivalent to the deficit in energy provided to the brain by glucose in people who are genetically at risk for Alzheimer's.

In other words, regular consumption of coconut oil and/or MCT oil could potentially provide a nutritional prevention strategy to decrease the risk of developing Alzheimer's, or at least delay onset of the disease. The ketone ester, which can raise ketone levels to 5 mmol/l or even higher, could provide as much as 60 percent of the energy requirement of the brain, potentially halting or even reversing the process of Alzheimer's disease.

Therapeutic Implications of the Ketone Ester

One of the earliest studies looking at the effects of ketones, entitled "The Metabolism of Bovine Epididymal Spermatozoa," was published in the *Archives of Biochemistry* in 1945 by H. A. Lardy, R. G. Hansen, and P. H. Phillips. They looked at the effects of sixteen different substances that might be used as fuel by cow sperm, including various sugars, lipids, and other metabolites. They found that the ketone bodies beta-hydroxybutyrate and acetoacetate were unique among these sixteen substances in that they increased the motility of the sperm while at the same time reducing the amount of oxygen consumed to accomplish this. Fifty years later, Dr. Richard Veech and his associates at the NIH were able to work out how this happens.

"WHAT A RIDE!"

After Dr. Veech received his degree in medicine and completed a one-year research fellowship at Harvard University, he had a two-year research fellowship at the NIH. In 1966, he went to Oxford University to work in the lab of the Nobel Prize–winning physician and biochemist/researcher Hans Krebs of "Krebs cycle" fame. For more than three years, he honed his skills there as a biochemist, working out details of certain chemical reactions that occur within mitochondria, among other things. Dr. Veech has told me that this work is so complex that most humans cannot begin to understand it. After Dr. Veech left Oxford, Dr. Krebs visited his lab at the NIH to review past studies and future projects every year until he died in 1981.

In a paper written by Dr. Veech in 2006 for the "Mini Series: Paths to Discovery" in *Biochemistry and Molecular Biology Education,* he relates how he came to study the effects of ketones:

> By the mid-1980s, review processes at NIH became more bureaucratized and centralized by NIH administrators along the lines of the 'peer-reviewed' process in which 'experts,' usually grantees of the institute under review, reviewed the intramural NIH laboratories. The work of our lab went from being a "national treasure" to a "waste of money," depending upon the eye of the beholder. By 1991, the work of the laboratory at NIH was judged to be inadequate, and I was notified that the laboratory would be shut down in two years' time. I decided that I would spend the last available two years studying a subject that I thought would be important and to take no notice whatever of programmatic goals set by administrators without actual laboratory experience. To their great credit, the laboratory members, who were all to be terminated at the end of this period, accepted my explanation that this was a "Birkenhead drill" [defined as "courage in the face of hopeless circumstances"] and stayed at their posts, completing the work outlined during the remaining two years.
>
> The problem chosen was to determine the effects of changes caused by the ketone bodies (beta-hydroxybutyrate and acetoacetate), insulin, and their combination on the working perfused rat heart.

Dr. Veech and his associates proceeded to study ketone bodies intensely to learn more about what they do. The first article about their study of ketones, "Control of Glucose Utilization in Working Perfused Rat Heart," appeared in the October 14, 1994, issue of the *Journal of Biological Chemistry.* Glucose was the focus of this very complex study, specifically how the enzymes involved in glucose metabolism in the working rat heart are affected by various substrates, one of which was the addition of ketone.

The second paper, entitled "Insulin, Ketone Bodies, and Mitochondrial Energy Transduction," was published in the *FASEB Journal* in May 1995. The study involved perfusing working rat hearts with a solution containing glucose. To this solution they added insulin, or the ketones beta-hydroxybutyrate and acetoacetate, or a combination of insulin and the ketone-body mixture. The ketone levels were consistent with those that occur during starvation. They found that the addition of either insulin or ketone bodies increased the efficiency of the hearts by about 25 percent, and the combination of insulin and ketone bodies increased the efficiency by about 36 percent. *The hearts pumped harder using less oxygen.* They learned that ketone bodies were able to duplicate nearly all the acute effects of insulin.

Understanding the Metabolic Effects of Ketones

The effects of insulin or ketones on the ability of the heart to work more efficiently is the result of increased production within the mitochondria of acetyl-CoA, the coenzyme from which the energy molecule ATP is made. This increased production of acetyl-CoA results in the generation of more ATP. The researchers were able to work out the biochemical details of exactly how this occurs. Ketones actually cause a sixteenfold increase in the production of acetyl CoA, similar to the effect of insulin. These findings indicate that during starvation, when glucose is not readily available and insulin levels are low, ketones can substitute for both glucose and insulin to ensure that cells continue to survive and function normally.

Ketones do not require insulin to enter the cell. Instead, ketones require a monocarboxylate transporter to cross the cell membrane. Ketones bypass several steps in the process normally used by glucose to enter the mitochondria and start the process of making acetyl-CoA and eventually ATP. This is particularly important in the brain, since insulin cannot cross the blood/brain barrier. For example, in the brains of people with Alzheimer's, which have become deficient in insulin and resistant to insulin, ketones can provide an alternative source of fuel. Ketones can also carry out many of the effects that are carried out by insulin in the normal, healthy brain. Ketones can even stimulate the production of glycogen, the stored form of glucose, a function normally provided by insulin.

Dr. Veech learned that by increasing the efficiency of ATP, ketones have the added benefit of increasing the efficiency of how cells use sodium, potassium, and calcium, the three major electrolytes in our bodies. These electrolytes are very important to the transport of substances into and out of the cell. Sodium, potassium, and calcium must be maintained within very specific ranges both inside and outside the cell, or there will be dire consequences. For example, when a brain cell is injured, let's say by trauma to the head, potassium leaks out of the cell and too much sodium and calcium enter the cell. This causes the cell to swell and lose its ability to function normally. Ketones prevent or correct this problem of electrolyte imbalance by increasing ATP. Thus, injuries to the brain by direct trauma or lack of oxygen could be treated by administering ketones.

One can envision that an intravenous solution containing ketones could be given immediately to an injured soldier, an accident victim, or a newborn who has suffered a lack of oxygen during delivery to reduce damage to the brain and other organs. (Successful studies of this will be discussed later in the chapter.) Dr. Veech has proposed in one of his ketone hypothesis papers from 2003 (discussed later) that the ketogenic diet might reduce seizures in people with epilepsy through the effect of ketones on ATP and the major electrolytes.

Dr. Veech has also found that ketones are able to reduce

the amount of damage from free radicals within the tiny energy-generating mitochondria by their action on coenzyme Q_{10} (also called CoQ_{10}). Coenzyme Q_{10} is another important coenzyme required for making ATP and also acts as an antioxidant. Ketones can also decrease damage to the cell by reducing the amount of hydrogen peroxide in the cytoplasm (the fluid within the cell). The antioxidants in fruits and vegetables that we hear so much about are other examples of substances that can reduce damage from oxygen free radicals.

In the discussion section of his 1995 paper, Dr. Veech states: "Provision of acetyl moieties within mitochondria has been suggested to reverse many age-related defects in mitochondrial ATP synthesis. Use of ketones may therefore provide unexpected benefits in the treatment of elderly patients or others suffering from oxidative damage to mitochondria." He also states in the abstract summary: ". . . the moderate ketosis characteristic of prolonged fasting or type 2 diabetes appears to be an elegant compensation for the defects in mitochondrial energy transduction associated with acute insulin deficiency or mitochondrial senescence." Simply put, raising the levels of ketones could be beneficial to people with diseases that involve a problem with damaged or aging mitochondria.

Developing the First Ketone Ester

By the time this work was published in 1995, Dr. Veech states in his 2006 paper:

> My lab had been closed, and its workers and techniques had been dispersed. As an over-age civil servant, I could not be "fired" but had no other visible means of support. I used this sabbatical in the closet to reflect on the implications of our findings on the remarkable effects of ketone bodies on mitochondrial redox potentials. Ketosis, resulting from either prolonged fasting or feeding a high fat, low-carbohydrate diet, has been used to treat refractory

epilepsy for over 100 years. An in-depth understanding of the bio-chemical details of the mechanism of action of ketone metabolism led to other and more widespread potential applications. What emerged from a detailed biochemical analysis of the effects of ketone metabolism was a surprising array of disease phenotypes, including specific rare monogenetic diseases and common polygenic diseases that might be benefited by mild ketosis. . . . Fortunately for my research, other sources of non-traditional funding became available that allowed us the chance to determine whether our hypotheses about the therapeutic benefit of alteration in metabolic substrates in a number of disease phenotypes were true. If these hypotheses prove to be correct, it will be ironic that the funding was provided by the Department of Defense, not the Department of Health and Human Services. Little did I know in 1966, when Krebs assigned me the task of determining the redox state of the NADP (nicotinamide adenine dinucelotide phosphate) system, that I would still be working on the problem forty years later. What a ride!

Thus, interest in his work with ketones and subsequent funding on the part of the Department of Defense allowed Dr. Veech to continue this research in his laboratory at the NIH.

In 1997, Dr. Veech, Dr. Yoshihiro Kashiwaya, and Todd King published another paper in the *American Journal of Cardiology,* further elaborating on the effects of ketones and their similarity to the actions of insulin in their effects on the working rat heart. In the summary, he states, "The ability of a physiologic ratio of ketones bodies to correct most of the metabolic defects of acute insulin deficiency suggests therapeutic roles for these natural sub-strates during periods of impaired cardiac performance and in insulin-resistant states."

The week before the paper was published, Dr. Veech filed a patent application simply entitled "Therapeutic Compositions" that enabled him to produce a form of the naturally occurring ketone body beta-hydroxybutyrate. The patent application has been regularly updated since then. The opening summary states:

Compositions comprising ketone bodies and/or their metabolic precursors are provided that are suitable for administration to humans and animals and which have the properties of, *inter alia,* (i) increasing cardiac efficiency, particularly efficiency in use of glucose; (ii) for providing energy source, particularly in diabetes and insulin-resistant states; and (iii) treating disorders caused by damage to brain cells, particularly by retarding or preventing brain damage in memory associated brain areas such as found in Alzheimer's disease and similar conditions. These compositions may be taken as nutritional aids, for example by athletes, or for the treatment of medical conditions, particularly those associated with poor cardiac efficiency, insulin resistance and neuronal damage. The invention further provides methods of treatment and novel esters and polymers for inclusion in the composition of the invention.

For many conditions, this ketone ester could be taken as a food that is capable of achieving levels of ketones that occur during starvation and on the classic ketogenic diet. At such levels, the ketone ester should be well tolerated and not result in untoward complications. In addition, the compound could be given intravenously to people with traumatic brain injury or who lack oxygen and who would not be able to take the substance by mouth.

While developing the ketone ester, Dr. Veech has continued to research the effects of ketones. As a result of his findings on the heart, it occurred to Dr. Veech that ketones might protect neurons in Parkinson's and Alzheimer's diseases. To prove this hypothesis, neurons were taken from the areas of the brain associated with both diseases and grown separately in culture. The cells were subjected to a substance known to cause these diseases. The ketone body beta-hydroxybutyrate was added to some of the cell cultures at levels found during starvation. The researchers found that *addition of the ketones significantly increased the survival of the neurons.* In addition, researchers found that the size of the cells was larger and had a greater outgrowth of neurites (axons and dendrites that connect neurons with other cells), suggesting that ketones can act as growth factors to neurons in culture.

Therefore, not only do ketones protect the neurons by providing more energy within the mitochondria, but they also appear to increase the growth and development of neurons. In the conclusion of his report on this study, "D-Beta-Hydroxybutyrate Protects Neurons in Models of Alzheimer's and Parkinson's Disease," published in the May 9, 2000, issue of the *Proceedings of the National Academy of Sciences,* Dr. Veech states:

> . . . elevation of ketones may offer neuroprotection in the treatment or prevention of both Alzheimer's disease, where therapy is lacking, and Parkinson's disease where therapy with L-dopa is time limited. The high-fat diet used in childhood epilepsy may not be suitable because of its atherogenic [arterial plaque-forming] potential; however, alternative dietary sources of ketones produced biotechnologically may overcome this difficulty and provide benefit without the undesirable effects of current ketogenic diets.

Dr. Veech's three important papers regarding the potential use of ketones to treat and prevent disease followed in 2001 and 2003.

- The first paper, entitled "Ketone Bodies, Potential Therapeutic Uses," appeared in the *International Union of Biochemistry and Molecular Biology (IUBMB) Life* in 2001 and was co-authored with Britton Chance, Yoshihiro Kashiwaya, Henry A. Lardy, and George F. Cahill Jr., the physician who discovered that neurons can use ketones as an alternative fuel to glucose.

- A second paper entitled "Ketoacids? Good Medicine?" was published in 2003 following a presentation by Dr. Cahill for the American Clinical and Climatological Association, and was co-written by Dr. Veech. This paper emphasized the importance of ketones in the evolution of humans with our large brain relative to other creatures.

- A third paper published in 2004, "The Therapeutic Implications of Ketone Bodies: The Effects of Ketone Bodies in Pathological Conditions," written solely by Dr. Veech for *Prostaglandins, Leukotrienes and Essential Fatty Acids,* explains the metabolic effects of ketones in exquisite detail: how ketones function as a fuel in the cell and in mitochondria and how they actually provide a more potent fuel than glucose; how ketones replace insulin during starvation, carrying out the same effects but in a more primitive way; and how ketones reduce oxygen free radical damage.

Supportive Research from Colleagues

Another important paper, "Ketones: Metabolism's Ugly Duckling," mentioned in Chapter 16, which appeared in the October 2003 *Nutrition Reviews,* was written by Dr. Theodore VanItallie, longtime colleague of Dr. Veech, along with Thomas H. Nufert. Dr. VanItallie was involved in the early work with medium-chain triglycerides, confirming that these fatty acids are partly converted in the liver to ketones. He also found that the classic ketogenic diet appears to be beneficial to people with Parkinson's disease. The article provides an elegant discussion of how ketones work, along with the basis for treatment with ketones of certain neurodegenerative diseases, with an emphasis on Alzheimer's and Parkinson's diseases.

One of the most exciting studies I have read about potential reversal of neurodegenerative disease by ketones was published in April 2003 in the *Lancet* entitled "D, L-3-Hydroxybutyrate Treatment of Multiple Acyl-Coa Dehydrogenase Deficiency." Johan Van Hove, M.D, Ph.D., and his associates reported successful treatment of three young children with a sodium salt of the ketone body beta-hydroxybutyrate. The three children each had a very rare enzyme defect called multiple acyl-CoA dehydrogenase deficiency (MADD).

People with this defect are unable to use fat to produce energy once they have used up their stores of glucose. One of the three was paralyzed and near death at two years of age and had a nearly complete reversal to walking and talking nineteen months after beginning treatment with ketones. Similar improvements occurred in the other two children who were treated with the ketone compound. This study provided important evidence that ketones can be used to treat a life-threatening disease and even reverse the effects of this disease without side effects. It is important to note that while some improvements occurred during the first days, other improvements occurred over many months. Another exciting point is that the levels of ketones reached in this study are relatively low—0.3 millemoles per liter (mmol/l)—similar to the levels we measured in Steve after consuming coconut oil and MCT oil.

Multiple Purposes of the Ketone Ester

In summary, as stated in Dr. Veech's patent application to make the ketone ester (World Intellectual Property Organization/1998/041200), ketones could be used to treat disease by:

- Acting as a substitute for insulin in conditions such as insulin deficiency and insulin deficiency, where the normal insulin signaling path is disordered. (Alzheimer's, also called diabetes type 3, is one disease process that would benefit from such treatment.)

- Bypassing the block in the use of glucose by the brain that occurs in Alzheimer's disease and many other conditions and providing an alternative source of energy to the brain, thereby preventing cell death. (This slows the progress of memory loss and dementia.)

- Increasing energy production in certain types of heart failure in which part of the problem is the inability of heart muscle cells to produce enough energy to function normally. (Ketones have been found to increase the efficiency of the heart by 25 percent, while reducing the amount of oxygen required in the process.)

- Increasing the supply of acetylcholine in the brain of people with Alzheimer's by increasing acetyl-CoA in the mitochondria. (Drugs such as Aricept and Exelon work to increase acetylcholine by blocking the enzymes that break it down rather than increasing the amount of acetylcholine made by the brain.)

- Increasing blood flow to the brain.

- Decreasing cerebral edema (swelling in the brain) and improving brain function after lack of oxygen, injury to the brain, or lack of blood flow to an area of the brain.

- Increasing cell survival, improving cell function, and encouraging growth of new cells and connections between cells.

- Stimulating the production of nerve growth factors and other substances that may result in the growth of neurons and nerves and also improve how well they function.

Dr. Veech also suggests that the ketone ester could be started as soon as a predisposition to Alzheimer's disease is determined, such as when a person is found to have a gene mutation known to carry a high risk of Alzheimer's.

DISEASE PROCESSES THAT COULD BENEFIT FROM ELEVATION OF KETONES WITH THE KETONE ESTER

Because of their properties, ketones could be used to treat a number of diseases in addition to Alzheimer's.

Alzheimer's Disease

Currently, an estimated 5.3 million people in the United States suffer from Alzheimer's disease at a cost of $148 billion per year. Treatments with medications that increase certain brain chemicals do not cure the disease but appear to slow its progress. Billions of dollars have been invested worldwide to learn the exact cause of this disease, with the expectation of finding a cure, but the answer has eluded researchers. Unless a means of preventing and treating this disease becomes available, as the Baby Boomers age, a projected 15 million people in the United States will have this horrific disease by the year 2050. The ketone ester of beta-hydroxybutyrate could be the light at the end of the tunnel.

In summary, a major hallmark of Alzheimer's disease is progressive insulin deficiency and insulin resistance in the brain. Ketones can be used by all brain cells as an alternative fuel to glucose and therefore could allow insulin-resistant brain cells to function more normally and survive. Ketones actually bypass several of the steps needed to use glucose as a fuel, entering directly into the chemical chain of events that leads to making acetyl-CoA and then ATP. In addition, ketones have many of the same effects as insulin in the brain. Ketones can provide fuel to the mitochondria, which then increase the production of the various metabolites needed to make ATP. In addition, ketone bodies can reduce damage to the mitochondria from free radicals.

It is possible, with the introduction of ketones in the body, that some repair and reversal could occur in Alzheimer's disease, since ketone bodies were shown in Dr. Veech's 2000 *PNAS* paper to increase the neurite outgrowths in hippocampal cells exposed to ketones. It seems likely that ketones can stimulate the growth and survival of neurons as well as the extensions from neurons (axons and dendrites), thereby increasing the connections between brain cells (synapses). The decrease in synaptic density is likely the primary pathological defect in Alzheimer's disease.

The ester of the ketone body beta-hydroxybutyrate, if used by people who are at risk, could potentially prevent Alzheimer's disease.

In addition, for people who already have the disease, this ketone ester could potentially halt the progress of the disease and perhaps even reverse some of the damage that has already occurred. Like insulin for the person with type 1 diabetes, the ketone ester could provide an effective treatment—a cure—for Alzheimer's disease.

Other Dementias

The patent application for the ketone ester lists a number of other less common and rare dementias that could potentially respond to treatment with ketone bodies, including:

- Bovine spongiform encephalopathy (BSE, or "mad cow disease")
- Corticobasal degeneration
- Creutzfeldt-Jakob Disease (CJD)
- Dementia associated with Pick's disease
- Dementia of Parkinson's with frontal atrophy
- Down syndrome associated Alzheimer's
- Frontal temporal lobe
- Lewy body dementia
- Posterior cortical atrophy (PCA)
- Progressive supranuclear palsy
- Vascular dementia

In addition, I know of one person with PCA who had a dramatic improvement after consuming oils with medium-chain triglycerides and has continued to show benefit nearly two years later.

Parkinson's Disease

About 500,000 people in the United States suffer from Parkinson's disease, another progressive neurodegenerative disease that is classified as a movement disorder. People with this disease gradually develop slowness of movement (bradykinesia), become stiff, and develop tremors. About 30 percent of people with Parkinson's eventually develop dementia. In Parkinson's, neurons that make a substance called dopamine are affected in a part of the brain called the substantia nigra. Dopamine acts as a hormone and as a neurotransmitter, a chemical that allows neurons to communicate at the synapses. Dopamine plays an important role in behavior and cognition, voluntary movement, sleep, mood, attention, working memory, and learning.

Like Alzheimer's, the disease process in Parkinson's involves dysfunction of mitochondria. The exact cause of this dysfunction is unknown in most cases, but it is thought to be related to damage from oxygen free radicals. The neurons that produce dopamine contain a high iron content, which makes them particularly susceptible to this type of damage. Similar to Alzheimer's, there is decreased glucose uptake on FDG-PET scans in the affected area of the brain.

Dopamine cannot cross the blood/brain barrier, but its precursor L-dopa can. So people with Parkinson's can obtain some relief by taking L-dopa. As the disease progresses, these neurons die, and eventually this treatment no longer works or the side effects begin to outweigh the benefits.

The ketogenic diet has been shown to help people with Parkinson's. In 2005, Dr. Theodore VanItallie reported results of a feasibility study in which he tested a hyperketogenic diet on seven volunteers who had idiopathic (cause unknown) Parkinson's (VanItallie, 2005). A test called the Unified Parkinson's Disease Rating Scale (UPDRS) was administered before and at the end of the study. The five people who completed the twenty-eight-day study had improvements ranging from 21 to 81 percent on the UPDRS, for an average improvement of 43.4 percent.

The ketone ester could provide treatment for Parkinson's disease by reducing free radical damage to the very important dopamine-producing neurons. Ketones could provide energy to malfunctioning mitochondria. Also, in one of Dr. Veech's studies, ketone bodies prevented death in neurons that were subjected to a substance that causes Parkinson's disease.

Other Diseases with Insulin Deficiency and/or Insulin Resistance

In addition to Alzheimer's disease, sometimes called type 3 diabetes, many other diseases involve a deficiency of insulin and/or insulin resistance. Ketones can act as an alternative fuel for all tissues with the exception of the liver and could prevent progressive damage to multiple organs over time.

In addition to Alzheimer's disease, here are some examples of insulin-deficient and insulin-resistant conditions that could benefit from treatment with ketones:

- Alcohol abuse

- Chronic stress

- Conditions requiring steroid use

- Cushing's disease

- Diabetes mellitus types 1 and type 2

- Diseases with chronic inflammation

- Leprechaunism, also called Donohue syndrome (rare genetic mutation that affects insulin receptors)

- Metabolic syndrome (abdominal obesity, elevated cholesterol, and high blood pressure)

- Polycystic ovarian syndrome

- Prediabetes (insulin resistance)

- Rabson-Mendenhall syndrome (rare genetic mutation that affects insulin receptors)

Other Conditions with Decreased Glucose Uptake in the Brain

A number of other conditions share this problem of decreased glucose uptake as demonstrated by abnormal PET scans and could benefit from treatment with ketone ester:

- Age-related memory impairment

- Amyotrophic lateral sclerosis (ALS or Lou Gehrig's disease)

- Birth asphyxia

- Cushing's disease

- Huntington's disease (also called Huntington's chorea)

- Mild cognitive impairment (precursor to Alzheimer's)

- Multiple sclerosis

- Some types of autism (many children respond to gluten-free or carbohydrate-specific diet)

- Stroke

- Sudden lack of oxygen

- Traumatic brain injury

Genetic Defects in Glucose Transport and PDH Activity

Some rare genetic defects involving a block in glucose transport into cells or in metabolism of glucose could benefit from treatment with the ketone ester:

- GLUT-1 deficiency syndrome (currently treated with the ketogenic diet) and other glucose transporter diseases

- Glycogen storage diseases

- Leigh's syndrome

Other Diseases Involving Mitochondrial Dysfunction

Diseases that involve mitochondrial dysfunction could also respond to this treatment:

- Friedreich's ataxia

- Mitochondrial myopathies

- Multiple sclerosis

- Muscular dystrophy

- Myasthenia gravis

- Diseases involving mitochondria in other organs

Diseases Involving Problems with Fatty Acid Metabolism

- Multiple acyl-CoA dehydrogenase deficiency (MADD)

Refractory Epilepsy

The classic ketogenic diet and several modifications of it have been used successfully for nearly 100 years to eliminate or reduce the frequency of epileptic seizures in children and some adults who do not respond to treatment with anticonvulsants. When the diet is rigidly adhered to, the levels of ketone bodies are in the 2 to 5 micromoles per liter (mmol/l) range, comparable to those in starvation. However, a single deviation in the diet, such as consuming too many carbohydrates for a single meal, can suddenly reduce the level of ketones and cause seizures to reoccur. Currently, it is not known with certainty whether it is the high level of ketones and/or the extremely low level of carbohydrate in the diet that is responsible for controlling seizures. If the high level of ketone bodies is the primary factor in controlling seizures, then treatment with the ketone ester to maintain these high levels could replace the ketogenic diet, a big relief for many families dealing with this disease.

Until the ketone ester is available, incorporating MCT oil into the ketogenic diet could make the process somewhat easier.

Diseases Associated with Hypoglycemia (Low Blood Sugar)

- Diabetes mellitus types 1 and 2 (Even though high blood sugar is the hallmark of these diseases, diabetics are prone to attacks of low blood sugar if too much insulin is available in relation to how much sugar is consumed; this can occur, for example, by overestimating how much insulin is needed).

- Hypoglycemia of the newborn (affects about 10 percent of newborns)

- Infant of diabetic mother syndrome

- Russell Silver syndrome

Eye Diseases Involving Defects in Neurons

The eye is an extension of the brain, and certain eye diseases are the result of degeneration of the highly specialized neurons in the optic nerve or in the retina. It is then conceivable that providing circulating ketone bodies could bring about improvement in these conditions, including certain forms of:

- Glaucoma

- Optic atrophy

- Optic neuropathy

Other Diseases

The above lists are far from inclusive of all the diseases and conditions that could benefit from treatment with ketones. Any disease should be considered for treatment with ketones that involves insulin resistance, decreased glucose transport into neurons or other cells, abnormal release of glycogen from cells resulting in hypoglycemia, and/or mitochondrial dysfunction, as well as certain rare genetic defects. For instance, the ketogenic diet has been shown to be beneficial for people with certain types of cancerous tumors, which use only glucose for energy and cannot use ketones. Several studies in animals and in humans show that elevation of ketone levels through the ketogenic diet can cause astrocytomic tumors in the brain to shrink, by as much as 80 percent in a mouse study (Seyfried, 2005).

It is very important that such treatment is discussed with the person's physician to determine if it is justified and would not be harmful or possibly worsen the disease.

CURRENT STATUS OF THE KETONE ESTER

Since the mid-1990s, Dr. Veech and his associates have worked tirelessly at the NIH to study ketone bodies and to find the chemical formulation of the ketone ester that will produce results. About three years ago, he hit upon a successful formulation of the ketone ester. He and his associates have been making this, day in and day out, producing about nine to ten pounds per week. Because certain components needed to make the ester are quite expensive, Dr. Veech has been working on methods to produce the ester inexpensively. He is now very close to meeting the goal of making the ketone ester affordable so that everyone who needs it will be able to get it.

However, the amount that can be produced in his lab would

provide enough ketone for only four or five people on an ongoing basis. Thus, a much larger facility is needed to mass-produce the ketone ester. This, of course, requires considerable funding. Dr. Veech has suggested that a viable option would be to convert one of the bankrupt ethanol plants to make the ketone ester, which involves a similar process. There are many of these plants across the country.

In the summer of 2009, about fifty normal, healthy adults were recruited to participate for several months in toxicity testing of the ketone ester. The dosage was gradually increased until levels were achieved in the range that occurs with starvation and the classic ketogenic diet. *There were no adverse effects.* Dr. Veech and his associates launched a pilot study of people with Parkinson's disease in Oxford, England. He explains that within twenty-eight days it should be apparent whether a person with Parkinson's responds to the ketone ester or not, whereas studies involving Alzheimer's typically require a year or longer to determine if a compound is effective, due to the nature of the disease process. A study of the effects of ketone esters on physiological and cognitive performance in normal subjects and elite athletes is now underway at Oxford University under the direction of Dr. Veech's longtime collaborator, Professor Keiran Clark.

At this point, those of us who have loved ones with Alzheimer's can encourage the people who make funding decisions to consider the potential of the ketone ester and provide the moneys needed to begin the study of ketone esters in people with Alzheimer's disease as well. After all, we and our loved ones are running out of time.

Making the Transition to a Healthy Diet That Includes Medium-Chain Fatty Acids

20

Dietary Guidelines: Getting Started

Shortly after my article "What If There Was a Cure for Alzheimer's and No One Knew?" began to circulate, I started to receive telephone calls and e-mails from people who wanted to learn if this could help their loved one and, if so, how to go about incorporating this dietary intervention into their everyday diet. Since many people have the same questions, I put together a set of dietary guidelines that have been revised several times. The short version is available on the website www.coconutketones.com. Here, in Part Three, is an overview on how to make the transition to a healthy diet that includes coconut oil and other foods rich in medium-chain fatty acids, as well as answers to some of the many questions I have received. Patience, persistence, and consistency are key to making this intervention work.

PATIENCE

When I bought my first jar of coconut oil, I wondered exactly how we would use this relatively hard, white "stuff" in our diet. At the same time, I picked up a pamphlet on coconut oil to learn the basics and found out that it melts at 76°F. So the first time we used it, I mixed a little over two tablespoons into oatmeal and saw that it readily turned to a clear liquid as soon as it touched the hot cereal. We continued to use coconut oil for breakfast in oatmeal for several months, until Steve advised me that he was tired of oatmeal! In the meantime, we learned that there were many other ways to use coconut oil and were already taking advantage of those ideas at other meals.

I know of many people who take coconut oil straight out of the jar on a spoon, and while convenient, this could get old in short order, particularly if the oil is taken several times a day. It is relatively tasteless and melts in your mouth, so most people find it is not hard to swallow. On the other hand, since it is a food, it seems logical to try to incorporate it into the diet by substituting it for other fats and oils.

How to Use This Hard, White "Stuff"

During the first couple of weeks that we used coconut oil, I found a number of good recipes online at some of the coconut oil vendor sites, which also contain considerable information about coconut oil in general. I also researched coconut oil cookbooks and ordered several. My favorite cookbook is written by Bruce Fife, N.D., *Coconut Lovers Cookbook* (2008), which contains the basics about cooking with coconut oil and a multitude of wonderful ideas and recipes for using coconut oil and other coconut products in drinks, salads, salad dressings, sauces and gravies, soups, breads, cakes, and other desserts, as well as complete Asian and traditional American meals. In many cases, it is simply a matter of using coconut oil instead of other oils, butter, or margarine in a recipe.

One of the interesting features of coconut oil is that it tends to enhance the flavor of many different foods. We no longer find it necessary, for example, to drown sweet potatoes in brown sugar and butter, using one or two teaspoons of coconut oil instead, with very nice results. We eat salmon once or twice a week and coat the filet with a tablespoon of coconut oil, and the salmon comes out moist and flavorful every time. Our younger daughter, Joanna, made a chocolate birthday cake with chocolate genache icing for

Steve and me (our birthdays are a week apart), substituting coconut oil for the other fats in the batter and icing. She did not tell our older daughter, Julie, who was not yet sold on the idea of using it herself. After eating a large piece, Julie remarked that she could eat that cake for "breakfast, lunch, and dinner." That was one of the best cakes I have ever eaten. (See for yourself with the recipe on page 360.)

After more than three years of using coconut oil, it has become a staple in our diet, as normal for us now as using olive oil and butter in the past. We still use olive oil and butter, just not as often.

Common Problems Encountered

A common problem that people encounter with coconut oil is intestinal upset. We were fortunate that Steve did not experience this problem, considering that we started with more than two tablespoons at one meal. I do not have a gall bladder, so I had some indigestion the first few times I ate the oil, but this problem disappeared after several days. Some people have diarrhea after taking just one teaspoon of coconut oil, and it can be rather urgent and explosive, usually happening within one or two hours of consuming the oil. I advise people to begin very slowly and start on a day when they are not planning to leave the house for several hours, to spare possible embarrassment. As the oil is increased, there is a level at which this will happen for nearly everyone. Some measures can be taken to reduce the likelihood of diarrhea, and I will address this in Chapter 24.

PERSISTENCE

I hear from some people who are very discouraged because they do not see improvement in their loved one with Alzheimer's soon after starting this dietary intervention. There are a number of reasons why this might happen.

Extent of Cell Damage

People with Alzheimer's, and perhaps other less common forms of dementia as well as other types of neurodegenerative diseases, have a problem of insulin resistance in neurons that prevents glucose transport into the cells. Since glucose is the primary fuel for cells, if there is no such fuel available or a very limited supply, the cells malfunction and will eventually die. There is evidence that this process has been occurring in the brain for many years, perhaps even decades, before there are obvious symptoms. Some people with a certain genetic make-up could have a problem from infancy.

Given how long it takes for the Alzheimer's process to affect the brain, it could likewise take considerable time to undo its effects with medication or diet. When there is already extensive damage, the neurons and pathways of neurons in the brain that are already dead can't be resurrected. Neurons that are not functioning normally due to lack of energy related to insulin resistance are likely candidates to improve. These neurons may also be depleted of other substances needed to produce the final energy molecule ATP (adenosine triphosphate). In this case, providing the other missing substance(s) may result in improved functioning of such neurons (discussed later in chapter).

A Mix of Memory Conditions

Another issue is that many people with Alzheimer's do not have pure Alzheimer's disease. In fact, most people with late-onset dementia have a mixture of vascular and Alzheimer's type abnormalities, and some also have Lewy bodies, which are abnormal accumulations of proteins inside the neuron, more often associated with Parkinson's disease and Lewy body dementia.

Vascular abnormalities are those related to problems with blood vessels, such as inflammation and blood clots. Some defects are so small they can only be seen with a microscope and may result in minimal loss of brain cells. At the other extreme, some defects can involve a very large stroke with widespread shrinkage of the brain. Memory issues can also occur as a result of conditions including, but not limited to, hypothyroidism, sleep apnea, head injury, brain tumor, vitamin B12 deficiency, lead or mercury toxicity (or other heavy metals), low pressure hydrocephalus, depression (although depression can be a symptom of Alzheimer's), and they can even be a side effect of certain medications, such as lipid-lowering statins. Since these processes are not one of insulin resistance or decreased uptake of glucose into the brain, the affected cells are not likely to respond directly to the addition of medium-chain fatty acids in the diet.

Keep in mind too that the role of ketones in the brain is very complex and appears to be more than just fuel for cells. It is possible that ketones may encourage growth of new neurons and connections between neurons by increasing certain proteins in the brain that promote this growth. Considering that the brain as a whole is made up of trillions of neurons, the process of repair could take considerable time. In other conditions, where diet has been used to treat or reverse disease, such as in autism, the process may take several years or longer. In the Van Hove study discussed in Chapter 19, which used the sodium form of ketones for children with the rare enzyme defect multiple acyl-CoA dehydrogenase deficiency (MADD), it took many months for the symptoms to reverse.

Age at Onset

The age of the person with Alzheimer's and the extent and location of the existing damage could certainly play a role in the speed and amount of improvement. Some people expect an overnight miracle reversal of this disease process, but this has to be put into perspective. Improvement is relative. Steve is young compared to the average person with dementia, and the process in early onset may include factors that may or may not be present in late onset disease.

That may account for why Steve had a dramatic improvement on the first day, with an increase in his score on the MMSE from 14 the prior day to 18 out of 30 points, but this is far from the normal score of 30. During the first two weeks of taking coconut oil, his clock drawing also improved remarkably from an amorphous entity to something one would recognize as a clock. But, still, the average person without dementia would be able to draw a considerably better clock and be able to position the hands to indicate the time, which Steve was unable to master. Steve continued to have other improvements very gradually over the course of many months. Some did not become obvious until we realized that he had not experienced a particular symptom for a period of time.

Some people improve rather slowly; over two to three months the changes may become more apparent, or perhaps you will see that things are not worse. So the strategy of adding coconut oil to the diet may be worthwhile continuing even if results are not obvious in the beginning. At some point, if you are thinking of giving up, you might consider the possibility that this strategy could at least stabilize or slow down the process for your loved one.

Remember that the improvements in the Accera studies were documented using a test of cognition, the ADAS-COG. But as I have learned from a number of people who have reported a positive response in their loved ones, many of the improvements are of the type that cannot be measured on a standardized test, such as increase in energy, interaction with others, recognition of people they had forgotten, return of the personality and sense of humor, and resumption of activities that appeared to be lost. Such things are difficult to quantify but certainly represent important and welcome changes for the person with the disease and their loved ones.

Dietary Deficiencies

Hopefully, we will be able to learn why some people improve more rapidly than others and why others do not improve at all. After attending the American College of Nutrition Conference in October 2009, I have additional insight about why this happens. It could be that the cells are so depleted of the various substances they need to make energy within the mitochondria that they don't recover simply by providing ketones.

In a presentation by cardiologist Stephen Sinatra, I learned more about other disease processes that involve a problem with energy production in the mitochondria. When a fuel, such as glucose or ketones, enters the mitochondria, this sets off a chain reaction that involves a number of enzymes and other substances. The end result is the generation of ATP, which is constantly and rapidly created and then broken down to allow the cell to perform its functions. Some of the substances that are required in the chain reaction to make ATP, such as CoQ10, L-carnitine, magnesium, and D-ribose, can become depleted for various reasons, so that less and less ATP is made. If these substances are provided to the cell in the form of food or supplements, it may be possible to increase production of ATP once again. Dr. Sinatra has written a number of books on this subject that explain in detail how these substances are used by cells and how supplementation can help replenish the supply of ATP in the cell. (See Suggested Reading in the Resources section.)

CONSISTENCY

Another issue that can affect how well a person responds to medium-chain fatty acids is consistency of staying with this dietary intervention. The more medium-chain fatty acids are included in the diet, the more ketones will be produced by the liver. After considerable experimentation, we learned that ketones are available in Steve's circulation for only about three hours after Steve consumes medium-chain triglyceride (MCT) oil and for as long as seven to eight hours after eating coconut oil. This no doubt varies somewhat from person to person. It is unknown how long ketones are available after production for use by neurons and whether they are used immediately or can be stored for later use in the cell. At this point, I am assuming, until proven otherwise, that ketones are used as quickly they become available to the brain.

Timing and Dosing

The brain requires a very high level of energy to operate efficiently. In order to have ketones available all the time to the brain, Steve receives a specific amount of MCT oil and coconut oil with each meal three times a day, at the minimum. We have also incorporated other foods into our diet that contain medium-chain fatty acids, such as goat milk, goat cheese, and other coconut products. (See Table 23.1 for a listing of these foods.)

This dietary intervention probably will not help very much if medium-chain fatty acids are given in a hit-or-miss fashion, such as every few days for a couple of days and then forgotten for two or three more days. Consistency is very important. One can think of it as "fuel in the tank;" if there is no fuel in the tank, the car will not run. It is as simple as that.

In addition, there may be a minimum amount of medium-chain fatty acids that will provide enough energy to the brain to make a difference. Taking one teaspoon a day of coconut oil is a good place to start to avoid certain side effects, such as diarrhea, but that may not be enough to provide the energy needed by the neurons in the brain that are insulin resistant and cannot use glucose. This is why I encourage people to gradually increase to an amount they can handle without diarrhea and to use it at each meal, three times a day. I have heard from caregivers who have tried once-a-day dosing and clearly see an improvement in alertness and other symptoms shortly after taking the oil in the morning, only to see the effect wear off in the afternoon.

For best results, I suggest that medium-chain fatty acids become part of each meal and that they be given consistently every day. It is not unusual in some parts of the world for coconut or coconut oil to be a part of every meal. It is a staple in the diet for many people in the Philippines and in other parts of Asia, Africa, Hawaii, and the Caribbean Islands.

If, after several months of trying this dietary intervention, the caregiver feels there has been no improvement whatsoever and wants to stop, I suggest that it be discontinued slowly and with caution. When certain substances are available to our cells, there is a tendency for the cell to make more of the enzymes needed to use it, a sort of "gearing-up" process. In this way, the body and brain will have a chance to adjust. If your loved one is receiving a significant amount of the oils, I advise decreasing slowly over a week or longer. I have heard from several people who did not realize how much the medium-chain fatty acids were helping until they were discontinued and they saw a nearly immediate decline in their loved one. In this case, do not hesitate to restart the oils, and be prepared that it may take some time to recover.

Keep a Journal

To help you decide if use of medium-chain fatty acids is effective, it can be very helpful to keep a journal. Shortly after it became obvious that Steve was improving, my sister Angela suggested that I start a journal, and this has been invaluable. About two weeks after Steve's first dose of coconut oil, as he improved, it occurred to me I might forget what he was like before he started taking it. I wrote several pages describing my observations about his symptoms, not only related to memory and cognition, but also effects on each of his senses, physical symptoms, our interactions with each other, and some of the rather odd things he would do. In the beginning, I made notes every day about how much oil he was taking, how we were using it in food, some interesting recipes, and of course, how he was doing, generally and specifically. (Chapter 5 includes some of these early journal entries.)

I also used the journal to keep track of information related to getting the message out and my questions, the people I talked with about this, thoughts and ideas about Alzheimer's disease, use of medium-chain fatty acids, and other things I learned along the way that might be helpful to treating this disease. At this point, three years later, I make journal entries about once a week, summarizing how Steve is doing, any changes, and important events.

For people trying this dietary intervention, a journal could be very useful to gauge how the person is responding over a period of time. I suggest that you record at the very least:

- The dates of your entries in the journal

- General and specific observations about the person's symptoms prior to adding medium-chain fatty acids to the diet

- The starting dose, including how much and how often

- Each increase in dose

- Any side effects, such as diarrhea or indigestion, and anything unusual for that person

- How you are using it, such as cooking with the oil and what foods you are putting it into

- Your observations about changes in the individual for better or worse

At any point in time, you can look back at your journal entries and have a better idea of whether your loved one has improved, seems to be about the same, or has gotten worse. With or without formal testing, this will help you decide whether this intervention is helpful or not.

21

The Saturated Fat and Cholesterol Issue

In general, it is a good idea to discuss any significant change such as adding coconut oil to the diet with your physician to make sure there are no contraindications. I hope that physicians everywhere will become aware of the potential for medium-chain fatty acids to help in certain conditions and will get past the misconception that coconut oil is an unhealthy fat.

Prior to making the effort to learn as much as possible about coconut oil, I saw it in natural food stores and wondered why it was on the shelf. Like many other people, including physicians, I was told somewhere along the way that coconut oil is an "artery-clogging fat." How the theory (called the lipid hypothesis) that a diet high in fat and cholesterol increases the risk of death from heart disease came about is the subject of an article written by biochemist and internationally renowned authority on fats Mary Enig, Ph.D., titled "The Oiling of America." Her article recounts how the edible oil industry engineered the dietary change that took place during twentieth-century America from natural oils like butter, lard, and coconut oil to mostly highly processed vegetable oils. Even though there were many contradictory studies, saturated fats came to be considered harmful and polyunsaturated fats healthy.

While it is true that coconut oil is high in saturated fat, this fact does not tell the whole story. Are all saturated fats and cholesterol truly bad for us or not? In order to discuss this question, a short course in coconut oil and fats is warranted.

COCONUT OIL BASICS

Coconuts are nutrient rich. They are a good source of iron, phosphorus, zinc, and other minerals and vitamins. They are also a rich source of protein and fiber, while containing few naturally occurring sugars. They have been widely used in African, Asian, and Pacific countries for hundreds of years, and it is estimated that one-third of the world's population depends on the coconut for food. Its oil, milk, juice, and meat are staples in the diet.

Coconut oil is made from pressing the meat of fresh coconuts. About 86 percent of the oil is saturated fat; the remaining fat is a mixture of 6 percent monounsaturated fat, 2 percent polyunsaturated fat, and a small amount of phytosterols, which are one of the components of statins used for lowering cholesterol. Coconut oil also contains a small amount of omega-6, an essential fatty acid.

In America, in the 1950s, you could buy coconut oil at your local grocery store. Everyone cooked with it. People used butter, lard, and coconut oil to fry in, and it was also used in baking. Unlike most other oils, natural coconut oil is solid at room temperature, does not easily become rancid due to the relatively high amount of saturated fat, and has a shelf life of at least two years.

As the use of partial hydrogenation to turn a liquid fat into a solid one to further extend the shelf life and versatility of other vegetable oils became more prevalent, products such as Crisco were heavily marketed to the public, and coconut oil was viewed as the primary competition. Tariffs were placed on coconut oil to make it more expensive and encourage people to use the less expensive, partially hydrogenated oils. Many physicians and researchers expressed concerns at that time about these manufactured fats, questioning whether they were truly safe, but their voices were not heard for many years.

FATTY ACID BASICS

Fat is one of the three macronutrients in our diet, along with protein and carbohydrates. Nearly all foods contain one or more of these three basic components. But fat is by far the richest energy source. In addition, we need fat to cushion many of our internal organs and to provide insulation to protect us against cold.

The Chemical Structure of Fatty Acids

Fats are comprised of three different types of atoms: carbon, hydrogen, and oxygen. These atoms chemically bond to create a fatty acid molecule. A fatty acid can be short, medium, long, and very long, depending on how many carbon atoms are in the chain.

- A short-chain fatty acid has less than six carbon atoms.

- A medium-chain fatty acid has six to twelve carbon atoms.

- A long-chain fatty acid has fourteen to twenty-two carbons.

- A very-long-chain fatty acid has more than twenty-two carbon atoms.

In all fatty acid chains, there are two possible sites for a hydrogen atom to attach to each carbon atom. At one end of the chain, the carbon atom has an additional hydrogen atom attached to it. At the other end of the chain, the carbon atom is attached to an oxygen atom and a hydroxyl molecule, which is composed of an oxygen and a hydrogen atom. All fatty acids have a hydroxyl group plus an oxygen atom attached to the carbon at one end (see Figure 21.1 on the following page).

Each type of fatty acid chain behaves a little differently in regard to how much, if any, is converted to ketones and what its functions are in the body. Short- and medium-chain fatty acids are digested faster and more easily than long-chain and very-long-

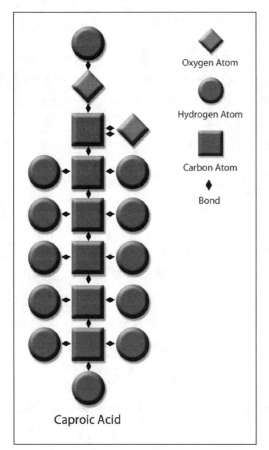

Caproic Acid

Oxygen Atom

Hydrogen Atom

Carbon Atom

Bond

Figure 21.1. Structure of a medium-chain fatty acid. This particular fatty acid is caproic acid, also called C:6, a fatty acid with six carbons in the chain. Diagram by Joanna Newport.

chain fatty acids. They are absorbed directly from the bowel after they are freed from the food by digestive enzymes and taken directly to the liver. In the liver, part of the fatty acid is converted to ketones and part is released directly into the circulation (blood or lymphatic systems) to be delivered to other tissues to use as energy.

Unlike the other fatty acids, medium-chain fatty acids are not made from scratch for use in our bodies except in the case of the lactating woman, in which they are made in the mammary glands as a component of breast milk. They are easily absorbed by the infant and used for energy. Human milk has about 60 percent of its energy calories as fat. About 35 percent of that fat is saturated. So if we are to have any medium-chain fatty acids available to us, they must come from foods in our diet that contain these types of fatty acids. As we know, medium-chain fatty acids are mainly found in coconut oil, palm kernel oil, and the fat of dairy and goat-milk products. After learning what I have about how medium-chain fatty acids can potentially bring about improvement in people with dementia and other neurodegenerative diseases, I have come to the conclusion that these fats may be essential fatty acids at least for some people. (See Table 23.1 for a list of other foods that contain medium-chain fatty acids.)

Most fats are comprised of long- and very-long-chain fatty acids, including soybean oil and canola oil, the most commonly used vegetable oils in the United States at the present time. These fats are not digested as quickly and easily as short- and medium-chain fatty acids. In addition, medium-chain fatty acids are not stored, but are used immediately for energy, whereas the longer-chain fatty acids tend to be stored as fat when an excessive number of calories are eaten at a given meal.

In addition to its chain length, a fatty acid can be either saturated or unsaturated, depending on the number of hydrogen atoms it contains and the number of bonds between the carbon atoms.

All short- and medium-chain fatty acids are saturated fats, meaning that the fat is considered "saturated," or completely filled with hydrogen ions; therefore, other types of atoms or molecules cannot attach to them. Some long- and very-long-chain fatty acids are saturated; some are monounsaturated. This means that they have one pair of carbon atoms that are each missing a hydrogen ion. So effectively, a pair of hydrogen ions are missing from the chain. When this occurs, a double bond forms between the two affected carbons; a double bond has twice as many negatively charged particles (electrons), which makes it shorter and stronger than a single bond. Some long-chain fatty acids are polyunsaturated, which means they have multiple sites that are not occupied by hydrogen atoms and form more than one double bond between carbons. These double bonds are very reactive, and potentially damaging oxygen free radicals can attach at these unoccupied sites (see Figure 21.2).

Just as the chain length of a fatty acid determines how it behaves and functions in our bodies, so too does the saturated,

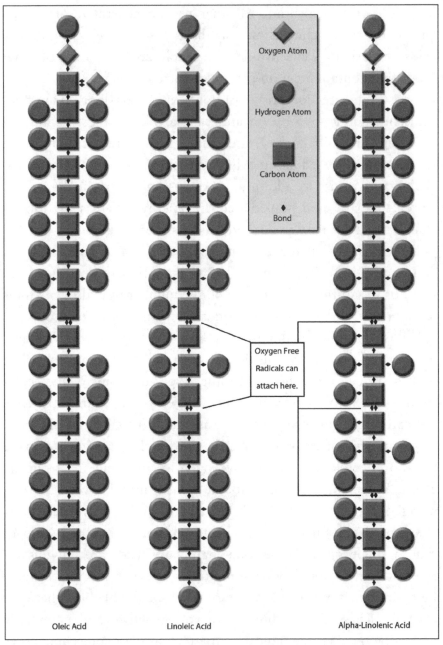

Figure 21.2. Diagrams of monounsaturated and polyunsaturated fatty acids. Oleic acid is a monounsaturated omega-9 fatty acid; linoleic acid, an omega-6 polyunsaturated fatty acid; and alpha-linolenic acid, an omega-3 polyunsaturated fatty acid. Diagram by Joanna Newport.

monounsaturated, and polyunsaturated chemical makeup of each fat, as we'll now see.

SATURATED FATS: MYTHS AND FACTS

There is a misconception that saturated fats found primarily in meat and dairy products are all bad and should be avoided at all cost. Saturated fats are also made naturally by the body. For example, palmitic acid, one of the most common long-chain saturated fats, is a major fatty acid in normal lung surfactant, a substance made inside each of the alveoli (air sacs) in the lung that keeps the alveoli open. Without surfactant, the lungs would collapse and we would die in short order. Very-long-chain saturated fatty acids are important components of cell membranes, especially in the brain. Certain saturated fats are important to white blood cell function, a major component of our response to infection; they are also used by the body to stabilize many different proteins, including those in the immune system, and to fight tumors. Certain other saturated fatty acids are important to signaling of hormones.

There is another misconception that oils such as soybean, olive, and canola contain no saturated fats, when in fact they do. These fats contain no short- or medium-chain fatty acids; however, they do contain long-chain saturated fatty acids. Table 21.1 on the following page shows the percentage of total fat in long- and very-long-chain saturated fatty acids in common oils and fat-containing foods.

One important feature of saturated fat is that because all its carbon atoms are attached to hydrogen atoms, it is more stable than monounsaturated or polyunsaturated fats. That means it stays fresher longer and doesn't become rancid or succumb to oxidation as quickly as unsaturated oils. Oxidation is a process in which fats, left exposed or subjected to heat sources, interact with oxygen and create oxygen free radicals. Oxygen free radicals, also called oxidants or reactive oxygen species, are natural byproducts

TABLE 21.1. COMMON OILS AND FATS AND THEIR PERCENTAGE OF LONG-CHAIN AND VERY-LONG-CHAIN SATURATED FATTY ACIDS

OILS AND FATS	% LONG-CHAIN AND VERY-LONG-CHAIN SATURATED FATTY ACIDS
Butter	61.6
Cocoa butter	60.0
Cow's milk fat	48.5
Heavy cream	48.5
Goat milk fat	40.5
Lard	38.6
Egg	37.0
Human milk fat	35.0
Salmon (% of total fat)	33.0
Coconut oil	27.8
Palm kernel oil	27.3
Cod liver oil	22.6
Fish oil	19.9
Peanut oil	16.9
Soybean oil	15.6
Margarine (% of total fat)	15.2
Olive oil	13.8
Corn oil	12.9
Sunflower oil	9.9
Flaxseed oil	9.4
Walnut oil	9.1
Canola oil	7.4
Safflower oil	6.2

Source: Agricultural Research Service. USDA National Nutrient Database for Standard Reference (Release 23) 2010, www.ars.usda.gov/nutrientdata.

in some chemical reactions in the body, but when released and present in excess can cause damage to cells and tissues. Oils that are high in saturated fats, such as coconut oil, tend to be stable at room temperature and will not become rancid for a considerable period of time. In addition, due to the presence of saturated fats, heating coconut oil to medium heat (350°F) or less will not alter the structure of the fat.

As pointed out earlier, all short- and medium-chain fatty acids like coconut oil are saturated fats, and they behave differently than long- and very-long-chain saturated fats. They are not stored as fat, but instead are partly converted in the liver to ketones or are used directly by tissues for energy. So while it is true that coconut oil has a high percentage (86 percent) of saturated fats, 70 percent of its saturated fat content is medium-chain fatty acids. In addition, contrary to popular belief, coconut oil and palm kernel oil contain no cholesterol. Most doctors who advise their patients to stay away from coconut oil are not aware of these facts.

At present, we are encouraged by groups such as the American Heart Association (AHA), Centers for Disease Control and Prevention (CDC), and World Health Organization (WHO) to limit our saturated fat intake to between 7 and 10 percent (depending on the group) of total calories. This represents 140 to 200 calories in a 2,000-calorie diet. This recommendation is based on some studies in which diets high in saturated fat have been correlated with an increased incidence of atherosclerosis (hardening of the arteries) and heart disease.

Early Studies on Saturated Fat and Heart Disease

During the first half of the twentieth century, deaths from athero-sclerosis (hardening of the arteries) and coronary artery disease (heart attacks) increased dramatically and much research was dedicated to determining why this was taking place. The basis for the lipid hypothesis (mentioned earlier) came to prominence with a 1953 study by Ancel Keys, Ph.D. (Keys, 1953), which was first presented at a meeting at Mt. Sinai Hospital. Dr. Keys presented data from six countries derived from the 1949 Food and Agriculture Organization (FAO) of the United Nations report that appeared to show that the number of deaths in men from "degenerative heart disease" increased as the percentage of fat in the diet increased (Figure 21.3). Keys' work was publicized widely in the lay press as well as in the scientific literature at that time, and he rose to a position of influence in related government policy making. Keys went on to publish a study of seven countries showing a relationship between high saturated fat intake and deaths from heart disease (Keys, 1970).

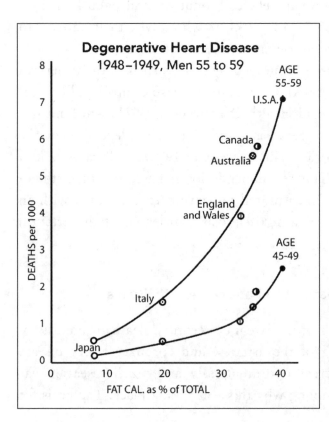

Figure 21.3. In a 1953 study by Keys, data for six countries from a 1949 FAO report appear to show that the risk of degenerative heart disease in men increases as the percentage of fat increases in the diet. Data adapted by Joanna Newport from Keys, 1953.

While many applauded Key's work and embraced it, other scientists and epidemiologists refuted Keys' study in articles written in the latter part of the 1950s (Mann, 1959; Yudkin, 1957; Yerushalmy, 1957). They pointed out that, at the time Keys presented his paper, data were actually available from the FAO for twenty-two countries and that if all twenty-two were used in a similar graph, the numbers were randomly scattered and did not show any relationship between dietary fat and deaths from heart disease. They accused Keys of cherry-picking the six countries to try to prove his hypothesis. In fact, Mann pointed out that a similar figure would appear if the amount of animal protein was considered instead of fat (Figure 21.4).

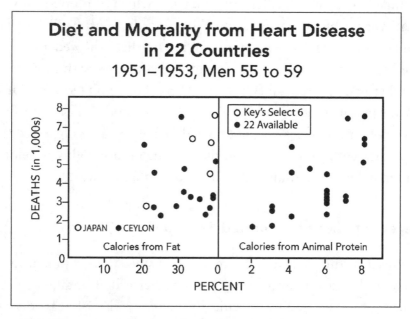

Figure 21.4. Disputing Keys' hypothesis that a high-fat diet causes degenerative heart disease, George Mann plotted data for all twenty-two countries available from the 1949 FAO report showing that there was no correlation between percent of fat intake and heart disease; furthermore, a graph of percent of animal protein intake versus heart disease produced a similar random pattern. Data adapted by Joanna Newport from Mann, 1959.

Yudkin showed that if the amount of meat and milk fats was considered, the available data did not support a connection with deaths from heart disease, nor did the evidence support high intakes of butterfat and cheese as culprits. In fact, when he looked at protein and sugar intake, Yudkin found there was a "better relationship" of heart disease with intake of sugar than any other nutrient they studied. It is important to know here that the trend in smoking also closely paralleled the rise in coronary artery deaths.

Two epidemiologists, Jacob Yerushalmy and Herman Hilleboe, in order to challenge Keys' data, performed similar studies looking at the data from the twenty-two countries. As in the Mann article, they showed there was no connection between mortality and percentage of fat in the diet when all twenty-two countries were included. They handpicked six countries, which, if plotted showing deaths from blood vessel lesions affecting the central nervous system (stroke) versus percent of fat in the diet, showed the exact opposite trend that Keys had found; the countries with more fat in the diet had less mortality (Figure 21.5). They pointed out that by no means did they consider Keys' a valid study since data from many other countries was not considered. They also suggested that countries with more abundant diet are also more highly developed and may be better equipped to diagnose cause of death.

Recent Studies on Saturated Fat and Heart Disease

Numerous studies have been undertaken since then with contradictory results, so the argument over whether a high intake of fat in general, or saturated fat specifically, increases risk of heart disease, stroke, and/or dementia continues to this day. In 2002, James Le Fanu challenged the validity of information in a textbook (Brisson, 1982) showing a trend of increasing mortality from heart attacks with increasing fat intake in twenty countries. Looking at the same data from another angle, Le Fanu noted that, for example, even

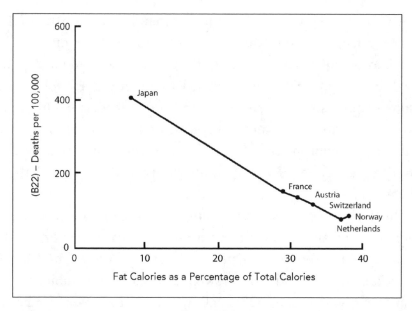

Figure 21.5. To illustrate the folly of hand-picking data to prove a point, Yerushalmy chose data for six of the twenty-two countries available from the 1949 FAO report to show that mortality from blood vessel lesions affecting the central nervous system (stroke) decreased as the percentage of fat in the diet increased. Data adapted by Joanna Newport from Yerushalmy, 1957.

though the percentage of fat intake was about the same (30 to 35 percent), the mortality rate was more than four times greater in Finland, Australia, and the United States than in France, which had the second lowest mortality rate of the twenty countries studied, with Japan ranking the lowest.

Large epidemiologic studies such as the fifty-year Framingham Heart Study, the WHO MONICA Project (monitoring worldwide trends and determinants in cardiovascular disease), and the Multiple Risk Factor Intervention Trial (a national study of primary prevention of coronary heart disease) have not found a connection between fat or saturated fat intake and increased risk of heart disease or stroke.

A number of saturated fat studies attempted to ascertain what specific effects the individual fatty acids might have on HDL or LDL cholesterol levels by adding disproportionate amounts to the diet (Tholstrup, 1994; Zock, 1994; Kris-Etherton, 1997). But the results of such studies are skewed and do not reflect eating in the real world. Natural fats and oils consist of a mixture of many fatty acids and the purportedly "bad" effect of one fatty acid may be offset by the "good" effect of another fatty acid, so that a balance is achieved.

This lack of consensus has prompted a number of articles and studies on the subject of saturated fats and the effects of low-fat diets. One study, published in the *American Journal of Clinical Nutrition,* may provide an answer. The authors combined data from twenty-one studies, which allowed them to look at the health effects of saturated fats on nearly 350,000 people over a period of five to twenty-three years: more than 11,000 developed heart, vascular (blood vessel) disease, or stroke (Siri-Tarino, 2010). This analysis showed that there is no significant evidence for concluding that saturated fat is associated with an increased risk of heart disease, stroke, or cardiovascular disease.

If anything, over the recent decades that Americans have been encouraged to eat a low-fat diet and to avoid saturated fats, conditions such as obesity, diabetes, and dementia *have been on the rise.*

Studies on Saturated Fat and Dementia

A great many studies over the past sixty years have looked at the effects of fat consumption and/or saturated, mono- and polyunsaturated fats on cardiovascular disease, stroke, or dementia. Specifically when looking at dementia, there are again contradictory studies. As just one example, the Rotterdam study of dementia versus fat intake in nearly 5,400 people over six years found no association between development of dementia with a high intake of fat, high intake of saturated fat, or low intake of mono- or poly-unsaturated fats (Engelhart, 2002). In 2009, Solfrizzi and others looked at a number of trials and likewise concluded that they could make "no definitive dietary recommendations on fish and unsaturated fatty acid consumption, or lower intake of saturated fat, in relation to the risk for dementia and cognitive decline" (Solfrizzi, 2009).

When I attended the Alzheimer's Association's International Conference on Alzheimer's Disease in Chicago in 2008, I had the opportunity to speak with many scientists presenting their research on posters. One of these was Michal Schnaider-Beeri, Ph.D., who, along with her associate, Uri Goldbourt, Ph.D., performed a study begun in the mid-1960s that looked at the relationship between saturated fat intake at midlife and the development of dementia three decades later. The subjects were nearly 10,000 Israeli men who were civil and municipal employees, ages forty to sixty-five, who were part of a long-term study of incidence and risk factors for cardiovascular disease, which included analysis of food intakes. The results were the opposite of what they expected. They divided the saturated fat intake into four quartiles and found that there was an inverse relationship between saturated fat intake and dementia. Those in the quartile with the lowest intake of saturated fat (an average of 14 percent) had the highest rate of late-life dementia, and those with highest intake of saturated fat (an average of 23 percent) had the lowest rate of dementia. They also found that the percent of calories from mono- and polyunsaturated fats were not related to late-life dementia (Goldbourt, 2008). Dr. Beeri had no explanation for these unexpected findings.

WHAT'S UNIQUE ABOUT MONOUNSATURATED FATS

As we know, monounsaturated fatty acids found in olive, canola, and peanut oils have one ("mono" means one) double bond between their carbon atoms. Because of this one double bond, monounsaturated fats are more stable than their polyunsaturated counterparts (discussed next). They are less prone to oxidation and are able to resist rancidity at higher temperatures than polyunsaturated oils.

One reason olive oil, in particular, is considered so healthy is due to its high concentration of monounsaturated fats. Studies have reported that adhering to the Mediterranean diet, popularized in the 1990s, may lower the risk for dementia and/or heart disease (Sofi, 2008; Gu, 2010). Nicolaos Scarmeas, M.D., found that adherence to the Mediterranean diet not only reduces the risk for Alzheimer's disease, but also alters the course of the disease by delaying mortality. People living in this region are also known for having a low incidence of coronary artery disease. Researchers attribute this to their diet, a combination of vegetables, grains, fish, and olive oil, the last of which makes up about 30 percent of their daily caloric intake.

Olive oil is about 73 percent monounsaturated fats, most notably omega-9 oleic acid, which epidemiological studies suggest may reduce the risk of coronary heart disease. There is also some evidence that the antioxidants in olive oil may improve cholesterol regulation, reduce LDL cholesterol, lower blood pressure, and fight inflammation, which is now being recognized as a factor in heart disease (Covas, 2007). Once again, while some studies support these statements, others argue that longevity found in the populations could be related to other factors such as genetics or high vitamin D levels related to sun exposure (Brown, 2007; Wong, 2008).

Olive, canola, and peanut oils are not the only oils that contain monounsaturated fats. Table 21.2 provides a list of common fats and oils with their percentage of monounsaturated fatty acids.

TABLE 21.2. COMMON OILS AND FATS AND THEIR PERCENTAGE OF MONOUNSATURATED FATTY ACIDS

OILS AND FATS	% MONOUNSATURATED FATTY ACIDS
Sunflower oil	83.7
Olive oil	73.0
Canola oil	63.3
Cod liver oil	46.7
Peanut oil	46.2
Lard	45.1 (or higher depending on animal's diet)
Margarine (% of total fat)	38.9
Egg (% of total fat)	38.2
Human milk fat	37.9
Salmon (% of total fat)	33.1
Cocoa butter	33.0
Fish oil (salmon)	29.0
Flaxseed oil	29.0
Cow's milk fat	28.9
Heavy cream (heavy, % of total fat)	28.9
Corn oil	27.5
Goat milk fat	26.8
Butter	25.9
Soybean oil	22.8
Walnut oil	22.8
Cod liver oil	22.6
Safflower oil	14.4
Palm kernel oil	11.4
Coconut oil	5.8

Source: Agricultural Research Service. USDA National Nutrient Database for Standard Reference (Release 23) 2010, www.ars.usda.gov/nutrientdata.

WHAT'S UNIQUE ABOUT POLYUNSATURATED FATS

As we know, polyunsaturated fatty acids are those in which there is more than one site ("poly" means many) on the carbon chain that does not have hydrogen ions, and therefore, there is a double bond between two of the carbons at more than one location. As such, these fatty acids are more volatile than saturated and monounsaturated fats. They have a tendency to oxidize and become rancid. As part of this process of oxidation, they can pick up oxygen free radicals. Certain free radicals play an important role, such as killing off bacteria within certain cells and in cell signaling, but when present in excess can result in cell damage, leading to cancers, atherosclerosis, alcohol-induced liver damage, and emphysema. Free-radical damage to mitochondria has been implicated in the development of Parkinson's and Alzheimer's diseases (see Chapter 14). Nevertheless, concerns about eating an excess of certain polyunsaturated fatty acids have not received as much attention as concerns about saturated fats.

Polyunsaturated fats also come in two forms: *cis* and *trans* forms. When fats have double bonds in the normal cis geometry, meaning that the hydrogen atoms are on the same side of the double carbon bond, the result is a cis fat. This gives the molecule a "bend" in the carbon chain and a lower melting point so that it interacts with other molecules. When the hydrogen atoms are on opposite sides of the carbon bond, the result is a trans fat. Trans fats are more stable than cis fats; they are easier to cook with and less likely to spoil than naturally occurring oils, which is why food manufacturers like using them. Trans fats, however, wreak havoc in our bodies (discussed next).

Polyunsaturated fats, found mostly in plant-based foods and oils, are some of the most common fats in our diet. Like all natural fats, they have their benefits. The body relies on polyunsaturates to create a special class of fatty acids known as omega fats. Certain omega-3 and omega-6 fatty acids are considered essential fatty acids (EFAs), because the body is unable to manufacture these types of fatty acids on its own and so they must be obtained from foods.

These essential fats are necessary for the body and brain to grow and develop normally and are critical in many important functions involving cell membranes and blood cells such as platelets, which help in clotting. Docosahexaenoic acid (DHA), for example, is an omega-3 fatty acid that makes up 50 percent of the weight of the neuron's plasma membrane; a deficiency of DHA could therefore have profound ramifications. In addition, both omega-3 and omega-6 supply our bodies with the raw material to produce certain hormones such as prostaglandins—powerful substances used throughout the body to regulate a wide range of functions, including blood pressure and inflammation.

Table 21.3 presents a list of common fats and oils and their percentages of total polyunsaturated fatty acids, as well as omega-6 and omega-3 fatty acids.

TABLE 21.3. COMMON FATS AND OILS AND THEIR PERCENTAGE OF POLYUNSATURATED FATTY ACIDS

OILS AND FATS	% POLYUNSATURATED FATTY ACIDS	% OMEGA-6 FATTY ACIDS	% OMEGA-3 FATTY ACIDS
Safflower oil	74.6	74.6	0
Flaxseed oil	66.0	12.7	53.3
Walnut oil	63.3	52.9	10.4
Soybean oil	57.7	51.0	6.8
Corn oil	54.7	53.5	1.2
Fish oil (salmon)	40.3	1.5	35.3
Salmon (% of total fat)	40.0	2.7	31.8
Peanut oil	32.0	32.0	0

OILS AND FATS	% POLYUNSATURATED FATTY ACIDS	% OMEGA-6 FATTY ACIDS	% OMEGA-3 FATTY ACIDS
Margarine (% of total fat)	30.1	27.6	2.4
Sunflower oil	29.0	29.0	trace
Canola oil	28.1	19.0	9.1
Cod liver oil	22.5	0.94	19.7
Egg (% of total fat)	13.6	11.5	7.4
Human milk fat	11.3	8.5	1.2
Lard	11.2	10.2	1.0
Olive oil	10.5	9.8	0.8
Cow's milk fat	3.7	2.3	1.4
Cream (heavy)	3.7	2.3	1.5
Butter	3.7	3.4	0.4
Goat milk fat	3.5	2.6	1.0
Cocoa butter	3.0	2.8	0.1
Coconut oil	1.8	1.9	0
Palm kernel oil	1.6	1.6	0

Source: Agricultural Research Service. USDA National Nutrient Database for Standard Reference (Release 23) 2010, www.ars.usda.gov/nutrientdata.

The key to getting the most of EFAs is a properly balanced intake of omega-6s to omega-3s. The typical polyunsaturated vegetable oils commonly used at home and in restaurants, usually soybean or safflower oils, especially when they are partially hydrogenated, have an excess of omega-6 relative to omega-3 fatty acids, often a ratio of between 20:1 and 40:1. The ideal ratio of omega-6 to omega-3 fatty acids is 4:1, and some experts recommend 2:1 or even 1:1.

Without a balanced intake of omega-6s to omega-3s, the benefits of these fats turn harmful. Omega-6 fatty acids tend to favor inflammation, vasoconstriction (narrowing of arteries that results in high blood pressure), and blood clotting. If you think about it, these are the very same factors that set a person up for a heart attack. Omega-3 fatty acids favor anti-inflammation, vasodilation (opening up blood vessels,) and decreased clotting or blood thinning. It is important that these two types of essential fatty acids are eaten in an appropriate ratio to balance these effects. The partially hydrogenated forms of soybean and canola oil have the added impact of raising cholesterol, particularly LDL, due to higher levels of trans fatty acids, which replace essential fatty acids. During partial hydrogenation, the omega-3 fatty acids disappear first, then the omega-6s, then the monounsaturated fatty acids.

Coconut oil has considerably less omega-6 fatty acid than soybean or canola oils, but contains no omega-3 fatty acid. By incorporating coconut oil into the diet in place of soybean or canola oil, excessive intake of omega-6 fatty acids can be avoided. At the same time, the ideal ratio of omega-6 to omega-3 fatty acids can be easily achieved by eating salmon once or twice a week or taking flax oil, fish oil, and/or cod liver oil supplements. Some other foods that contain omega-3 fatty acids include walnuts, chia grain, and flax meal. To learn more about these beneficial fats, I highly recommend *Fish, Omega-3, and Human Health* (2005) by William Lands, Ph.D., and *The Omega-3 Connection,* a very comprehensive treatment of this subject by Andrew Stoll, M.D.

THE PROBLEM WITH TRANS FATS

Trans fats are made up of trans fatty acids. Trans fats occur naturally in some foods, especially those from animals. But most trans fats are made during food processing through partial hydrogenation of polyunsaturated fats and are found in many processed and fast foods, most margarine, and many vegetable oils.

Pressure created by government guidelines on the American public to reduce saturated fat in the diet resulted in greater consumption of trans fatty acids, since they are the most suitable alternatives for the food industry when semi-solid and solid fats are used in a food product. In the hydrogenation process, a polyunsaturated oil is subjected to high heat and pressure while hydrogen is introduced into the oil. Hydrogen atoms are added to some of the bonds as a result. Sometimes the fats will become completely saturated with hydrogen atoms and are identical to the saturated fats found in nature. On the other hand, some of the fats will be only partly saturated with the hydrogen atoms (producing a partially hydrogenated fat), and these will contain some trans bonds. The trans double bond gives the molecule a straighter shape, a higher melting point, and a more rigid structure.

The problem for humans is that our cells and cell membranes are not programmed through evolution to use these altered fats. Normally, in the cell membranes, the lipid molecules line up like tiny magnets end to end and side to side, called lipid bilayers (Figure 21.6). They repel water on the inside, which keeps the contents of the cell inside the cell, and they repel the watery fluids on the outside of the cell, which keeps the outside world from entering the cell. When a cell membrane tries to incorporate a trans fat molecule, which is differently shaped, it is like trying to put a square peg into a round hole (Figure 21.7). It doesn't line up normally with the other lipid molecules, which can affect the fluidity and the functioning of the cell membrane and even the lifespan of the cell.

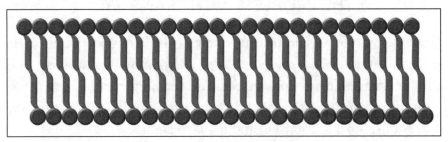

Figure 21.6. Lipid bilayer of cell membrane with naturally occurring fatty acids. Diagram by Joanna Newport.

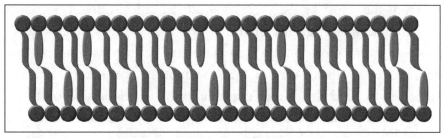

Figure 21.7. Lipid bilayer of cell membrane with naturally occurring and trans fatty acids. Trans fatty acids are more rigid and can interfere with the fluidity and normal function of the cell membrane. Diagram by Joanna Newport.

The well-known Nurses' Health Study, which looked at many aspects of health related to diet and other lifestyle factors, shows why it is very important to stay away from partially hydrogenated fats. In 1993, Walter Willet, M.D., and others collected dietary data from questionnaires completed in 1980 by 85,095 women who were not diagnosed at that point with coronary heart disease, stroke, diabetes, or high cholesterol levels. During the next eight years, there were 431 new cases of fatal and non-fatal heart attacks. After controlling for weight and caloric intake, the only difference the researchers found in diet was a higher intake of trans fatty acids in the affected women. Their intakes of saturated fat, mono- or polyunsaturated fat, and dietary cholesterol did not change their risk of developing heart disease (Willett, 1993).

In 1999, many years after the problems with trans fats were recognized and reported by lipid biochemists, the federal government began the process of enacting a rule to require labeling on foods of trans fats. In about 2003, this process went into effect, and many of the food manufacturers and fast-food chains made a switch from using partially hydrogenated oils to natural oils in their products. Up to that time, a large order of fries at one of the major fast food chains could contain as much as 25 grams, nearly two tablespoons, of trans fatty acids.

Trans fats must be listed on food labels, unless one serving contains less than 0.5 grams of trans fats. This is deceptive because food may very well contain trans fats and yet the serving size can be adjusted to make certain that the label lists no trans fat. My advice is to read the list of ingredients on labels and avoid anything that contains hydrogenated or partially hydrogenated oils. You will be very surprised to see how many foods contain these unhealthy fats.

Physicians who tell their patients to avoid coconut oil rarely suggest that they should also avoid the trans fatty acids in partially hydrogenated vegetable oils. They may not even be aware of the true artery-clogging potential of these manufactured fats in very many kitchens, convenience foods, and fast-food restaurants. A large number of physicians consume partially hydrogenated fats themselves on a regular basis without batting an eye. I know because I used to be one of them!

CHOLESTEROL BASICS

Cholesterol is not actually a fat itself, but rather a steroid of fat. All cholesterol is made from the basic energy molecule acetyl CoA, and most of it is made in the body rather than consumed in the diet. The major dietary sources of cholesterol are found in foods of animal origins such as cheese, egg yolks, beef, pork, poultry, and shrimp. Concern that elevated cholesterol levels may have something to do with heart disease originated in about 1910, when the German chemist Adolf Windaus (1876–1959) reported that atherosclerotic plaques from the aortas (the main artery from the heart to the body) of human subjects with heart disease contained twenty to twenty-sixfold higher concentrations of cholesterol than normal aortas (Goldstein, 2003).

There has been much debate ever since as to whether cholesterol causes these plaques to form and, therefore, causes cardiovascular disease, stroke, and dementia, as opposed to playing a very different role, which is discussed below.

Cholesterol: Myths and Facts

The cholesterol issue, in general, focuses on levels that are considered to be too high. But low cholesterol levels also appear to play a role in disease. Extremely low cholesterol levels are associated with higher risk of death from cancer, for example, and are associated with higher mortality in general (Schatz, 2001). High levels of cholesterol may even be protective against Alzheimer's disease (Seneff, 2011).

There is much to be learned about the true role of cholesterol in the body, including grave misconceptions that all cholesterol is bad. Cholesterol is so vital, in fact, that it is contained in practically every cell in the body and performs a long list of beneficial functions. The body uses cholesterol to produce adrenal and sex hormones, aid in the manufacture of bile acids needed for the digestion of fats, help keep the skin healthy, and provide a source of vitamin D, a necessity for calcium absorption.

Cholesterol is required in infancy for normal brain development (large amounts of cholesterol are present in human breast milk). It makes up from 30 to 40 percent of the cell membrane, which helps create the cell's shape and protects it from being bent or deformed. It is a critical component of some cell receptors, which bind to specific chemicals to allow transport of certain substances into the cell, and it also forms a protective coating around the myelin sheaths of the nerves in the brain and central nervous system. Cholesterol also protects our cells from free-radical attack, therefore acting as an antioxidant.

We need a certain amount of cholesterol every day to perform these many essential functions. According to Dr. Enig (mentioned earlier), the total body cholesterol for the average 150-pound man is equal to 145,000 milligrams (mg), or about one-third of a pound. About 10,000 to 14,000 mg of this cholesterol is circulating in the bloodstream. What we don't eat is otherwise produced in large part by the liver and intestines and can be produced inside nearly every properly functioning cell. If we take in too much cholesterol, the liver will make less; if we do not take in enough cholesterol in food, the liver will make more. This is why reducing dietary intake of cholesterol has relatively little, if any, impact on lowering total cholesterol levels. The liver is reported to make as much as 5 grams (5,000 mg) of cholesterol a day, so if a person consumes the currently recommended 300 mg, of which only half is absorbed by the intestines, the small amount eaten will have very little effect on the total cholesterol level.

Until not too many years ago, elevated cholesterol was considered unhealthy without regard to the components of cholesterol known as high-density lipoprotein (HDL) cholesterol and low-density lipoprotein (LDL) cholesterol. The HDL cholesterol is considered "good" cholesterol because it carries cholesterol away from the arterial walls, thus preventing the buildup of cholesterol in the blood vessels. LDL cholesterol, on the other hand, is considered harmful since it is a component of the plaques in the arterial walls that may result in decreased blood flow and artery blockages.

As it turns out, LDL cholesterol may not be completely bad after all; it is part of the body's response to infection and inflammation and is involved in repair of damaged artery walls. LDL cholesterol works with white blood cells to kill bacteria that have invaded the wall of the artery when it is damaged. LDL cholesterol then becomes part of a plaque, a sort of patch, applied to wounds in artery walls. In addition, researchers have learned that high blood pressure, which damages the walls of the arteries, may be a greater risk factor for a heart attack than elevated total cholesterol levels. Total cholesterol levels include both HDL and LDL cholesterol.

An HDL level of less than 40 milligrams per deciliter (mg/dl) is considered to be a major risk factor for heart disease, according to the National Cholesterol Education Program 10-Year Risk Assessment Calculator, which uses information from the Framingham Heart Study (Adult Treatment Panel III, 2004 Update). However, this assessment tool does not mention LDL cholesterol level as a risk factor. The Framingham Heart Study, which was initially designed to explore the risk factors in the development of heart disease, found that obesity, inactivity, and type A (high-strung) behavior were all shown to contribute to heart disease risk, but found no correlation between diet with supposed high cholesterol foods and heart disease. Moreover, about half of people who suffer from heart attacks have total cholesterol levels in the normal range under 200 mg/dl.

Recent studies are looking more closely at very small particles of cholesterol called VLDL, or very-low-density lipoproteins, that are not measured with the standard lipid profile as possible suspects (Ren, 2010). Also, researchers have discovered that people with elevated C-reactive protein levels, a marker of often hidden inflammation, are at much greater risk of a heart attack than people who have normal C-reactive protein levels (Ridker, 2002). Is cholesterol the actual culprit in heart disease, or is it merely at the scene of the crime? This is still not fully understood. Scientists do not fully understand cholesterol and the role it plays in disease. Should we be trying to lower cholesterol, or should we be paying more attention to the underlying processes, such as inflammation and inflammation-triggers, that raise purportedly bad cholesterol? Hopefully the answers to these questions will be forthcoming.

What Role Does Cholesterol Play in Dementia?

One of the major unanswered questions is what role, if any, cholesterol plays in the development of dementia. Again, studies support both sides of the issue. Cholesterol performs critical functions in the brain. It is a critical component of cell receptors that bind to specific chemicals to allow transport of certain substances into the cell; it forms a coating around the myelin sheaths that protect the nerves; and it is required for "membrane fusion," which is required for release of neurotransmitters at the synapses and can affect the data-processing and memory functions in the brain (Tong, 2009). Considering how important cholesterol is in the basic structure of every cell, we might question whether we really want to take a medication like statins that will remove cholesterol from the brain. Perhaps we should know more about what effects lowering cholesterol has on the brain, how much cholesterol is removed, and exactly what changes take place in the brain when a person takes statins.

The brain makes up only about 2 percent of the total body mass. However, about 25 percent of the total cholesterol in the body is found in the brain (Seneff, 2011). Cholesterol does not cross the blood/brain barrier, except a small amount of LDL on special transporters, and so the brain must make nearly all of its own cholesterol. According to Stephanie Seneff, Ph.D., "Cholesterol is required everywhere in the brain as an antioxidant (in order to prevent ion leakage), an electrical insulator, as a structural scaffold for the neural network, and a functional component of all membranes."

Apolipoproteins are involved with transport of cholesterol throughout the body, and people who are ApoE4+ tend to have high cholesterol levels. There is evidence that a defect in metabolism of cholesterol in the brain may play a role in the development of Alzheimer's disease. It has also been found that in people with Alzheimer's disease, the cerebrospinal fluid, which bathes the brain and spinal cord, is depleted of lipoproteins, cholesterol, triglycerides, and fatty acids compared to the fluid in people without Alzheimer's. In fact, the fatty acid levels in the spinal fluid are depleted by a factor of six compared to that in normal controls

(Mulder, 1998). Dr. Seneff, who also addresses the problem of high-carbohydrate intake, concludes, "Simple dietary modification toward fewer highly processed carbohydrates and relatively more fats and cholesterol is likely a protective measure against Alzheimer's disease."

Papers written by Beatrice Golomb, M.D., who studies adverse effects of statins at University of California San Diego, are very enlightening (Golomb, 2005 and 2008; Evans 2009). She has reviewed the literature extensively and states that the only group of people who appear to benefit from taking statins with reduced rates of heart attack and related mortality are middle-aged men up to age sixty-five who have elevated cholesterol *and* other risk factors for cardiac disease. She says women don't benefit at any age, and men and women over age seventy do not benefit. They have no decrease in mortality from heart disease, even if they have existing cardiac disease. Dr. Golomb also says that the incidence of side effects is about 45 percent, and for some people, these involve problems with memory and cognition (Wagstaff, 2003; Evans 2009). Some people even develop Parkinson's disease.

An article published in 2009, which received a lot of press, claimed that people with dementia had higher levels of cholesterol at midlife (Solomon 2009). The article entitled "Midlife Serum Cholesterol Levels and Increased Risk of Alzheimer's and Vascular Dementia Three Decades Later" appeared in *Dementia and Geriatric Cognitive Disorders*. If you read the complete article, the average total cholesterol level at midlife for people who did not develop dementia three decades later was 224 mg/dl; with Alzheimer's, 228 mg/dl; and with vascular dementia, 226 mg/dl. (Vascular dementia is a general term describing problems with reasoning, planning, judgment, memory, and other thought processes caused by brain damage from impaired blood flow to the brain.) Due to the large number of people in the study (9,884), this tiny difference was considered statistically significant.

When the groups were looked at in terms of total cholesterol levels less than 200 mg/dl (considered normal), levels of 200 to 239 mg/dl (considered borderline), and high levels of 240 mg/dl or above, there was considerable overlap between the three groups. Of the people with Alzheimer's disease, 23 percent fell into the normal range, 40 percent in the borderline range, and 37 percent in the high range. Of people with vascular dementia, 23 percent had values in the normal range, 46 percent were borderline, and 31 percent had high levels. Of the people *without* dementia, 27 percent fell into the normal range, 41 percent were in the borderline range, and 32 percent were in the high range.

Interestingly, people with vascular dementia and people with no dementia had essentially the same rate of high total cholesterol levels. No data were collected on HDL or LDL levels, nor on whether the people were receiving lipid-lowering agents (statins). I wonder how a difference of four points in cholesterol, which can fluctuate that much day to day, could make the difference between having dementia and not having dementia three decades later? If anything, I believe this study shows that elevated cholesterol levels may not have much of an impact on Alzheimer's, or even on the development of vascular dementia, except perhaps when the person has a relatively rare genetic predisposition to extremely high cholesterol levels, known as familial hypercholesterolemia.

When statins first became available to treat elevated cholesterol levels, treatment was started at levels considerably higher than the current recommendations. Over the years, the level for treating cholesterol has gradually dropped to 200 mg/dl, and many physicians automatically begin statin treatment at this level without regard to the values of HDL and LDL, the ratio of HDL to LDL, or the ratio of LDL to total cholesterol, which may be more important. In addition, other risk factors for heart attack should be considered when deciding whether statins should be initiated, such as a history of high blood pressure, diabetes, strong family history of cardiac disease, such as heart attacks at mid-life and whether the individual is male or female, and whether there is evidence of inflammation, such as an elevated C-reactive protein. When we block production of cholesterol with a statin, it affects not only the cholesterol level (mostly LDL), but also the levels of sex and steroid hormones and production of other substances in the same pathway, including ketones. People taking statins may also become deficient in CoQ10, a very important enzyme in energy production. It is possible that some people taking statins may not respond as well to a dietary intervention with medium-chain fatty acids as those who are not taking statins. This has yet to be confirmed.

After everything I have read about cholesterol since Steve started using coconut oil, and weighing the known risks and benefits, we made a decision in the summer of 2009 to take Steve off simvastatin (Zocor), which is known to decrease production of cholesterol and actually remove cholesterol from the brain. It was not an easy decision, since we don't really know what the long-term consequences are of either keeping him on the drug or taking him off.

I am not suggesting that everyone discontinue statins or any other medications they are taking. I do suggest that each medication be carefully looked at by the physician with regard to whether each is necessary and whether the benefits outweigh the risks. Every treatment, every medication, carries risks and benefits. In the case of someone with advanced dementia, it is far more likely that the person will die of the dementia than of heart disease related to a new dietary change.

Does Coconut Oil Have an Effect on Cholesterol?

If the evidence related to the effect, or lack of effect, of saturated fats and cholesterol on disease seems cloudy, the evidence related to effects of coconut oil on cholesterol is even murkier. For many years, coconut oil has been called the artery-clogging fat due to its high saturated fat content, but as discussed in the previous pages, about 70 percent of the saturated fats in coconut oil are medium-chain fatty acids, which behave differently than the longer-chain saturated fatty acids.

As interest in the possible effects of cholesterol on human health grew in the 1950s and 1960s, numerous animal studies and small human studies were undertaken to try to learn about the effects of various oils singly or in combination with each other. Cocoa butter, palm oil (which contains considerable saturated fat but minimal medium-chain fatty acids), and coconut oil or palm kernel oil (different than palm oil) were often included in these studies when trying to compare saturated versus mono- or polyunsaturated fats. In some studies, the saturated fats were combined with polyunsaturated fats such as safflower or soybean oil in various proportions to try to learn something about how much each might influence the cholesterol level. Some studies used hydrogenated or partially hydrogenated fats. By feeding people diets of hydrogenated fats, with and without essential fatty acids, one study determined that the increases in total cholesterol and triglyceride fats and the lowering of HDL cholesterol that appeared to occur with the hydrogenated forms of saturated fats were actually the result of an EFA deficiency and not the saturated fat in the diet (Williams, 1989).

The early human studies were usually performed on a small number (two to twenty) of men, who were most often young, healthy college students, but sometimes older men with hypercholesterolemia and coronary artery disease (Cater, 1997), prisoners (Erickson, 1964), or schizophrenics on a psychiatric unit (Hegsted, 1965; Keys, 1957). The diets often consisted of carefully measured frozen meals and/or liquid formulas, with each subject serving as his own control, as they consumed each of several different diets in succession for three to five weeks at a time. Measurements of the cholesterol profile and triglycerides were taken at the onset of the study and at appropriate intervals as subjects were changed from one diet to another.

When the first large computers became available, attempts were made to construct formulas that could predict the cholesterol level based on the amount of saturated fat and the number of carbons in the chain of the fatty acids in the diet, but these were later found to be flawed (Keys, 1957, 1966; Grande, 1961; Hegsted, 1965). As the technology grew to make it possible to extract a particular fatty acid from oils, it was then possible to design studies to look at what effect an individual fatty acid might have on the lipid profile if added in excess to the diet (Tholstrup, 1994).

There were inherent differences in the diet formulations from study to study, and the results were often contradictory and didn't reflect eating in the real world, since the diet formulas were highly controlled and the people studied were in confined settings for many weeks. By 2003, with hundreds of such studies available, Ronald Mensink and others performed a meta-analysis (a statistical synthesis of related studies), combining results of sixty such studies of more than 1,600 individuals, performed between 1970 and 1998 that met strict criteria and, therefore, eliminated many poorly designed studies. They primarily focused on the effects of saturated, monounsaturated, and polyunsaturated fats, as well as individual fatty acids, partially hydrogenated fats, and trans fats on the level of HDL cholesterol and the ratio of total to HDL cholesterol (a lower number is better).

In relation to coconut oil, researchers found that lauric acid (a medium-chain fatty acid that comprises 50 percent of the fat in coconut oil) increased total cholesterol, but much of its effect was the result of raising HDL cholesterol. Lauric acid had a more favorable effect on the ratio of total cholesterol to HDL cholesterol than any other fatty acid, saturated or unsaturated, including the monounsaturate omega-9 oleic acid, the primary fatty acid in olive oil (Mensink, 2003). A trans-monounsaturated fatty acid (a trans fat left with just one double bond as a result of partial hydrogenation) was found to have the greatest negative effect of all the fatty acids, including the saturated fats, on HDL and total cholesterol to HDL ratio. Also of interest in this study, substituting an equal amount of calories of carbohydrate for any type of fat in the diet produced the most negative effect, more than double that of the most negative fatty acid, on HDL and the total cholesterol to HDL ratio.

People living in areas of the world such as the Philippines, Sri Lanka, Thailand, and the Pacific islands, when they include coconut and coconut oil as staples in their diet, have a low risk of cardiovascular disease compared to people in other areas of the world where coconut oil is not part of the diet (Dayrit, 2003; Lindeberg, 1993; Shorland, 1969). In one area of India where coconut and coconut oil are used extensively, an analysis of 124 patients admitted to a teaching hospital with signs and symptoms of dementia found that Alzheimer's represented less than 5 percent of these dementias (Jha, 2004).

One of the most striking studies is a population study performed by Ian Prior and others in 1981 on the Polynesian atolls Pukapuka and Tokelau, where coconut is a staple of the diet and part of every meal in one form or another. All of the men and women ages fifteen to sixty-four years old were included in these studies, 436 on Pukapuka and 948 on Tokelau. The researchers collected data over eight weeks to determine the average consumption of the various components of the diets. In both groups, the total cholesterol and triglyceride levels increased with age. For the Pukapukans, who consumed 34 percent of the calories in their diet as coconut, the average cholesterol level was 149 mg/dl in the youngest men and 180 mg/dl in the oldest men in the study; for the women, those levels were 170 and 194 mg/dl. The Tokelauans consumed almost twice as much coconut as the Pukapukans, an astounding 63 percent of their diet, and had higher levels. However, they varied from a low of 184 mg/dl in the teenage men to 217 mg/dl in the oldest men, and in the females, 197 mg/dl in the teens to 245 mg/dl in those aged fifty-five to sixty-four. None of these islanders had elevated triglyceride levels. At the time of this study, coronary heart disease was rare in these populations (Prior, 1981).

Until 2004, a cholesterol level of 240 was considered the cutoff for treating patients with statins here in the United States and only for people with other risk factors for heart disease. Only the oldest female Tokelauans would have qualified for such treatment, assuming they might have had any other risk factors. Also of interest, one might also expect that people eating 63 percent of their diet as coconut would be downright obese, but the heaviest Tokelauans were 173-pound middle-aged men. In both groups of islanders, coconut is also a staple in the diet of some of their other favorite foods, pigs and chickens, and such fats are incorporated into the adipose tissue of whatever animal or human consumes them, resulting in even more saturated fat intake for these people.

Prior also noted that immigrants from Tokelau to New Zealand experienced changes in their diet amounting to an actual decrease in saturated fat to around 41 percent of their total calorie intake, still very high by government standards. They also had increases in dietary cholesterol, carbohydrate, and sugar intake, and experienced increases in their total cholesterol levels, higher LDL cholesterol and triglyceride levels, and lower HDL cholesterol levels.

A similar, albeit smaller, five-year study was conducted of 100 men ages twenty to fifty with coronary disease whose average cholesterol levels were in the 235 to 250 mg/dl range (Bierenbaum, 1967). The men were instructed to eliminate certain dairy products (such as ice cream), rich desserts, pastries, fried foods, and fatty meats, and their diets were somewhat controlled by providing them with five frozen dinners per week. Otherwise they were free-living, working men. The men all received 28 percent of their diet as fat, but were divided into two groups, one receiving a mixture of corn-safflower oil (about 11 percent saturated fat) and the other a mixture of coconut-peanut oil (about 21 percent saturated fat and much lower in polyunsaturated fat). The important aspect of this study was the duration. The men were studied for twelve months and then followed up at five years. Although the cholesterol levels dropped by as much as 10 percent in some of the men during the early months, the levels returned to baseline by the end of the year. Researchers found no difference in the cholesterol levels between the two groups at twelve months and at five years, even though the second group consumed twice as much saturated fat, primarily from coconut oil.

Does Medium-Chain Triglyceride Oil Have an Effect on Cholesterol?

There have also been a number of studies looking at the effect of medium-chain triglyceride (MCT) oil on cholesterol levels. One small study showed an increase in cholesterol related to MCT oil (Cater, 1997). Nine male subjects with coronary artery disease, ages fifty-five to seventy-five, were studied on a metabolic ward, divided into three groups, and given one of three fats (palm oil, sunflower oil, or MCT oil) as the only fat in the diet for three weeks; then they were crossed over to the other diets in succession. When the men received the MCT oil or palm oil, they had higher levels of total cholesterol levels, mostly due to increases in LDL levels. A significant problem with this study is that neither MCT oil nor palm oil contains any omega-3 essential fatty acids, and MCT oil contains no omega-6 essential fatty acids. As discussed earlier in this chapter, EFA deficiency would be expected to produce these findings. Other studies of MCT oil have shown a neutral effect, or even a favorable effect on cholesterol levels when essential fatty acids are also added to the diet (Beveridge, 1959; Bourque, 2003; St-Onge, 2008).

Using Common Sense and Safeguards

The proponents and detractors of coconut oil can each point to small studies that favor their point of view. Many of these studies do not reflect eating in the real world. A large-scale study of the effects of prolonged coconut oil consumption in men and women of all ages, and especially in the elderly, is needed to answer this question once and for all. Such a study needs to look at people consuming their usual diet, and the use of coconut oil should be considered in the context of other aspects of the diet. Care would be required to ensure that non-hydrogenated coconut oil is used and that an appropriate balance of omega-3 fatty acids is included. Such a study would not be an easy undertaking, since the diet as a whole can vary significantly from person to person.

Until we know conclusively the relationship between coconut oil and cholesterol, I suggest physicians monitor the lipid profile. Where elevated total cholesterol with low HDL levels is a concern, it behooves the physician to look closely at other elements of the patient's diet that may contribute to this problem, particularly the use of partially hydrogenated oils and fats, as well as high-sugar or high-carbohydrate intake, and high-caloric intake. Low-carbohydrate diets have been found to normalize blood lipids such as triglycerides and LDL while increasing HDL. Triglycerides are formed by combining a glycerol molecule with three molecules of fatty acid and are always present in the bloodstream. Abnormally high triglyceride levels have been linked to atherosclerosis (hardening of the arteries), which can further lead to a higher risk of heart disease and stroke.

There is a misconception that elevated triglyceride levels come from eating too much fat, when, in fact, they are related in general to an excess of calories and in particular to an excess of carbohydrates (sugar) in the typical American diet. For those with elevated triglyceride levels, the physician or dietician should inquire about how much and what types of high carbohydrate foods are in the diet. It is surprising, for example, how many people consume a half-gallon or more of soda pop in a day. Each 12-ounce can of the leading brands of cola contain 40 grams of carbohydrate, the equivalent of 8 teaspoons of sugar. A half-gallon of soda contains about 213 grams, or 43 teaspoons of sugar. Mind-boggling! Each time you consume a can of soda, a spike in blood sugar and insulin follows. This viscous cycle may contribute to the development of insulin resistance and eventually type 2 diabetes mellitus, which inflicts damage on the brain, eyes, kidneys, and other organs. As you learned in Chapter 14, people with diabetes are at considerably higher risk than the average person of developing dementia.

Any hydrogenated or partially hydrogenated oil, including coconut oil, will increase LDL cholesterol levels, so it is very important when incorporating coconut oil into the diet to use *non-hydrogenated* coconut oil. The government requires that if a food contains hydrogenated or partially hydrogenated fats that these words must appear on the label, so you can be assured that the oil is non-hydrogenated if it is not stated on the label. If you want reassurance, most labels have a toll-free number to call to learn more about the product. In addition, the less processed the coconut oil is, the more healthy nutrients it will contain, so it is worthwhile to use *organic, virgin* coconut oil.

Many who start incorporating coconut oil in their diet will be pleased to see an increase in HDL cholesterol and a decrease in triglycerides, particularly if coconut oil is *substituted for* other fats in the diet, rather than simply added to the diet. In addition, an even more positive effect is likely if hydrogenated and partially hydrogenated oils are eliminated from the diet. The best way to accomplish this is to look closely at labels of packaged foods and avoid certain fast-food restaurants.

MORE THOUGHTS ON FATTY ACIDS

The current Western diet has drifted very far from the diet of our ancestors just over the last fifty years. The major change in the types of fats we eat is just one important aspect of the difference between our diet and our grandparents' diet. By consuming oils that contain trans fats and an overabundance of omega-6 fatty acids that favor inflammation, we, as a society and as individuals, may be paying dearly with an exponential rise in avoidable diseases, such as high blood pressure, heart disease, diabetes, and neurodegenerative diseases. Other important changes in our diet, discussed in the next chapter, further compound this problem.

There is still a great deal to be learned about the exact roles that each fatty acid plays in our bodies, particularly in our brains. For an extensive discussion of everything you may want to know about fats and fatty acids, I highly recommend a book by Dr. Enig called *Know Your Fats* (2000). I read this book cover to cover shortly after embarking on my Internet frenzy related to coconut oil to help Steve. This is the most highlighted and dog-eared book in my library. Another excellent series of books for those who want to learn more about coconut oil are those written by Bruce Fife, N.D. His books are very thoroughly researched and documented. My favorite is *Coconut Cures* (2005), which includes an extensive discussion of the various research studies related to coconut oil and the questions related to the saturated fat/cholesterol issue and heart disease.

22

Why Diet Makes a Difference

Diet is something that is within our complete control. Except in infancy and very unusual circumstances, we determine every bite we put into our mouths and how much we eat. For many years, I was extremely overweight and felt that this was the one area of my life (at least until Steve developed dementia) that I was going to have to accept as my fate. I was somehow born to be fat—it was in my genes. When I came to accept that, in fact, I have complete control over my diet, I adopted a healthier way of eating and began to incorporate exercise into my hectic life. I was finally able to the lose weight that was holding me back.

In 2005, I was very overweight, on the verge of type 2 diabetes, my heart was enlarged, and I had osteoporosis. I was mystified in particular about the osteoporosis, since I consumed at least three to four servings of dairy every day and even took calcium supplements. I recently learned from Beverly Teter, Ph.D., a lipid biochemist at the University of Maryland, that short-chain fatty acids in dairy products optimize the absorption of calcium from the intestine into the circulation. Unless you consume whole-fat dairy, the calcium in these foods will not be fully absorbed. For decades, I thought I was doing myself a favor and saving calories by consuming fat-free dairy products. Use of fat-free milk didn't keep me from gaining weight, in fact, quite the contrary.

The phrase "you are what you eat" may seem trite and over-used, but it is a fact. We should think about this every time we eat.

FOOD: FRESH AND WHOLE VS. PACKAGED AND PROCESSED

Food is many other things to people, but when it comes right down to it, nearly everything we put into our mouths is broken down to be used immediately by our bodies or stored for future use. The cells of our bodies are extremely complex and dynamic. We are constantly making new cells to replace old cells. What we eat will affect the quality (how well they function) and the life span of the new cells we make.

Much of what we eat is used to fuel the cells in the body either now or later. This is true of the major components of food, which are carbohydrate, protein, and fat—all of which can be used for fuel. These macronutrients, along with thousands of other micro-nutrients, are needed to make new cells by providing the required energy and building blocks. These include the numerous vitamins and minerals that we are all familiar with, but also many we may not be so familiar with, such as the phytonutrients.

Phytonutrients are compounds found in plants that may affect our health. In recent years, hundreds of phytonutrients have been discovered, and we are learning new things every day about what they do for us. Many of these phytonutrients work in conjunction with vitamins and minerals to carry out various processes in the body. Some phytonutrients prevent damage to cells, while others help keep us healthy by reducing our chances of developing infec-tions or certain cancers. One good reason to eat a variety of fresh, or freshly frozen, fruits and vegetables is to take in as many of these nutrients as possible every day, since they are often lost when food is canned or otherwise processed.

Food as a Foreign Substance

When we eat processed foods not only do our bodies miss out on the natural substances they need to function at their fullest potential, but we also end up consuming an abundance of chemicals that are used to enhance color and taste, inhibit the growth of bacteria, and increase the shelf life of these goods. The use of these methods of manufacturing food has come about as a result of the huge population growth in recent history. All these people must be fed, and advances in technology have made it possible to mass-produce food and deliver it wherever it is needed. The downside is that much of our food has become overly processed and laden with these additives and potentially harmful artifical ingredients.

Many of the substances in our foods are foreign to our bodies. They were not part of the fresh, unprocessed food eaten by humans for our entire history as a species until the past century. We are not programmed to use many of these chemicals, but they will be used, one way or the other, by our bodies. Some of these substances, such as partially hydrogenated fats, trans fats, and high-fructose corn syrup, may very well be used in ways that are harmful to us. For example, in the past, humans consumed milk that was fresh from the cow, without pasteurization and homogenization. Now, primarily to extend shelf life and feed the masses, most of the milk we drink has been seriously tinkered with. The fat is removed from the milk and homogenized to allow it to mix uniformly so the cream does not separate and rise to the top. Then this processed fat is placed back into the other components of the milk in various percentages to make fat-free, low-fat, or whole-fat milk. Do the fats in milk behave the same way once they are processed this way? According to Dr. Teter and others, they do not.

Fresh, unprocessed milk tastes quite different, in a good way, from the processed stuff. It is illegal to sell raw milk in many states due to the fear of infection, a realistic concern, since milk must be stored and transported to feed so many. In Florida, where we live, raw milk cannot be sold for human consumption and must be labeled "for pet consumption only!" (If you can get access to raw milk from a quality dairy farm, it may be well worth your efforts to do so. It is even possible in some areas to get raw goat milk, which contains a significant amount of medium-chain fatty acids.) This may seem radical but consider that less than a century ago, and for millennia before that, our ancestors drank raw milk. What has happened to *our* food is radical. Moreover, today, we have to worry about the pesticides, hormones, and antibiotics taken in by the animals and the products derived from them that we eat.

A WHOLE FOOD DIET

The easiest way to avoid consuming these substances is to stay away from packaged cookies, crackers, pastries, ready-to-eat foods and snacks, and other processed foods as much as possible and to embrace an organic, whole food diet. This type of diet includes a variety of different colored fresh fruits and vegetables, nuts and legumes, whole grains, natural unprocessed oils, wild rather than farm-raised fish, and full-fat dairy or goat's milk, eggs, poultry, and meat from free-range, grass-fed animals. In an ideal world we would all have access to these quality foods. If they are available, we will be better off making these choices whenever possible. If you have access to fruits and vegetables from local farmers, they may be smaller, but will probably taste better, and be better for you, than the larger, genetically engineered produce that has lost much of its nutrient content.

Read Labels

It is important to note that not all packaged foods are bad. Some food manufacturers are making the effort to provide products without an abundance of chemicals. Just look at the ingredients label to decide for yourself. If there is a list of chemicals that you don't recognize, consider putting it back rather than taking it home. Look for products that contain whole grains, such as whole grain rice or whole-wheat flour, rather than "refined" or "enriched" flours. Refined flours, for example, have been overly processed and much of the micronutrient content that we need has been removed. They are then "enriched" with a few essential vitamins to try to make up for this.

Packaging, however, can also be deceptive. You may see "contains whole grains" on the package, but bleached, enriched flour will come first on the list of ingredients. Also, you will see "100 percent virgin olive oil" on the front label of some salad dressings, and it is indeed one of the ingredients, but the product actually contains more soybean oil (a primarily polyunsaturated oil) than olive oil (a primarily monounsaturated oil), according to the order on the ingredients label. I am also willing to bet that most people don't know that the majority of peanut butters on grocery store shelves contain partially hydrogenated soybean oil. We have been eating these same brand-name products for decades without even thinking about it. Just look at the list of ingredients on the label! You will be very surprised to see how many foods contain unhealthy fats and foreign non-food substances.

It may not be possible to eliminate every type of processed food from your diet, depending on where you live and what you have access to, but any steps you can take in that direction will be beneficial to your health.

Can a Healthy Diet Prevent Alzheimer's Disease?

Steve and I are among the first generation to live most of our lives on the "convenience diet." We were the first in our families to buy a microwave oven when I was in medical school in the 1970s so that we could take advantage of packaged foods and otherwise speed up cooking. I did not believe that I had the time to cook the way our mothers did and embraced any opportunity to reduce the time I spent in the kitchen. I am afraid that we are paying for this now. The biochemistry classes I took in medical school taught me how food is metabolized but not how to eat.

In researching Steve's disease, I have learned more about nutrition in the last five years than in the previous thirty years of my medical training and practice. Since 2005, we have completely revamped our diet. If you had told me in 2004 that I would be frequenting whole food and natural food grocery stores, eating fresh fruits and vegetables, and cooking healthy meals every day, I would have looked at you cross-eyed. Do we ever eat packaged or processed foods? I would not be telling the truth if I said no to that question. However, these types of foods are now at the bottom of the list rather than the top of our food choices and probably make up less than 5 percent of what we eat. When I pick up a package in the store, I look at the ingredients list, and if I don't like what I see, I put it back.

With the convenience diet, we are taking in too many things that we don't need and we are not getting enough of important nutrients that we do need. Since we are what we eat, then it is very possible that something we are eating, or not eating, triggers and/or promotes the development of Alzheimer's and other neurodegenerative diseases. If you or a loved one are fighting a neurodegenerative disease, or want to avoid acquiring one, consider making the transition to a healthier whole food diet.

SUPPLEMENTS AND DIET

I know of many people who take a huge number of different supplements to try to undo the damage from Alzheimer's and other diseases, yet continue to eat an overly processed diet, stripped of nutrients and laden with additives and partially hydrogenated fats. It makes good sense to try to provide ourselves with nutrients our bodies will recognize and use the way evolution has programmed us to use them. While certain supplements, such as omega-3 fatty acids, may help us in the fight against disease, supplements alone may not be able to overcome the ongoing damage that we may inflict upon ourselves by continuing to consume a convenience food diet. I have spoken with many caregivers who provide their loved ones with an abundance of different supplements, but pay very little attention to their diet. They cannot be convinced how important it is for them to stop drinking soda pop or binging on other sugary, highly processed foods that promote insulin resistance.

Many important nutrients are not absorbed into the body unless there is fat in the meal. For example, vitamins A, D, and E are fat-soluble vitamins, meaning that, unless they are in an oil-based substance or at least emulsified so they can mix with water, they will not be absorbed. It may be pointless to try to get your daily requirement of these vitamins in the form of a dry pill. It is more beneficial to get these vitamins in an oil-based product, and even better, in an actual food in which they naturally occur, such as cod liver oil, whole-fat dairy products, and eggs.

There is considerable evidence now that vitamins do not act alone. Hundreds of phytonutrients accompany the vitamin in natural foods and support the absorption and use of the vitamin in the body. So, in the best of all worlds, we will get our vitamins naturally. In the case of vitamin D, we can achieve this with relatively small doses of exposure to the sun, and for the other vitamins from consuming the foods in which they typically occur.

Remember, to derive the best level of nutrition, eat unprocessed food with nothing added or taken away. Eat beef, fish, and poultry and the other products derived from these animals, such as dairy and eggs, from animals that are allowed to eat their own natural diet, rather than an excess of grain that they would not normally consume if they were in the wild. Incorporate a variety of colors of fresh produce to ensure you take in a variety of antioxidants, vitamins, and other nutrients, and drink whole-fat milk, or better yet, raw milk if available.

There is clearly a role for dietary supplements in the fight against Alzheimer's and other such diseases. However, there is no medication or supplement that can undo the ill effects of an unhealthy diet or take the place of a healthy diet. The primary role of dietary supplements should be literally to supplement the healthy diet as secondary insurance to make sure that certain important nutrients are provided.

23

Questions and Answers about Coconut Oil

Until a commercial ketone ester is available to us, the next best strategy we can undertake is to incorporate medium-chain fatty acids into our diet. Medium-chain fatty acids are taken up directly from the intestine into the liver, where they are partially converted to ketones. These ketones are then taken up quickly by cells that can use them, including those in the brain, and can serve as an alternative fuel for cells that are unable to use glucose effectively. In addition, medium-chain fatty acids can be used directly as fuel by mitochondria, the tiny organelles inside of cells that generate ATP.

There are several ways to incorporate medium-chain fatty acids into the diet: with coconut oil, medium-chain triglyceride (MCT) oil, and foods and products rich in these medium-chain fatty acids. This chapter focuses mainly on answering frequently asked questions about coconut oil and coconut oil in foods. The following chapter will answer questions concerning MCT oil and products that contain MCT oil.

COCONUT OIL

Who Should Try Dietary Intervention with Coconut Oil?

People who have a neurodegenerative disease that involves decreased glucose uptake in neurons may benefit from taking higher amounts of coconut and/or MCT oil to produce ketones, which may be used by brain cells and other organs as energy. These diseases include Alzheimer's and other dementias, Parkinson's, Lou Gehrig's disease (amyotrophic lateral sclerosis, or ALS), multiple sclerosis, Duchenne muscular dystrophy, autism, Down syndrome, and Huntington's chorea. There are a number of uncommon conditions that also involve decreased glucose uptake in the brain or other organs that could respond (for a list of the conditions, see page 262). Your physician should be able to help you learn if this dietary intervention is appropriate for you or your loved one.

If you are at risk for one of these diseases due to family history, you might consider making this dietary change to try to prevent or at least delay the onset and lessen the effects of the disease.

Some rare conditions involve a problem of fat metabolism in which the use of coconut oil and/or MCT oil *may not be appropriate and may even worsen the condition.* Therefore, consultation with your physician is very important.

What Are Some Benefits of Coconut Oil?

Coconut oil is easily absorbed by the body and increases absorption of certain vitamins and minerals and other important nutrients. This also holds true for coconut milk and coconut meat, whether wet or dry, such as flaked or grated coconut. The fiber in coconut meat may be especially beneficial for people with Crohn's disease, other types of inflammatory bowel disease or other malabsorption syndromes, and for people who have diarrhea from coconut or MCT oil.

All cell membranes and about 60 to 70 percent of the brain are largely made up of fats. Many cell functions take place within the cell membrane. The majority of the fats most of us consume today are vegetable oils, usually soybean or canola oil. These oils often contain hydrogenated and partially hydrogenated polyunsaturated fats and trans fats, which can carry potentially damaging oxygen free radicals into cell membranes. Even nonhydrogenated polyunsaturated fatty acids can become oxidized (rancid) and pick up oxygen free radicals. If you begin to substitute coconut and other natural oils, such as olive oil and even butter, along with omega-3 fatty acids in your meals, you may be able to undo some of the damage. Most of the cells in the body turn over within three to six months, and you may notice a nicer texture to your skin and a decrease in certain problems such as yeast and fungal infections.

Coconut oil is a wonderful moisturizer and is used in tanning lotions and other skin care products. In the tropics and areas where coconut oil is readily available, it is often applied to the skin before going out in the sun. Some people use coconut oil in their hair as a natural conditioner. Coconut oil feels soothing, is not sticky, and is absorbed readily into the skin. For dry skin, it can be applied while still damp after showering; then the skin can be blotted dry.

For a lengthy discussion of the many other benefits of coconut oil, I highly recommend the book *Coconut Cures* (2005) by Bruce Fife, N.D.

What If My Loved One with Alzheimer's Is Apoe4+? Should We Bother Trying This?

Yes! In the Accera studies (the makers of Axona, the prescription powdered form of MCT oil), even though the ApoE4+ people as a group did not show improvement, many of the individuals with that genetic make-up did have improved scores on cognitive testing. This was not noted in the article in which the study results were published, but I learned this in conversation with one of the authors. In addition, Steve is ApoE4+ and responded to treatment with medium-chain fatty acids.

How Much Coconut Oil Should I Take?

If you take too much oil too fast, you may experience indigestion, cramping, or diarrhea. To avoid these symptoms, take coconut oil with food and start with one teaspoon per meal, increasing slowly as tolerated over a week or longer.

If diarrhea develops, drop back to the previous level and stay at that level for at least a few days before trying to increase again. See more ideas for reducing the problem of diarrhea later in this chapter.

For most people, the goal is to increase gradually to four to six tablespoons a day, depending on the size of the person, spread over two to four meals. Not everyone will be able to tolerate this much oil.

Mixing MCT oil and coconut oil could provide higher levels and a steady level of ketones. One formula is to mix 16 ounces MCT oil plus 12 ounces coconut oil in a quart jar and increase slowly as tolerated, starting with one teaspoon. This mixture will stay liquid at room temperature. See more about MCT oil in Chapter 24.

How Can Coconut Oil Be Used in the Diet?

Coconut oil can be substituted for any solid or liquid oil, lard, butter, or margarine in baking or cooking on the stove, and it can be mixed directly into foods already prepared. Some people take it straight with a spoon, but many people may find it hard to swallow this way and more pleasant to take with food.

Use coconut oil instead of butter on toast, English muffins, bagels, grits, corn on the cob, potatoes, sweet potatoes, rice, vegetables, noodles, and pasta. When stir-frying or sautéing on the stove, coconut oil smokes if heated to more than 350°F or medium heat. You can avoid this by adding a little olive or peanut oil. Coconut oil can be used at any temperature in the oven when mixed in foods. Mix coconut oil into your favorite soup, chili, or sauce. It can also be basted onto foods such as fish as long as the oven temperature is 350°F or below.

Coconut oil tends to become hard when exposed to cold foods. For example, if used as a salad dressing, it will turn into hard little chunks if the vegetables in the salad come straight out of the refrigerator. Some people actually like this effect and call them "crunchies." If not, try adding equal amounts of coconut oil to another favorite salad dressing that has been warmed slightly. Also, the mixture of MCT and coconut oil tends to stay liquid and works well in this situation. This also enables you to add it to smoothies, yogurt, or kefir.

For those who cannot handle coconut oil, grated or flaked coconut, coconut milk, and fresh coconut may be good substitutes, as they are digested much more slowly. Ideas for incorporating these foods into the diet are discussed later in the chapter. Caregivers have found very creative ways to get coconut oil into the diet of their loved ones. Two of my favorite recipes are for coconut macaroons (page 361) and coconut fudge (page 362). Also check the Resources section for cookbooks containing many more great ideas and recipes.

What Is the Nutrient Content of Coconut Oil?

Coconut oil has about 117 to 120 calories per tablespoon, about the same as other oils. It contains 57 to 60 percent medium-chain fatty acids, which are absorbed directly from the intestine without the need for digestive enzymes. This portion of the coconut oil is not stored as fat. Coconut oil is about 86 percent saturated fats, most of which are the medium-chain fats that are metabolized differently than animal saturated fats. The oil contains no cholesterol and no trans fat as long as it is nonhydrogenated. An advantage of a saturated fat is that there is nowhere on the molecule for free radicals or oxidants to attach. About 6 percent of coconut oil is monounsaturated fats and 2 percent polyunsaturated fats. Coconut oil also contains a small amount of phytosterols, which are one of the components of the statins used for lowering cholesterol.

Coconut oil contains a small amount of omega-6 fatty acids but *no* omega-3 fatty acid, so this must be taken in addition to coconut oil. You can obtain all the essential fatty acids required by using just coconut oil and omega-3 fatty acids. If you were to use coconut oil as your primary oil, the only other oil you would need is one that contains omega-3 fatty acids. You can get this by eating salmon twice a week; taking liquid fish oil or cod liver oil, which also contains significant amounts of vitamins A, D, and E; or taking fish oil or flax oil capsules, at least two to three per day. Some other good sources of omega-3 fatty acids are ground flax meal, chia (a fine grain), walnuts and walnut oil, lingonberry, and purslane. Soybeans, soybean oil, and canola oil contain small amounts of omega-3 fatty acids. It is important to note here that the basic omega-3 fats found in vegetable sources, alpha-linolenic acid (ALA), may not readily convert to the very important docosahexaenoic acid (DHA) and eicosapentaenoic acid (EPA) omega-3 fatty acids that are also essential. DHA makes up 50 percent of the neuron's plasma membrane, and low levels of DHA have been associated with Alzheimer's disease as well as many other conditions. DHA is so important that very strong consideration should be given to getting this fatty acid directly from a marine source.

Lauric acid is a medium-chain fatty acid that makes up almost half of coconut oil and is a saturated fat. Scientific studies show that lauric acid has antimicrobial properties and may inhibit growth of certain bacteria, fungi/yeast, viruses, and protozoa. It is one of the components of human breast milk that prevents infection in a newborn. Coconut oil and/or palm kernel oil, which have a similar composition of fats, are added to nearly every infant formula to try to duplicate the important fatty acids, such as lauric acid, found in human breast milk. It is quite remarkable that coconut oil is considered so very safe and even important for the human newborn and yet considered by many to be dangerous for the adult human. The inconsistency here is mind-boggling.

What Kind of Coconut Oil Should I Use?

Be sure to examine the label on the back of the jar or container. Look for coconut oils that are nonhydrogenated with no trans fat. Avoid coconut oils that are partially hydrogenated or super-heated because these processes change the chemical structure of the fats. In the United States, food manufacturers are required to state on the product label if there are hydrogenated or partially hydrogenated oils and trans fats. One caution is that they can state on labels that there are no trans fats if a serving contains less than 0.5 grams. This can be deceptive, since the serving size is often adjusted accordingly.

Two types of coconut oil are on the market: unrefined and refined. The label for unrefined coconut oil normally reads "virgin" or "extra virgin," may read "raw," and most often also reads "organic." These unrefined oils are generally pressed from freshly harvested coconuts and are rarely exposed to high levels of heat. As a result, they are more flavorful and nutritious than refined coconut oils, and tend to be more expensive, largely because the nature of the equipment and the process used in removing the oils from the meat are more costly to the manufacturer.

There are quality differences with more than six different ways of making virgin coconut oil. Generally, some type of mechanical process, such as a press or a centrifuge is used rather than chemicals to separate the oil from the coconut meat; one example is the process called direct micro-expelling (DME) developed by Dan Etherington of Kokonut Pacific in Australia. DME is a cold (low-heat) process of pressing the oil from the fresh meat within one hour of opening the coconut.

Refined coconut oil is made from copra (dried coconut flesh), which, in the drying process and transit time to the oil mills often picks up mold and off-flavors, thus it needs to be refined to be palatable. The label usually reads "regular," "all natural," or "RBD" (refined, bleached, and deodorized). The dried coconut is soaked in bleach and solvents are used to leech out the oils, which are subjected to high temperatures to further purify and liquefy the oils. Refined coconut oils have virtually no coconut taste or aroma.

Coconut oil can be found at your local health food stores and natural food markets, most Asian markets, some traditional grocery stores, as well as large department stores with grocery sections. You can also use the Internet to find other quality brands of coconut oil and at a wide range of prices not available at your local retailers, however, the quality can vary enormously; don't expect the highest quality for the lowest price.

Check the Resources section for a listing of websites offering coconut oil and coconut oil products.

What about Using Coconut Oil Capsules?

Using coconut oil capsules is not an efficient way to give the oil since the capsules are relatively expensive and nearly all contain only 1 gram of oil per capsule, whereas there are 14 grams in one tablespoon of oil. Some products state there are 4 grams per serving; however, the serving size is four capsules. It would require taking about fourteen capsules to equal one tablespoon of coconut oil, so it may not be practical and could be expensive to use capsules. On the other hand, for people who will not use the oil in liquid form and have no problem with swallowing capsules, this may offer an alternative. (See the Resources section.)

Why Does Coconut Oil Look Cloudy?

Coconut oil is a clear or slightly yellow liquid above 76°F but becomes solid at 76°F and below. If your house is kept right around 76°F, you may even see partly liquid oil with solid clouds floating in it. If your home is generally kept at 75°F or below, the oil will tend to be a white or slightly yellow, and soft to semi-solid.

What Other Coconut Products Contain Coconut Oil?

- Coconut milk is a combination of the oil and the water from the coconut, and most of the calories are from the oil. Look for brands with 10 to 13 grams of fat in 2 ounces. Coconut milk also contains some protein and a small amount of carbohydrate, which gives it a slightly sweet taste. Coconut milk can generally be found in natural foods stores, Asian stores, and the Asian and/or Hispanic sections of traditional grocery stores. Look at the fat content closely on the label, and be aware that some less expensive brands are considerably diluted with water. You can dilute condensed coconut milk yourself with water, or even better, with coconut water, which is loaded with vitamins and other nutrients. Organic coconut milk products are also available. Some coconut milks are also labeled "light" or "lite." Much of the oil has been removed, and using these lower fat products defeats our purpose of including coconut oil in the diet. Coconut milk blends very well into smoothies and is a tasty substitute for cow's milk on cereal or right out of the glass. Coconut milk can be substituted for some or all of the milk in many recipes.

- Some wonderful ice creams are now available in a variety of flavors made with coconut milk as the first ingredient. Coconut milk ice creams are available at Asian markets, many natural food stores, and some traditional grocery stores. There are even some ice cream products labeled "gluten free." Coconut ice cream may be one way to encourage coconut oil intake for someone with a sweet tooth or for an otherwise uncooperative loved one.

- Coconut cream is mostly coconut milk, often has added sugar, and comes in liquid and powdered forms.

- Flaked or grated coconut can be purchased unsweetened or sweetened and is a very good source of coconut oil and fiber. Grated coconut has about 15 grams of oil and 3 grams of fiber in one-fourth cup; in fact, about 70 percent of the carbohydrate content is fiber. The oil in grated coconut can help with absorption of certain vitamins and other nutrients as well. Flaked or grated coconut can be bought in bulk, usually for less than three dollars per pound, at many natural food stores, and can be added to cold or hot cereals, smoothies, soup, ricotta or cottage cheese, and used as a topper for ice cream. Flaked coconut is often found in trail mix, and some people snack on unsweetened flaked coconut. Homemade or store-bought macaroons are a delicious source of coconut.

- Frozen or canned coconut meat often has a lot of added sugar and not much oil per serving. Coconut meat can also be found in jars as coconut balls and "coconut sport," which is large strands of coconut. These products are especially nice for adding to fruit salads.

- A fresh coconut can be cut up into pieces and eaten raw. A 2-inch square piece has about 160 calories with 15 grams of oil (equivalent to about one tablespoon oil) and 4 grams of fiber. Removing the meat from the coconut can be quite a challenge, however. In Bruce Fife's *The Coconut Lover's Cookbook* (2008), he suggests heating the whole coconut in an oven for twenty minutes at 400°F after poking two holes in the eyes of the coconut and draining the coconut water. I like to strain off the coconut water, and then Steve and I share it, since it has significant nutrients as well. After the coconut cools down, it can be opened with a hammer or whatever tool you can think of. To avoid shattering anything important, we take the coconut outside and crack it open on newspapers covering the garage floor. The meat can usually be pried from the shell with a blunt knife.

This is quite a process and can be time consuming, but some consider it well worth it. Pieces of coconut meat can be saved for a week or longer in the freezer.

- Coconut water does not usually contain coconut oil, but does contain many other nutrients and has other health benefits. The electrolyte composition is similar to human plasma and is useful to prevent or treat dehydration. Coconut water has been used as intravenous fluid in Asia and was even used by our American troops when supplies of standard intravenous fluids were low. Coconut water is coming into its own now as a sports drink.

- MCT oil is part of the coconut oil and can also be purchased in some natural food stores or on the Internet. (Check the Resources section for listings.) This may be useful for people who are on the go and do not have much time to cook. MCT oil can also be mixed with coconut oil as described in the next chapter. MCT oil is used as energy and not stored as fat, so it may be useful for someone who wants to lose weight if it is substituted for some other fats in the diet.

What Are Some Coconut Oil Equivalents?

The following coconut foods contain the equivalent of 1 tablespoon of coconut oil:

- Coconut milk (undiluted): $4^1/_2$ tablespoons
- Coconut meat: 2- x 2- x $^1/_2$-inch piece
- Coconut grated: $^1/_3$ cup
- Coconut oil capsules (1 gram): 14 capsules

How Should Coconut Products Be Stored?

Coconut oil is extremely stable with a shelf life of at least two years when stored at room temperature. The container should have an expiration date on it. In the refrigerator, coconut oil becomes quite hard, so you may need a chisel to get it out of the jar! If you wish to keep it in the refrigerator, you can measure out one or two tablespoons into each section of a plastic ice cube tray. The coconut oil pops easily out of the tray. Refrigeration is not necessary, but some people may be more comfortable storing it this way.

Coconut milk is mostly coconut oil and can be substituted for the oil in many ways. Coconut milk must be refrigerated after opening, and should be used within a few days or tossed out.

Grated or flaked coconut can be stored at room temperature, but may last longer if stored in a refrigerator.

A freshly cut coconut can be stored in the refrigerator for a few days or freezer for a couple of weeks.

What Other Foods Contain Short- and Medium-Chain Fatty Acids?

Some other foods contain short- and medium-chain fatty acids that are worth mentioning, including whole cow's milk, goat's milk, and cheeses. Table 23.1 shows the content (in grams per ounce) of short- and medium-chain fatty acids contained in these and other foods. Short-chain fatty acids behave similarly to medium-chain fatty acids in that they are also converted to ketones in the liver. In general, the amounts are considerably less than in coconut oil. However, using these foods may contribute to the overall production of ketones. In other parts of the world, certain oils listed in Table 23.1 may be more available than in the United States.

As a point of reference about how important medium-chain fatty acids are to humans, a ten-pound breastfeeding baby gets about 3.12 grams medium-chain fatty acids per quart of breast milk. Extrapolated to a 150-pound adult, that would be the equivalent of 47 grams of medium-chain fatty acids and would require eating five and a half tablespoons of coconut oil.

To try to duplicate what is in human breast milk, infant formulas contain medium-chain triglyceride oil as well as coconut and/or

TABLE 23.1. FOODS WITH SHORT- AND MEDIUM-CHAIN FATTY ACIDS

FATS AND OILS	GRAMS PER 0.5 OUNCE (approximately 3 tsp/15 ml)
Coconut oil	8.3
Babassu oil	7.7
Palm kernel oil	7.5
Goat butter	2.4
Ucuhuba butter	1.8
Cow butter	1.6
Nutmeg butter	0.4
Shea nut butter	0.24
Lard	0.04

CREAM AND CHEESE	GRAMS PER OUNCE (approximately 6 tsp/30 ml)
Goat cheese	2.0
Feta cheese	1.4
Cream (heavy)	1.3
Cream cheese	1.0
American cheese	0.85
Mozzarella	0.78

MILKS AND COTTAGE CHEESE	GRAMS PER 8 OUNCES (approximately 1 cup/240 ml)
Goat milk	1.7
Infant formula	1.0
Cow milk (full-fat)	0.9
Human breast milk	0.78
Cottage cheese	0.78

Note: The following commonly eaten fats and oils contain no short- and medium-chain fatty acids: canola, cod liver, corn, fish, flaxseed, olive, peanut, safflower, soybean and sunflower oils, as well as margarine.

Source: USDA National Nutrient Database for Standard Reference, Release 23. Agricultural Research Service (www.ars.usda.gov/nutrientdata), 2010.

palm kernel oil. When children are weaned from the breast and from infant formulas, the usual next step in the United States is to transition to cow's milk. In recent years, there has been a push to encourage feeding even small children low-fat or fat-free milk and milk products, which would eliminate virtually every potential source of medium-chain fatty acids from the diet of the average child.

It may interest some readers to know that the mother of a child with autism contacted me because she had observed that the seizures and other neurologic symptoms related to her disease began to occur shortly after she was weaned off infant formula. After she read my July 2008 article, it occurred to her that perhaps the medium-chain fatty acids in the formula had delayed the onset of the disease. Some parents of children with autism believe that a vaccine triggers the disease. Many children receive a "junior" formula until fifteen to eighteen months of age, at which point they are weaned to cow's milk. It just so happens that certain vaccines are given at the same visits at which the pediatrician suggests it is time to come off formula. Could there be a relationship between the lack of medium-chain fatty acids in the diet and autism?

At this point, I must repeat that medium-chain fatty acids may be essential fatty acids, not only for adults but also for children. Many people with Alzheimer's have a life-long history of memory problems. Could consuming these fatty acids beginning in childhood lessen this problem? I also believe there is an autism/ Alzheimer's connection.

Are There Any Commercial Products Available That Contain a Mixture of Coconut Oil and MCT Oil?

In its natural state at room temperature, coconut oil is usually solid and, as mentioned earlier, can be challenging to measure and mix with other foods. By the time this book is published, new products may be on the market to make the process of incorporating coconut oil in the diet considerably easier.

One such product under development is called Cocomul from Cognate Nutritionals, a company for which I serve as an advisor. It is a liquid nutritional supplement that is easily taken "as is" in measured amounts or can be mixed with other liquids or foods. Cocomul contains both coconut oil and MCT oil and therefore provides a large measure of medium-chain fatty acids in a delicious, convenient, and consistent formula that is very low in sodium and lactose and contains no artificial sweeteners. This product is composed exclusively of ingredients classified by the Food and Drug Administration (FDA) and the U.S. Department of Agriculture (USDA) as "generally recognized as safe" (GRAS). The availability of Cocomul will be particularly useful to anyone needing assistance, as well as those who want an easy, convenient way to add coconut oil and MCT oil to the diet. For more information, see www.cognatenutritionals.com.

Alpha Health Products is developing another new product in Canada called MCT Gourmet Salad Oil that combines MCT oil with DME virgin coconut oil in the 4:3 ratio that Steve and I have used. Unrefined chia seed oil is also added to provide omega-3 fatty acids, as well as vitamin E. This oil mixture is liquid and very stable at room temperature due to the high MCT content and will easily combine with lemon or vinegar to make salad dressing. It has a pleasant nutty taste and is a superior healthy oil for daily use. For more information, see www.alphahealth.ca.

Can Someone Who Is in Assisted Living Take Coconut Oil?

If your loved one is in assisted living, the doctor may be willing to prescribe coconut oil to be given at each meal and can order the oils to be increased gradually as tolerated. A number of people have reported success in this regard.

I know of one assisted living facility in which the cook was preparing some foods with coconut oil. She said the residents with Alzheimer's seemed more talkative and to have more energy. Hopefully, over time the directors of these facilities will consider allowing staff to cook with coconut oil.

If no such options are possible, another alternative is to ask the person's physician for a prescription for Axona (www.about-axona .com), a powdered form of MCT oil, manufactured by Accera. Also, a company called True Protein (www.trueprotein.com) offers a nonprescription powdered form of MCT oil combined with some carbohydrate that can be added to liquids or pureed foods.

What about Someone with Liver Disease Using Coconut Oil?

This dietary intervention may not be appropriate for someone with liver disease. A healthy liver is required to convert medium-chain fatty acids to ketones.

Partially hydrogenated oils, including partially hydrogenated coconut oil, can result in a fatty liver. Therefore, it is important to always use nonhydrogenated coconut oil or any other oil, for that matter.

Do I Need to Be Worried about Gaining Weight from the Extra Fat in the Diet?

No and yes! Some studies show that substitution of coconut oil for other fats in the diet can actually result in weight loss of ten to twelve pounds over the course of a year, because the medium-chain fatty acids are converted directly to energy and not stored as fat. However, if the fat is simply added to the diet and nothing subtracted, you can expect to gain weight. In general, if you consume more calories than you burn in the course of a day, the net result will be weight gain.

The best way to avoid gaining weight is to *substitute* coconut oil for most other fats and oils in the diet, and if that isn't enough, eliminate or cut back on portion sizes of carbohydrates, such as breads, rice, potatoes, cereals, and other grains. In general, it is a good idea to use whole-milk products, but if weight gain is a problem, you can compensate for some of the new fat in the diet by changing from full-fat to lower-fat dairy products, such as milk, cheese, cottage cheese, and yogurts, as well as to low-fat or fat-free salad dressings, to which you can add coconut oil. By the same token, if you decide to go with low-fat dairy, be aware that you may not absorb as much calcium and vitamin D through the intestine, compared to absorption when using full-fat dairy.

Also, some people overestimate portions substantially by dipping into the coconut oil jar with a kitchen tablespoon. You can avoid this problem by using a measuring spoon and removing the excess by leveling it off with a knife. This can make a big difference in the number of calories consumed.

Tiny glass measuring cups are available at grocery stores with markings for teaspoons, tablespoons, and milliliters. These little measuring cups are especially useful for combining salad dressing with coconut oil and for measuring out the liquid MCT/coconut oil mixture discussed elsewhere.

Can Coconut Oil Be Given to Animals?

One of the most unexpected emails I received was from a lady who wanted to know if coconut oil might improve cognition in her thirteen-year-old Welsh terrier. It is completely understandable that someone wouldn't want to see their beloved elderly pet suffer with dementia any more than another family member. It turns out that one of the Accera MCT oil studies involved elderly dogs, and they did in fact show improved cognition in response to consuming the oil (Studzinski, 2008; Taha, 2009). I relayed this information to her and suggested that she follow the guidelines for children: give one-quarter teaspoon for each ten pounds the dog weighed two or three times a day. Her dog weighed twenty pounds, so she decided to give her one-half teaspoon in her food twice a day. Several weeks later, she reported that her dog was getting up and around more and finding her way to her food bowl, which she was not able to do prior to consuming the oil.

Dogs can also get diarrhea from coconut oil. The lady reported that one of her friends decided to use twice the recommended amount, and her dog developed diarrhea. Apparently, it is a good idea to start with caution and increase gradually with animals as well as people.

24

Questions and Answers about Medium-Chain Triglyceride Oil

I knew for several decades that medium-chain triglyceride (MCT) oil existed, since it was in use in newborn intensive care units as early as the 1970s. I assumed it was only available to hospitals, but not long after Steve responded to coconut oil, I learned that it could easily be purchased over the counter. I was surprised to find it in several local natural food stores and to learn that it is commonly used by bodybuilders to increase lean body mass. Following are the most frequently asked questions I receive about using MCT oil.

MCT OIL

What Is Over-the-Counter MCT Oil?

Medium-chain triglyceride oil is derived from coconut oil or palm kernel oil. Most of the products that are readily available over the counter are a mixture of caprylic (C:8) and capric (C:10) acids, with small amounts of caproic (C:6) and lauric acids (C:12)—the four medium-chain triglycerides found in coconut oil. Coconut oil is about 60 percent medium-chain fatty acids and contains a much larger proportion of lauric acid compared to MCT oil. About 70 percent of the saturated fats in coconut oil are medium-chain fatty acids.

MCT oil can be used as an alternative to coconut oil to produce mild ketosis. The primary differences between using MCT oil and coconut oil are that a smaller volume of oil can be taken without the additional fatty acids found in coconut oil and that the levels of ketones may be slightly higher, although compared to coconut oil, they leave the circulation after a few hours.

Diarrhea is a common side effect of using MCT oil, so it is a good idea to start with a small amount, such as one-half or one teaspoon and gradually increase to an amount that is tolerated, such as one to two tablespoons two to four times a day. (More suggestions follow.) At higher levels of MCT oil, most people develop diarrhea, so when this happens, you may want to cut the dose back to the previous level.

How to Avoid Diarrhea?

The most common complaint with MCT oil is the problem of diarrhea, which usually occurs if too much is taken by someone who has not taken it before, or if the amount of oil is increased too quickly. MCT oil is more likely than coconut oil to produce this problem, which occurs in about 25 percent of people as they begin taking the oil.

Considering the amount of oil that one might consume in a day's time—upwards of six to eight tablespoons—most people will find the level at which they have diarrhea, which usually occurs within an hour or so of eating the oil. An occasional person will experience diarrhea with just one teaspoon, so caution should be exercised with the first dose.

Some strategies to help decrease the likelihood of developing diarrhea are:

1. Start with a small amount of oil, such as one teaspoon once or twice a day, and increase slowly as tolerated. Increase by one teaspoon every few days until reaching the desired amount, possibly as much as two or more tablespoons three times a day.

2. Always take the oil with other foods.

3. Take the oil slowly during the course of the meal, over twenty to thirty minutes. If the oil is mixed with food, this will be easier to accomplish.

4. Mixing the oil with cottage cheese may decrease the odds that diarrhea will occur, so it might be practical to take the oil with cottage cheese one or more times per day. Cottage cheese is also an excellent source of protein and provides a relatively small amount of carbohydrate.

5. If using even small amounts of oil persists in causing diarrhea, consider trying other coconut products such as coconut milk or even grated coconut, which contains a substantial amount of oil. The oil may be released more slowly in the course of digestion and therefore be less likely to set off diarrhea.

What Is Axona?

For those who want a method prescribed by their physician, Axona, from the Accera Company, is now on the market. This is a powdered form of MCT oil mixed with some other nutrients and emulsifiers that dissolve in liquids and can be taken as a drink. Current recommendations are to take Axona once a day in the morning. More frequent dosing has not been studied as of this writing, so the company is bound by Food and Drug Administration (FDA) rules to recommend just once-a-day dosing. (For more information, go to www.about-axona.com.) A video demonstrating how ketones work as an alternative fuel is available there.

A company called True Protein (www.trueprotein.com) offers a nonprescription powdered form of MCT oil combined with some carbohydrate.

Why Do You Mix MCT Oil and Coconut Oil?

About two months after starting Steve on coconut oil, after receiving results of his ketone levels, we began experimenting with mixing MCT oil and coconut oil. After Steve took just coconut oil in the morning, his ketone levels peaked at about three hours and were nearly gone after eight to nine hours, just before dinner time. Steve's ketone levels with just MCT oil were higher but gone within three hours. I reasoned that a mixture of MCT and coconut oil should result in higher levels and longer-lasting levels, so that some ketones are always circulating.

Why Not Use Just MCT Oil?

If you decide to take just MCT oil several times a day, the levels fluctuate up and down more than with coconut oil or with a mixture of coconut and MCT oils. Also, some fatty acids in whole coconut oil are not found in MCT oil, and I think they might contribute to the improvements seen in Steve and others. For example, the lauric acid in coconut oil kills certain types of viruses, such as those that cause fever blisters. At least one group of researchers has found evidence of the herpes simplex virus type 1 that causes fever blisters in the beta-amyloid plaques in the brains of people with Alzheimer's, especially those with the ApoE4 gene like Steve. Taking coconut oil seems to be working for Steve in that he was regularly fighting fever blisters, sometimes for several weeks at a time, and these episodes have become much less severe and less frequent, with just four episodes over two years.

Coconut oil is also reported to support the thyroid, and many people with dementia have or develop hypothyroidism at some point in the disease process. People with Down syndrome all develop Alzheimer's disease by the time they reach their thirties or forties, and they also have a problem with hypothyroidism. Coconut oil could have a beneficial effect in this regard.

Why Not Use Just Coconut Oil?

Many people have reported to me that they have seen improvements in their loved ones with Alzheimer's using just coconut oil. Steve had a dramatic improvement using just coconut oil for the first two months. I don't know for certain if there is any additional benefit to adding MCT oil, so I see no problem with using just coconut oil for this dietary intervention. One of the reasons to consider adding MCT oil would be to achieve higher levels of ketones. Only part of MCT oil is converted to ketones, so the remaining medium-chain fatty acids could potentially be used by neurons as an alternative fuel. So the more medium-chain fatty acids one can tolerate, the more will be available to brain. Much more needs to be learned about exactly what medium-chain fatty acids do.

Another point to consider is that by mixing MCT and coconut oil in a four-to-three ratio, the long-chain saturated fatty acids are reduced to about 10 percent of the total fat. For those worried about the possible health issues related to saturated fats (read Chapter 21), this offers an alternative to using an equivalent amount of coconut oil. See page 355 for a recipe to make this mixture.

25

What Have You Got to Lose?

For more than nine years, our family has been dealing with early onset Alzheimer's disease. As my husband declined, I fully expected to be a widow by the time I was sixty. In May 2008, I came across a dietary intervention completely by accident on the Internet that reversed Steve's downward spiral. Consuming oils with medium-chain fatty acids can bypass the problem of insulin resistance and insulin deficiency in the brain by providing the brain with ketones as an alternative fuel to glucose. Coconut oil contains large concentrations of these fatty acids, and even medium-chain triglyceride (MCT) oil is readily available over the counter.

ISSUES TO CONSIDER

I believed that if Steve improved, others would too, and I felt a moral obligation to get the message out. People should have the opportunity to learn about this dietary intervention and try it for their loved ones with Alzheimer's disease and other conditions that share the problems of insulin resistance and/or insulin deficiency. While not everyone responds, many people have reported positive improvements to me as a result of making this dietary change. For those who are responsive to ketones, patience, persistence, and consistency are key to making this intervention work. Some have improvements that are very obvious during the first few days, while others seem to stabilize, which may not be obvious for several months or longer. For this reason, I recommend keeping a journal of your loved one's symptoms, noting any changes that occur over time for better or worse.

Weigh the Risks and the Benefits

All treatments carry risks and benefits, and this one is no exception. So I strongly recommend that the patient and family discuss this dietary intervention with the physician before getting started. Many people have had a problem with getting their physician to even consider that this dietary intervention might work. These physicians need only review their freshman biochemistry to recall that medium-chain fatty acids are converted in the liver to ketones and that ketones can provide an alternative fuel for neurons and other cells. While this may seem too simple, it is simply true. I know of many physicians who have opened their minds to this concept and are now advising their patients to use coconut oil and/or MCT oil.

When weighing the risks and benefits, the physician should strongly consider that the brain is dying in Alzheimer's disease and should weigh any perceived risks of using coconut oil against this important fact. Where there are concerns about cholesterol and saturated fats, I suggest that the physician monitor the patient's lipid profile. Even more important, the physician should counsel the patient about other changes leading to a healthier diet, such as eating whole foods that contain antioxidants and many other important nutrients and avoiding partially hydrogenated oils and a high-calorie, high-carbohydrate diet.

EVERY DAY COUNTS

Dr. Richard Veech of the NIH has developed a ketone ester that has passed human toxicity studies with no adverse effects and will soon begin a pilot study for treatment of Parkinson's disease. Funding to mass-produce this ester has been lacking, and that has hampered efforts to begin clinical trials for Alzheimer's disease, which will be lengthy, due to the nature of the disease. One of my primary goals in writing this book is to bring attention to the ketone ester with the hope that funding will follow.

The levels of ketones after taking the ketone ester will be considerably higher than what can be achieved by taking large quantities of coconut oil or even MCT oil. Even greater improvement could potentially occur when people have access to the ketone ester. It will likely be several more years before the ester is approved by the FDA and available to those who need it, but those who have Alzheimer's disease now don't have years to wait. In the meantime, this dietary intervention with medium-chain fatty acids can potentially bring about a reprieve from Alzheimer's and possibly other diseases. Some people respond more dramatically than others and some not at all. I don't know how long the effect will last, but in Steve's case, we seemed to have gained at least two to three years in his fight against Alzheimer's disease.

For those who are considering this and aren't sure what to do, what have you got to lose?

Recipes

Here are some basic recipes to get started, along with some of our favorites.

MCT Oil/Coconut Oil Mixture

Yield: 28 ounces

• •

16 ounces MCT oil

12 ounces coconut oil

Directions: If coconut oil is solid, place container into a pot of warm water for fifteen to twenty minutes until it melts. Combine in a one-quart container with a tight lid and invert several times to mix. The quart-size bottles that MCT oil normally comes in are perfect for storing this mixture. Using a funnel will make it easier to pour the coconut and MCT oils into the bottle. Store at room temperature.

COCONUT MILK

YIELD: 4 ounces, or about 15 grams of coconut oil

• •

1 can of coconut milk (with 11 grams fat per 2 ounces)

$1/2$ can of water or coconut water

1 to 2 teaspoons of honey, agave syrup,
or other sweetener to taste

Pinch of salt

Directions: Place ingredients in a container and shake well before use. Store coconut milk in the refrigerator, and discard unused portion after four days. If used for children, discard after two days.

Variation: Add 1 teaspoon dolomite powder to mixture to add calcium supplementation to diet.

ORANGE-COCONUT MILK

YIELD: One serving

• •

4 ounces coconut milk (above)

8 ounces orange juice
or diet orange soda

Directions: Place coconut milk in a 12-ounce glass, then slowly add orange juice or diet orange soda and mix with a spoon.

Variation: Try diet grape soda or root beer instead of orange soda.

BERRY-COCONUT MILK SMOOTHIE

YIELD: About 12 ounces per serving

• •

$^1/_2$ cup crushed ice

1 cup frozen blueberries
or 4 large frozen strawberries

$^1/_3$ cup Fiber One Original, Smart Bran,
or GoLean Crunch cereal

1 teaspoon honey, agave syrup,
or equivalent sweetener such as stevia

$^1/_3$ cup coconut milk (above)

$^2/_3$ cup milk

1 hard-boiled or raw egg

$^1/_2$ scoop vanilla whey protein powder

Your usual "dose" of coconut oil (melted)
or MCT/coconut oil (optional).

Directions: Place all ingredients in a blender and blend on "liquify" speed for about 30 seconds. If mixture is too thick, add more coconut milk as needed.

Variations: Add $^1/_2$ banana and 2 large strawberries per serving; substitute equivalent amount of apple, blueberry, or pomegranate juice for part or all of the milk; or substitute $^1/_3$ cup sliced almonds for cereal.

Note: For those who are concerned about adding raw egg, microwave the egg for about 20 seconds to kill bacteria before adding to other ingredients.

BANANA-PEANUT BUTTER-COCONUT MILK SMOOTHIE

YIELD: About 12 ounces per serving

$^{1}/_{2}$ cup crushed ice

1 frozen banana (break into four pieces before freezing)

$^{1}/_{3}$ cup cereal such as Fiber One Original,
Smart Bran, or GoLean Crunch

1 tablespoon fresh ground or natural
peanut or almond butter

1 teaspoon honey, agave syrup,
or equivalent stevia or sweetener

$^{1}/_{3}$ cup coconut milk (above)

$^{1}/_{3}$ cup milk

1 hard-boiled or raw egg

$^{1}/_{2}$ scoop vanilla whey protein powder

Optional: Add your usual "dose" of coconut oil (melted)
or MCT/coconut oil.

Directions: Place all ingredients in a blender and blend on "liquify" speed for about 30 seconds. If mixture is too thick, add more coconut milk as needed.

Variation: Substitute $^{1}/_{3}$ cup sliced almonds for the cereal and/or nut butter.

Note: For those who are concerned about using raw egg, microwave the egg for about 20 seconds to kill bacteria before adding to other ingredients.

SIMPLE SALMON DINNER FOR TWO

YIELD: Two servings

• •

2 fresh whole sweet potatoes or yams

10 to 12 ounces salmon fillet, any size

1 bunch fresh asparagus

2 to 3 tablespoons coconut oil, melted

Garlic and herb or other favorite seasoning

Additional $1/2$ to 1 tablespoon coconut oil per potato

Directions: Preheat oven to 350°F. Wash, dry, and pierce sweet potatoes several times with a fork and place on the oven rack for about 25 to 30 minutes.

Place aluminum foil on a large cookie sheet or spray the cookie sheet with olive oil spray. On one side of the cookie sheet place a salmon fillet, skin side down, and on the other evenly distribute the asparagus spears. Melt about 2 to 3 tablespoons of coconut oil (or more for a very large fillet), and paint the oil onto the salmon and asparagus using a pastry brush. Sprinkle seasoning over fish and asparagus.

When sweet potatoes have been in the oven for 25 to 30 minutes, move them to the side and place the cookie sheet with fish and asparagus in the oven. Bake for 20 minutes longer. The salmon should be very moist and separate easily with a fork. Open each sweet potato, cut grooves with a knife, and spoon $1/2$ to 1 tablespoon coconut oil onto each potato.

ULTRA CHOCOLATE LAYER CAKE WITH CHOCOLATE GANACHE ICING

YIELD: Two 10-inch round layers
$1/_{16}$ of cake = 1 tablespoon coconut oil

• •

CAKE

3 ounces semi-sweet chocolate morsels

$1^1/_2$ cups hot brewed coffee

3 large eggs

$3/_4$ cup coconut oil

$1^1/_2$ cups buttermilk, well shaken

$3/_4$ teaspoon vanilla extract

3 cups sugar

$2^1/_2$ cups whole-wheat flour

$1^1/_2$ cups unsweetened dark cocoa powder

2 teaspoons baking soda

$3/_4$ teaspoon baking powder

$1^1/_4$ teaspoon sea salt

Directions: Preheat oven to 300°F. Spray two 10-inch round layer cake pans with a nonstick oil such as Baker's Joy, or line the pan bottoms with wax paper.

Melt chocolate morsels in hot coffee, stirring occasionally. In a large mixing bowl, beat eggs until smooth and slightly thickened, about 3 to 5 minutes. Slowly add, one at a time, oil, buttermilk, extract, and melted chocolate mixture and beat until well combined.

In a separate bowl, combine sugar, flour, cocoa powder, baking soda, baking powder, and salt with a large wire whisk. Slowly add dry mixture to wet ingredients and mix on medium speed until just combined.

Divide mixture evenly between two pans and bake in

center of oven for 1 hour to 1 hour 10 minutes, until a tooth-pick comes out clean. Place pans on a rack and allow to cool completely, then invert the layers onto rack, using a knife around edges of pan to loosen cake, if necessary. Remove wax paper, if used. After completely cool, apply ganache icing.

ICING

1 cup heavy cream

2 tablespoons sugar

2 tablespoons light corn syrup

16 ounces semi-sweet chocolate morsels

$1/4$ cup coconut oil

Directions: Using a $1^1/_2$-quart saucepan, bring cream, sugar, and corn syrup to a boil over moderately low heat, stirring constantly with a whisk until sugar is dissolved. Remove pan from heat and add chocolate, whisking until completely melted. Add oil and whisk until smooth. Allow mixture to cool until consistency allows for easy spreading. Apply ganache between layers and on top and sides of cake. Store in refrigerator and bring to room temperature before serving.

Variation: Top off slices of cake with strawberry or raspberry topping.

COCONUT MACAROONS

YIELD: 18 small cookies

• •

2 egg whites

Pinch of salt

$1/_2$ teaspoon vanilla, chocolate, or almond extract

$2/_3$ cup sugar

1 cup shredded coconut

Directions: Beat egg whites with salt and extract until soft peaks form. Gradually add sugar (or stevia if you prefer) and beat until stiff. Fold in coconut. Coat a cookie sheet with generous amount of butter. Drop batter by the rounded teaspoon onto cookie sheet. Bake at 325°F for 20 minutes. Each cookie contains approximately 4 grams of coconut oil.

Variation: Instead of $2/3$ cup sugar, add $1/4$ cup sugar and 1 to 2 dashes of stevia extract or equivalent sweetener.

COCONUT FUDGE

YIELD: About 16 ounces

• •

1 cup coconut oil

1 cup chocolate chips

Directions: Melt and thoroughly mix together the oil and chocolate chips in a bowl or a large measuring cup. Divide mixture equally into a plastic ice cube tray and place in the freezer. Chill until set. In a sixteen-cube tray, each cube will equal one tablespoon of coconut oil and will easily pop out of the tray. Store in refrigerator or freezer.

Variation: Add about $1/4$ cup grated coconut and/or nut pieces for variety.

Resources

SUGGESTED READING

The following books are good sources of information for those who wish to explore further the topics discussed in this book.

Calbom, Cherie. *The Coconut Diet*. New York, NY: Warner Books, 2005.

_____. *The Ultimate Smoothie Book*. New York, NY: Wellness Central/Hachette Book Group, Inc., 2006.

Enig, Mary, Ph.D. *Know Your Fats*. Silver Spring, MD: Bethesda Press, 2000.

_____ and Sally Fallon. *Eat Fat, Lose Fat*. New York, NY: Penguin Group, 2005.

_____ and _____. *Nourishing Traditions*. 2nd edition. Washington, DC: New Trends Publishing Inc., 2001.

Fife, Bruce, N.D. *Coconut Lover's Cookbook*. Colorado Springs, CO: Piccadilly Books, Ltd., 2008.

_____ and Conrado S. Dayrit, M.D. *Coconut Cures*. Colorado Springs, CO: Piccadilly Books, Ltd., 2005.

Freeman, John, M.D., Eric Kossoff, M.D., Jennifer Freeman, and Millicent Kelly, R.D. *The Ketogenic Diet*. 4th edition. New York, NY: Demos Medical Publishing, 2007.

Lands, William, Ph.D. *Fish, Omega-3 and Human Health*. 2nd edition. Urbana, IL: AOCS Press, 2005.

LeBlanc, Gary J. *Staying Afloat in a Sea of Forgetfulness: Common Sense Caregiving*. Bloomington, IN: Xlibris Corporation, 2010.

Lombard, Jay, M.D., and Carl Germano, R.D., C.N.S., L.D.N. *The Brain Wellness Plan*. New York, NY: Kensington Books, 2000.

London, Jan. *Coconut Cuisine: Featuring Stevia*. Summerton, TN: Book Publishing Company, 2006.

MacBean, Valerie. *Coconut Cookery*. Berkeley, CA: Frog Books, 2001.

Mace, Nancy, and Peter Rabins, M.D. *The 36-Hour Day*. New York, NY: Time Warner Book Group, 2001.

Price, Weston A., D.D.S. *Nutrition and Physical Degeneration*. 8th edition (first published in 1939). La Mesa, CA: The Price-Pottenger Nutrition Foundation, 2008.

Simopoulos, Artemis, M.D., and Jo Robinson. *The Omega Diet*. New York, NY: HarperCollins Publishers, Inc., 1999.

Sinatra, Stephen, M.D. *The Sinatra Solution: Metabolic Cardiology*. Laguna Beach, CA: Basic Health Publications, 2008.

Snowdon, David, Ph.D. *Aging with Grace*. New York, NY: Bantam Books, 2001.

Stoll, Andrew L., M.D. *The Omega-3 Connection*. New York, NY: Simon & Schuster, 2001.

Vanderhaeghe, Lorna, and Karlene Karst, R.D. *Healthy Fats for Life*. 2nd edition. Toronto, Canada: John Wiley & Sons, 2004.

VanRyzin, Christine. *Alzheimer's Averted: A Path to Survival*. Appleton, WI: Elemental Basic Publishing, 2004.

Zook, Sylvia, M.S., Ph.D. *Eatin' After Eden*. Tucson, AZ: Wheatmark, 2008.

RESOURCE ORGANIZATIONS

The following is a list of organizations and medical websites that can provide additional information on all aspects of Alzheimer's disease.

Alzheimer's Association: www.alz.org

Alzheimer's Disease International: www.alz.co.uk

Alzheimer's Family Organization: www.alzheimersfamily.org

National Institute on Aging Alzheimer's Disease Education and Referral Center: www.nia.nih.gov/Alzheimers

National Institutes of Health Clinical Trials Registry:
www.clinicaltrials.gov

FORUMS, BLOGS, AND MESSAGE BOARDS

Alzheimer's Association Message Board:
www.alz.org/living_with_alzheimers_message_boards_lwa.asp

Alzheimer's Research Forum: www.alzforum.org

The Alzheimer's Spouse: www.thealzheimerspouse.com

Dr. Newport's Blog: www.coconutketones.blogspot.com

SOURCES FOR COCONUT OIL
AND MEDIUM-CHAIN TRIGYLCERIDE OIL

The following websites offer an array of coconut oil and MCT oil products.

Alpha Health Products: www.alphahealth.ca

Amazon.com: www.amazon.com

Barlean's Organic Oils: www.barleans.com

Cheap Vitamins: www.cheapvitamins.com

Coconut Oil Online: www.coconutoil-online.com

Cognate Nutritionals: www.cognatenutritionals.com

Nature's Approved: www.naturesapproved.com

Niulife: www.niulife.com.au

Nutiva: http://nutiva.com

Spectrum: www.spectrumorganics.com

Swanson Health Products: www.swansonvitamins.com

Tropical Traditions: www.tropicaltraditions.com

True Protein: www.trueprotein.com

Wilderness Family Naturals: www.wildernessfamilynaturals.com

COCONUT OIL INFORMATION

Coconut Research Center: www.coconutresearchcenter.org

KETOGENIC DIET INFORMATION AND SUPPORT

The Charlie Foundation:
www.charliefoundation.org

Matthews Friends:
www.matthewsfriends.org

References
and Related Articles

Introduction

Mauer K, S Volk, H Gerbaldo. "Auguste D and Alzheimer's disease." *Lancet* Vol 349 (May 1997): 1546–1549.

National Institutes of Health/National Institute on Aging/Alzheimer's Disease Education and Referral Center, 2009 Progress Report on Alzheimer's Disease. Available online at: www.nia.nih.gov/Alzheimers/Publications/ADProgress2009.

Chapter 1: Steve Before the Fall

Reiman EM, K Chen, GE Alexander, et al. "Functional brain abnormalities in young adults at genetic risk for late-onset Alzheimer's dementia." *PNAS* Vol 101, No 1 (Jan 2004): 284–289.

Chapter 2: Steve's Descent

Flory JD, SB Manuck, RE Ferrell, et al. "Memory performance and the apolipoprotein E polymorphism in a community sample of middle-aged adults." *Am J Med Genet* Vol 96 (2000): 707–711.

Folstein MF, SE Folstein, PR McHugh. "Mini-Mental State: a practical method for grading the cognitive state of patients for the clinician." *J Psychiat Res* Vol 12 (1975): 189–198.

Klein WL, F De Felice, PN Lacor, et al. "Why Alzheimer's is a disease of memory: synaptic targeting by pathogenic A? oligomers (ADDLS)." In *Synaptic Plasticity and the Mechanism of Alzheimer's Disease* by DJ Selkoe, A Triller, Y Christen. Springer, 2008: 103–132.

Landau SM, D Harvey, CM Madison, et al. "Comparing predictors of conversion and decline in mild cognitive impairment." *Neurology* Vol 75, No 3 (Jul 2010): 230–238.

Reiman EM, K Chen, GE Alexander, et al. "Functional brain abnormalities in young adults at genetic risk for late-onset Alzheimer's dementia." *PNAS* Vol 101, No 1 (Jan 2004): 284–289.

Small GW, LM Ercoli, DHS Silverman, et al. "Cerebral metabolic and cognitive decline in persons at genetic risk for Alzheimer's disease." *PNAS* Vol 97, No 11 (May 2000): 6037–6042.

Zhao WQ, FG De Felice, S Fernandez, et al. "Amyloid beta oligomers induce impairment of neuronal insulin receptors." *FASEB Journal* Vol 22 (Jan 2008): 246–260.

Chapter 4: A Chance Discovery

De la Monte SM, JR Wands. "Review of insulin and insulin-like growth factor expression, signaling, and malfunction in the central nervous system: relevance to Alzheimer's disease." *J Alzheimers Dis* Vol 7 (2005): 45–61.

Klein WL, F De Felice, PN Lacor, et al. "Why Alzheimer's is a disease of memory: synaptic targeting by pathogenic A? oligomers (ADDLS)." In *Synaptic Plasticity and the Mechanism of Alzheimer's Disease* by DJ Selkoe, A Triller, Y Christen. Springer, 2008: 103–132.

Tantibhehyangkul P, SA Hashim. "Medium-chain triglyceride feeding in premature infants: effects on fat and nitrogen absorption." *Pediatrics* Vol 55 (Mar 1975): 359–370.

U.S. Department of Agriculture Nutrient Data Laboratory. "Nutrient analysis of coconut oil (vegetable)." (Dec 2010) Available online at: www.ars.usda.gov/nutrientdata.

Chapter 5: Climbing Out of the Abyss

Henderson ST. "High carbohydrate diets and Alzheimer's disease." *Med Hypotheses* Vol 62 (2004): 689–700.

Veech RL. "The therapeutic implications of ketone bodies: the effects of ketone bodies in pathological conditions: ketosis, ketogenic diet, redox states, insulin resistance, and mitochondrial metabolism." *Prostaglandins, Leukot Essent Fatty Acids* Vol 70 (2004): 309–319.

Chapter 6: Getting the Message Out

Newport MT. "What if there was a cure for Alzheimer's disease and no one knew?"

Available online at: www.coconutketones.com.

Reiman EM, K Chen, GE Alexander, et al. "Functional brain abnormalities in young adults at genetic risk for late-onset Alzheimer's dementia." *PNAS* Vol 101, No 1 (Jan 2004): 284–289.

Chapter 11: Two Overseas Trips

Newport MT. "What if there was a cure for Alzheimer's disease and no one knew?"

Available online at: www.coconutketones.com.

Zuccoli G, N Marcello, A Pisanello, et al. "Metabolic management of glioblastoma multiforme using standard therapy together with a restricted ketogenic diet." *Nutri Metab* Vol 7, No 33 (2010): 1–7.

Chapter 13: Caregiver Reports

Newport MT. "What if there was a cure for Alzheimer's disease and no one knew?"

Available online at: www.coconutketones.com

Studzinski CM, WA MacKay, TL Beckett, et al. "Induction of ketosis may improve mitochondrial function and decrease steady-state amyloid-? precursor protein (APP) levels in the aged dog." *Brain Res* Vol 1226 (2008): 209–217.

Taha AY, ST Henderson, WM Burnham. "Dietary enrichment with medium-chain triglycerides (AC-1203) elevates polyunsaturated fatty acids in the pareital cortex of aged dogs: Implication for treating age-related cognitive decline." *Neurochem Res* Vol 34, No 9 (Sept 2009): 1619–1625.

Chapter 14: Type 3 Diabetes and Alzheimer's Disease

Akomolafe A, A Beiser, JD Meigs, et al. "Diabetes mellitus and risk of developing Alzheimer disease: Results from the Framingham study." *Arch Neurol* Vol 63 (Nov 2006): 1551–1555.

De Felice F, M Vieira, T Bomfim, et al. "Protection of synapses against Alzheimer's-linked toxins: Insulin signaling prevents the pathogenic binding of A? oligomers." *PNAS* Vol 206, No 6 (Feb 2009): 1971–1976.

De la Monte SM, JR Wands. "Review of insulin and insulin-like growth factor expression, signaling, and malfunction in the central nervous system: Relevance to Alzheimer's disease." *J Alzheimers Dis* Vol 7 (2005): 45–61.

De la Monte SM, JR Wands. "Alzheimer's disease is type 3 diabetes—evidence reviewed." *J Diabetes Sci Technol* Vol 2, No 6 (Nov 2008): 1101–1113.

Hoyer S. "Brain metabolism and the incidence of cerebral perfusion disorders in organic psychoses." *Deutsche Zeitschrift für Nervenheilkunde* Vol 197, No 4 (1970): 285–292.

Hoyer S. "The abnormally aged brain: its blood flow and oxidative metabolism. A review-part II." *Archives of Gerontology and Geriatrics* Vol 1, No 3 (1982): 195–207.

Hoyer S. "Abnormalities of glucose metabolism in Alzheimer's disease." *Ann N Y Acad Sci* Vol 640 (1991): 53–58.

Hoyer S. "Brain glucose and energy metabolism abnormalities in sporadic Alzheimer disease. Causes and consequences: an update." *Exp Gerontol* Vol 35 (2000): 1363–1372.

Hoyer S. "Glucose metabolism and insulin receptor signal transduction in Alzheimer disease." *Eur J Pharmacol* Vol 490 (2004): 115–125.

Kim EJ, SS Cho, Y Jeong, et al. "Glucose metabolism in early onset versus late onset Alzheimer's disease: an SPM analysis of 120 patients," *Brain* Vol 128 (2005): 1790–1801.

Liu Y, F Liu, K Iqbal, et al. "Decreased glucose transporters correlate to abnormal hyperphosphorylation of tau in Alzheimer's disease." *FEBS Letters* Vol 582 (2008): 359–364.

O'Connor T, KR Sadleir, E Maus, et al. "Phosphorylation of the translation initiation factor eIF2? increases BACE1 levels and promotes amyloidogenesis." *Neuron* Vol 60 (2008): 988–1009.

Page KA, A Williamson, N Yu, et al. "Medium-chain fatty acids improve cognitive function in intensively treated type 1 diabetic patients and support *in vitro* synaptic transmission during acute hypoglycemia." *Diabetes* Vol 58, No 5 (May 2009): 1237–1244.

Pasquier F, A Boulogne, D Leys, et al. "Diabetes mellitus and dementia." *Diabetes Metab* Vol 32 (2006): 403–414.

Piert M, R Koeppe, B Giordani, et al. "Diminished glucose transport and phosphorylation in Alzheimer's disease determined by dynamic FDG-PET." *J Nucl Med* Vol 37, No 2 (Feb 1996): 201–208.

Steen E, BM Terry, EJ Rivera, et al. "Impaired insulin and insulin-like growth factor expressioin and signaling mechanisms in Alzheimer's disease: Is this type 3 diabetes?" *J Alzheimers Dis* Vol 7, No 1 (Feb 2005): 63–80.

Whitmer R, A Karter, K Yaffe, et al. "Hypoglycemic episodes and risk of dementia in older patients with type 2 diabetes mellitus." *JAMA* Vol 301 (Apr 2009): 1565–1572.

Chapter 15: What Causes Alzheimer's Disease?

Bishop NA, T Lu, BA Yankner. "Neural mechanisms of ageing and cognitive decline." *Insight* (2010): 529–535.

Blennow K, MJ de Leon, H Zetterberg. "Alzheimer's disease." *Lancet* Vol 368, No 9533 (Jul 2006): 387–403.

Bu G. "Apolipoprotein E and its receptors in Alzheimer's disease: pathways, pathogenesis and therapy." *Nature Review Neuroscience* Vol 10, No 5 (May 2009). Available online at: www.nature.com/nrn/journal/v10/n5/abs/nrn2620.html.

Casselli R, A Cueck, D Osborne, et al. "Longitudinal modeling of age-related memory decline and the APOE ?4 effect." *NEJM* Vol 361 (Jul 2009): 255–263.

De la Monte SM, A Neusner, J Chu, et al. "Epidemiologic trends strongly suggest exposures as etiologic agents in the pathogenesis of sporadic Alzheimer's disease, diabetes mellitus, and non-alcoholic steatohepatitis." *J Alzheimers Dis* Vol 17, No 3 (2009): 519–529.

De la Monte SM, M Tong. "Mechanisms of ceramide-mediated neurodegeneration." *J Alzheimers Dis* Vol 16, No 4 (2009): 704-714.

De la Monte SM, M Tong, M Lawton, L Longato. "Nitrosamine exposure exacerbates high fat diet-mediated type 2 diabetes mellitus, non-alcoholic steatohepatitis, and neurodegeneration with cognitive impairment." *Mol Neurodegener* Vol 4, No 54 (2009): 1–13.

De la Monte SM, L Longato, M Tong, et al. "The liver-brain axis of alcohol-mediated neurode-generation: role of toxic lipids." *Int J Environ Res Public Health* Vol 6 (2009): 2055–2075.

Dickerson FB, JJ Boronow, C Stallings, et al. "Infection with herpes simplex virus type 1 is associated with cognitive deficits in bipolar disorder." *Biol Phychiatry* Vol 55 (2004): 588–593.

Fleminger S, DL Oliver, S Lovestone, et al. "Head injury as a risk factor for Alzheimer's disease: the evidence ten years on; a partial replication." *J Neurol Neurosurg Psychiatry* Vol 74 (2003): 857–862.

Flory JD, SB Manuck, RE Ferrell, et al. "Memory performance and the apolipoprotein E polymorphism in a community sample of middle-aged adults." *Am J Med Genet* Vol 96 (2000): 707–711.

Holmes C, C Cunningham, E Zotova, et al. "Systemic inflammation and disease progression in Alzheimer disease." *Neurology* Vol 73 (2009): 768–774.

Itzhaki RF, MA Wozniak. "Herpes simplex virus type 1, apolipoprotein E, and cholesterol: a dangerous liaison in Alzheimer's disease and other disorders." *Prog Lipid Res* Vol 45 (2006): 73–90.

Itzhaki RF, MA Wozniak. "Herpes simplex virus type 1 in Alzheimer's disease: the enemy within." *J Alzheimers Dis* Vol 13 (2008): 393–405.

Kristmunsdottir T, SG Arnadottir, G Bergsson, et al. "Development and evaluation of microbicidal hydrogels containing monoglyceride as the active ingredient." *J Pharm Sci* Vol 88, No 10 (Oct 1999): 1011–1015.

McGrath N, NE Anderson, MC Croxson, et al. "Herpes simplex encephalitis treated with acyclovir: diagnosis and long term outcome." *J Neurol Neurosurg Psychiatry* Vol 63 (1997): 321–326.

Mortimer JA, CM Van Duijn, V Chandra, et al. "Head trauma as a risk factor for Alzheimer's disease: a collaborative re-analysis of case-controlled studies." *Int J Epidemiol* Vol 20, Suppl 2 (1991): S28–35.

National Institutes of Health/National Institute on Aging/Alzheimer's Disease Education and Referral Center, 2009 Progress Report on Alzheimer's Disease. Available online at: www.nia.nih.gov/Alzheimers/Publications/ADProgress2009.

Rossini AA, AA Like, WL Chick, et al. "Studies of streptozotocin-induced insulitis and diabetes." *Proc Natl Acad Sci* Vol 74, No 6 (Jun 1977): 2485–2489.

Sahin E, RA DePinho. "Linking functional decline of telomeres, mitochondria and stem cells during ageing." *Nature* Vol 484 (Mar 2010): 520–528.

Schwarz A. "Dementia risk seen in players in N.F.L. Study." *New York Times,* Sept 30, 2009.

Shipley, SJ, ET Parkin, RF Itzhaki, et al. "Herpes simplex virus interferes with amyloid precursor protein processing." *BioMed Central* Vol 5 (2005): 48.

Soscia SJ, JE Kirby, KJ Washicosky, et al. "The Alzheimer's disease-associated amyloid ?-protein is an antimicrobial peptide." *PLoS One* Vol 5, No 3 (2010): e9505.

Thormar H, CE Isaacs, HR Brown, et al. "Inactivation of enveloped viruses and killing of cells by fatty acids and monoglycerides." *Antimicrob Agents Chemother* Vol 31, No 1 (Jan 1987): 27–31.

Tong M, A Neusner, L Longato, et al. "Nitrosamine exposure causes insulin resistance diseases: relevance to type 2 diabetes mellitus, non-alcoholic steatohepatitis, and Alzheimer's disease." *J Alzheimers Dis* Vol 17, No 4 (2009): 827–844.

VanItallie TB. "Parkinson's disease: primacy of age as a risk factor for mitochondrial dysfunction." *Metabolism Clinical and Experimental* Vol 57, Suppl 2 (2008): S50–S55.

Wozniak MA, SJ Shipley, M Combrinck, et al. "Productive herpes simplex virus in brain of elderly normal subjects and Alzheimer's disease patients." *J Med Virol* Vol 75 (2004): 300–306.

Wozniak MA, RF Itzhaki, SJ Shipley, et al. "Herpes simplex virus infection causes cellular amyloid accumulation and secretase upregulation." *Neuroscience Letters* Vol 429 (2007): 95–100.

Wozniak MA, AP Mee, RF Itzhaki. "Herpes simplex virus type 1 DNA is located within Alzheimer's disease amyloid plaques." *J Pathol* Vol 217 (2009): 131–138.

Wozniak MA, AL Frost, RF Itzhaki. "Alzheimer's disease-specific tau phosphorylation is induced by herpes simplex virus type 1." *J Alzheimers Dis* Vol 16 (2009): 341–350.

Yao J, RW Irwin, L Zhao, et al. "Mitochondrial bioenergetic deficit precedes Alzheimer's pathology in female mouse model of Alzheimer's disease." *PNAS* Vol 106, No 34 (2009): 14670–14675.

Zhong N, K Weisgraber. "Understanding the Association of apolipoprotein E4 with Alzheimer disease: clues from its structure." *J Biol Chem* Vol 284, No. 10 (Mar 2008): 6027–6031.

Chapter 16: Ketone Basics

Blurton-Jones M, M Kitazawa, H Martinez-Coria, et al. "Neural stem cells improve cognition via BDNF in a transgenic model of Alzheimer disease." *PNAS* Vol 106, No 32 (Aug 2009): 13594–13599.

Bourgneres PF, C Lemmel, P Ferre, et al "Ketone body transport in the human neonate and infant." *J Clin Invest* Vol 77 (1986): 42–48.

Cahill GF Jr, TT Aoki. "Alternate fuel utilization by brain." In *Cerebral Metabolism and Neural Function* by JV Passonneau, RA Hawkins, WD Lust, et al, eds. Baltimore, MD: Williams & Wilkins, 1980, p. 234–242.

Cahill GF, Jr. "Fuel metabolism in starvation." *Annu Rev Nutr* Vol 26 (2006): 1–22.

Cahill GF, Jr. "Ketosis." *Kidney Int* Vol 20 (1981): 416–425.

Courtice FC, CG Douglas. "The effects of prolonged muscular exercise on the metabolism." *Proc R Soc* Vol 119B (1936): 381–439.

Fery F, EO Balasse. "Ketone body turnover during and after exercise in overnight-fasted and starved humans." *Am J Physiol Endocrinol Metab* Vol 245 (1983): 318–325.

Forssner G. "Über die einwirkung der muskelarbeit auf die acetonkörperausscheiding bei kohlenhydratarmer kost." *Skand Arch Physiol* Vol 22 (1909): 393–405.

Gilbert DL, PL Pyzik, JM Freeman. "The ketogenic diet: seizure control correlates better with serum beta-hydroxybutyrate than with urine ketones." *J Child Neurol* Vol. 15 (2000): 787–790.

Hasselbalch SG, PL Madsen, LP Hageman, et al. "Changes in cerebral blood flow and carbohydrate metabolism during acute hyperketonemia." *Amer J Physiol* Vol 270 (1996): E746–751.

Hoyer S. "Abnormalities of glucose metabolism in Alzheimer's disease." *Ann N Y Acad Sci* Vol 640 (1991): 53–58.

Johnson RC, SK Young, R Cotter, et al. "Medium-chain triglyceride lipid emulsion: metabolism and tissue distribution." *An J Clin Nutr* Vol 52 (1990) 502-8

Johnson RE, F Sargent II, R Passmore. "Normal variations in total ketone bodies in serum and urine of healthy young men." *Exp Physiol* (1958): 339–344.

Johnson RH, JL Walton, HA Krebs, et al. "Post-exercise ketosis." *Lancet* (December 1969): 1383–1385.

Kashiwaya Y, T King, RL Veech. "Substrate signaling by insulin: A ketone bodies ratio mimics insulin action in heart." *Am J Cardiol* Vol 80, No 3A (1997): 50A–64A.

Koeslag JH, TD Noakes, AW Sloan. "Post-exercise ketosis." *Physiol* Vol 301 (1980): 79–90.

Owen OE, AP Morgan, GF Cahill Jr, et al. "Brain metabolism during fasting." *J Clin Invest* Vol 46 (1967): 1589–1595.

Owen OE. "Ketone bodies as a fuel for the brain during starvation." *Biochem Mol Biol Educ* Vol 33, No 4 (2005): 246–251.

Passmore R, RE Johnson. "The modification of post-exercise ketosis (the Courtice-Douglas effect) by environmental temperature and water balance." *Exp Physiol* (1958): 352–361.

Preti L. "Die muskelarbeit und deren ketogene wirkung." *Biochem Z* Vol 32 (1911): 231–234.

Rennie MJ, S Jennett, RH Johnson. "The metabolic effects of strenuous exercise: a comparison between untrained subjects and racing cyclists." *ExpPhysiol* (1974): 201–212.

Turner N, K Hariharan, J TidAng, et al. "Enhancement of muscle mitochondrial oxidative capacity and alterations in insulin action are lipid species dependent: potent tissue-specific effects of medium-chain fatty acids." *Diabetes* Vol 48 (2009): 2547–2554.

VanItallie TB, SS Bergen, Jr. "Ketogenesis and hyperketonemia." *Amer J Med* Vol 31 (1961): 909.

VanItallie TB, TH Nufert. "Ketones: metabolism's ugly duckling." *Nutr Rev* Vol 61, No 10 (Oct 2003): 327–341.

Vaynman S, Z Ying, F Gomez-Pinilla. "Hippocampal BDNF mediates the efficacy of exercise of synaptic plasticity and cognition." *Eur J Neurosci* Vol 20, No 10 (Nov 2004): 2580–2590.

Wahren, J, Y Sato, J Östman, et al. "Turnover and splanchnic metabolism of free fatty acids and ketones in insulin-dependent diabetics at rest and in response to exercise." *J Clin Invest* Vol 73 (May 1984): 1367–1376.

Yamada K, M Mizuno, T Nabeshima. "Role for brain-derived neurotrophic factor in learning and memory." *Life Science* Vol 70, No 7 (Jan 2002): 735–744.

Chapter 17: The Discovery of Ketones and the Ketogenic Diet

Bough KJ, JM Rho. "Anticonvulsant mechanisms of the ketogenic diet." *Epilepsia* Vol 48, No 1 (2007): 43–58.

Gerhardt J. "Diabetes mellitus und aceton." *Wiener Medizinische Presse* Vol 6 (1865): 672.

Haces ML, K Hernández-Fonseca, ON Medina-Campos, et al. "Antioxidant capacity contributes to protection of ketone bodies against oxidative damage induced during hypoglycemic conditions." *Exp Neurol* Vol 211, No 1 (2008): 85–96.

Hartman AL, M Gasior, EPG Vining, et al. "The neuropharmacology of the ketogenic diet." *Pediatr Neurol* Vol 36, No 5 (2007): 281–292.

Heinbecker P. "Studies on the metabolism of Eskimos." *J Biol Chem* Vol 80, No 2 (1928): 461–475.

Henderson ST. "High carbohydrate diets and Alzheimer's disease." *Med Hypotheses* Vol 62 (2004): 689–700.

Hirschfield F. "Beobachtungen über die acentonurie und das coma diabeticum." *Z Klin Med* Vol 28 (1895): 176–209.

Huttenlocher PR, AJ Wilbourn, JM Signore. "Medium-chain triglycerides as a therapy for intractable childhood epilepsy." *Neurology* Vol 21 (1971): 1097–1103.

Lavau M, V Fornari, SA Hashim. "Ketone metabolism in brain slices from rats with diet induced hyperketonemia." *J Nutr* Vol 108 (1978): 621–639.

Maalouf M, JM Rhob, MP Mattson. "The neuroprotective properties of calorie restriction, the ketogenic diet, and ketone bodies." *Brain Res Rev* Vol 59 (2009): 293–315.

Prins ML. "Cerebral metabolic adaptation and ketone metabolism after brain injury." *J Cereb Blood Flow Metab* Vol 28 (2008): 1–16.

Prins M. "Ketogenic diet and treatments: diet, ketones, and neurotrauma." *Epilepsia* Vol 49 (2008): 111–113.

Rho JM. "Substantia(ting) ketone body effects on neuronal excitability." *Epilepsy Currents* Vol 7, No 5 (2007): 142–144.

Robinson AM, DH Williamson. "Physiological roles of ketone bodies as substrates and signals in mammalian tissues." *Physiol Rev* Vol 80, No 1 (1980): 143–187.

Van der Auwera I, S Wera, F Van Leuven, et al. "A ketogenic diet reduces amyloid beta 40 and 42 in a mouse model of Alzheimer's disease." *Nutr Metab* Vol 2, No 28 (2005): 1–8.

Wilder RM, "The effect of ketonemia on the course of epilepsy." *The Clinic Bulletin* Vol 2 (1921): 307–308.

Zhao Z, DJ Lange, A Voustainiouk, et al. "A ketogenic diet as a potential novel therapeutic intervention in amyotrophic lateral sclerosis." *BMC Neurosci* Vol 7 (2006): 29.

Chapter 18: Medium-Chain Triglycerides and Ketones

Bergen SS, Jr., SA Hashim, TB VanItallie. "Hyperketonemia induced in man by medium-chain triglyceride." *Diabetes* Vol 16, No 10 (Oct 1966): 723–725.

Costantini LC, JL Vogel, LJ Barr, et al. "Clinical efficacy of AC-1202 in mild to moderate Alzheimer's disease." Proceedings of the 59th Annual Meeting of the American Academy of Neurology Conference, Apr 28–May 5, 2007.

Costantini LC, LJ Barr, JL Vogel, et al. "Hypometabolism as a therapeutic target in Alzheimer's disease." *BMC Neurosci* Vol 9, Suppl 2 (Dec 2008): S16.

Cunnane S, S Nugent, M Roy, et al. "Brain fuel metabolism, aging, and Alzheimer's disease." *Nutrition* Vol 27, No 1 (Jan 2011): 3–20.

Das AM, T Lücke, U Meyer, et al. "Glycogen storage disease type 1: impact of medium-chain triglycerides on metabolic control and growth." *Ann Nutr Metab* Vol 56 (2010): 225–232.

Embden G, F Kalberlah. "Uber acetonbildung in der leber." *Beitr Chem Physiol, u Path* Vol 8 (1906): 121.

Hartman AL, M Gasior, EPG Vining, et al. "The neuropharmacology of the ketogenic diet." *Pediatr Neurol* Vol 36, No 5 (2007): 281–292.

Hashim SA, S Bergen Jr., K Krell, et al. "Intestinal absorption and mode of transport in portal vein of medium-chain fatty acids." *J Clin Invest* Vol 43 (1964): 1238.

Henderson ST (Inventor). "Combinations of medium-chain triglycerides and therapeutic agents for the treatment and prevention of Alzheimer's disease and other diseases resulting from reduced neuronal metabolism." Available online at: www.freepatentsonline.com United States Patent 20080009467.

Henderson ST. "Ketone bodies as a therapeutic for Alzheimer's disease." *Journal of the American Society for Experimental NeuroTherapeutics* Vol 5 (Jul 2008): 470–480.

Henderson ST, JL Vogel, LJ Barr, et al. "Study of the ketogenic agent AC-1202 in mild to moderate Alzheimer's disease: a randomized, double-blind, placebo-controlled, multicenter trial." *Nutri Metab* Vol 6, No 31 (Aug 2009): 1–25.

Kadish I, O Thibault, EM Blalock, et al. "Hippocampal and cognitive aging across the lifespan: a bioenergetic shift precedes and increased cholesterol trafficking parallels memory impairments." *J Neurosci* Vol 29, No 6 (Feb 2009): 1805–1816.

Mochel F, P DeLonlay, G Touati, et al. "Pyruvate carboxylase deficiency: clinical and biochemical response to anaplerotic diet therapy." *Mol Genet Metab* Vol 84 (2005) 305–312.

Mochel F, S Duteil, C Marelli, et al. "Dietary anaplerotic therapy improves peripheral tissue energy metabolism in patients with Huntington's disease." *Eur J Hum Genet* Vol 10 (2010): 1–4.

Page KA, A Williamson, N Yu, et al. "Medium-chain fatty acids improve cognitive function in intensively treated type 1 diabetic patients and support *in vitro* synaptic transmission during acute hypoglycemia." *Diabetes* Vol 58, No 5 (May 2009): 1237–1244.

Pi-Sunyer FX, SA Hashim, TB VanItallie. "Insulin and ketone responses to ingestion of medium and long-chain triglycerides in man." *Diabetes* Vol 18, No 2 (Feb 1969): 96–100.

Reger MA, ST Henderson, C Hale, et al. "Effects of ?-hydroxybutyrate on cognition in memory-impaired adults." *Neurobiol Aging* Vol 25 (2004): 311–314.

Schön H, I Lippach, W Gelpke. "Stoffwechsel untersuchungen mit einem mischglycerid der fettsäuren mitlerer kettenlänge. II. Untersuchungen über die veränderungen des ketonkörpergehmaltes von blut and urin nach zufuhr des mischglyderides." *Gasteroenterologia* Vol 91 (1959): 199.

Studzinski CM, WA MacKay, TL Beckett, et al. "Induction of ketosis may improve mitochondrial function and decrease steady-state amyloid-? precursor protein (APP) levels in the aged dog." *Brain Res* Vol 1226 (2008): 209–217.

Taha AY, ST Henderson, WM Burnham. "Dietary enrichment with medium-chain triglycerides (AC-1203) elevates polyunsaturated fatty acids in the parietal cortex of aged dogs: implication for treating age-related cognitive decline." *Neurochem Res* Vol 34, No 9 (Sept 2009): 1619–1625.

Tantibhedhyangkul P, SA Hashim. "Clinical and physiologic aspects of medium-chain triglycerides: alleviation of steatorrhea in premature infants." *Bull N Y Acad Med* Vol 47, No 1 (1971): 17–33.

Tantibhehyangkul P, SA Hashim. "Medium-chain triglyceride feeding in premature infants: Effects on fat and nitrogen absorption." *Pediatrics* Vol 55 (Mar 1975): 359–370.

Turner N, K Hariharan, J TidAng, et al. "Enhancement of muscle mitochondrial oxidative capacity and alterations in insulin action are lipid species dependent: potent tissue-specific effects of medium-chain fatty acids." *Diabetes* Vol 48 (2009): 2547–2554.

Chapter 19: The Therapeutic Implications of the Ketone Ester

Cahill GF Jr., RL Veech. "Ketoacids? Good medicine?" *Trans Amer Clin Climatol Assoc* Vol 114 (2003): 149–163.

Ciarmiello A, M Cannella, S Lastoria, et al. "Brain white-matter volume loss and glucose hypometabolism precede the clinical symptoms of Huntington's disease." *J Nucl Med* Vol 47, No 2 (Feb 2005): 215–222.

Cornille E, M Abou-Hamdan, M Khrestchatisky, et al. "Enhancement of L-3-hydroxybutyryl-CoA dehydrogenase activity and circulating ketone body levels by pantethine. Relevance to dopaminergic injury." *BMC Neurosci* Vol 11 (2010): 51.

Kashiwaya Y, K Sato, N Tsuchiya, et al. "Control of glucose utilization in working perfused rat heart." *J Biol Chem* Vol 269, No 41 (Oct 1994): 25502–25514.

Kashiwaya Y, T King, RL Veech. "Substrate signaling by insulin: A ketone bodies ratio mimics insulin action in heart." *Am J Cardiol* Vol 80, No 3A (1997): 50A–64A.

Kashiwaya Y, T Takeshima, N Mori, et al. "D-b-hydroxybutyrate protects neurons in models of Alzheimer's and Parkinson's disease." *PNAS* Vol 97, No 10 (May 2000): 5440–5444.

Masuda R, JW Monohan, Y Kashiwaya. "D-beta-hydroxybutyrate is neuroprotective against hypoxia in serum-free hippocampal primary cultures." *J Neuroscience Res* Vol 80, No.4 (May 2005): 501–509.

Nagahara AH, DA Merrill, G Coppola, et al. "Neuroprotective effects of brain-derived neurotrophic factor in rodent and primate models of Alzheimer's disease." *Nature Medicine* Vol 15, No 3 (March 2009): 331–337.

Sato K, Y Kashiwaya, RL Veech, et al. "Insulin, ketone bodies, and mitochondrial energy transduction." *FASEB Journal* Vol 9 (May 1995): 651–658.

Seyfried TN, P Mukherjee. "Targeting energy metabolism in brain cancer: Review and hypothesis." *NutrMetab* Vol 2, No 30 (2005): 1–9.

Smith SL, DJ Heal, KF Martin. "A potential metabolic approach to cytoprotection in major surgery and neurological disorders." *CNS Drug Rev* Vol 11, No 2 (2005): 113–140.

Suzuki Y, H Takahashi, M Fukuda, et al. "?-hydroxybutyrate alters GABA-transaminase activity in cultured astrocytes." *Brain Res* Vol 1268 (2009): 17–23.

Tieu K, C Perier, C Caspersen, et al. "D-?-hydroxybutyrate rescues mitochondrial respiration and mitigates features of Parkinson disease." *J Clinl Invest* Vol 112, No 6 (2003): 892–901.

Van Hove JLK, S Grünewald, J Jaeken. "D, L-3-hydroxybutyrate treatment of multiple acyl-CoA dehydrogenase deficiency (MADD.)" *Lancet* Vol 361 (April 2003): 1433–1435.

VanItallie TB, C Nonas, A Di Rocco, et al. "Treatment of Parkinson disease with diet-induced hyperketonemia: a feasibility study." *Neurology* Vol 64 (Feb 2005): 728–730.

Veech RL, B Chance, Y Kashiwaya, et al. "Hypothesis paper: ketone bodies, potential therapeutic uses." *IUBMB Life* Vol 51 (2001): 241–247.

Veech RL. "The therapeutic implications of ketone bodies: the effects of ketone bodies in pathological conditions: ketosis, ketogenic diet, redox states, insulin resistance, and mitochondrial metabolism." *Prostaglandins, Leukot Essent Fatty Acids* Vol 70 (2004): 309–319.

Veech RL. "The determination of the redox states and phosphorylation potential in living tissues and their relationship to metabolic control of disease phenotypes." *Biochem Mol Biol Educ* Vol 32, No 3 (2006): 168–179.

Chapter 21: The Saturated Fat and Cholesterol Issue

Abramson J, RJ Barnard, HC Barry, et al. "Petition to the National Institutes of Health seeking an independent review panel to re-evaluate the National Cholesterol Education Program Guidelines." (Sept 2004). Available online at http://cspinet.org/new/pdf/finalnihltr.pdf.

Ahrens EH. "Nutritional factors and serum lipid levels." *Am J Med* Vol 23 (1957): 928.

Ahrens EH, J Hirsch, W Insull Jr. "The influence of dietary fats on serum-lipid levels in man." *This Week's Citation Classic* Vol 1 (1957): 943–953.

American Heart Association. "Inflammation, heart disease and stroke: the role of C-reactive protein." AHA Scientific Statement (2002). Available online at www.americanheart.org/presenter.jhtml?identifier=4648.

Ascherio A, MB Katan, PL Zock, et al. "Trans fatty acids and coronary heart disease." *NEJM* Vol 25 (1999): 1994–1998.

Beveridge JMR, WF Connell, HL Haust, et al. "Dietary cholesterol and plasma cholesterol levels in man." *Canadian Journal of Biochemistry* Vol 37 (1959): 575–582.

Bierenbaum ML, DP Green, A Florin, et al. "Modified-fat dietary management of the young male with coronary disease." *JAMA* Vol 202, No 13 (1967): 59–63.

Bourque C, MP St-Onge, AA Papamandjaris, et al. "Consumption of oil composed of medium-chain triacyglycerols, phytosterols, and n-3 fatty acids improves cardiovascular risk profile in overweight women." *Metabolism* Vol 52, No 6 (2003): 771–777.

Brisson G. *Lipids in Human Nutrition*. Lancaster, England: MTP Press (1982): 98.

Brouwer IA, AJ Wanders, MB Katan. "Effect of animal and industrial trans fatty acids on HDL and LDL cholesterol levels in humans—a quantitive review." *PLoS One* Vol 5, No 3 (2010): e9434.

Brown JM, GS Shelness, LL Rudel. "Monounsaturated fatty acids and and atherosclerosis: opposing views from epidemiology and experimental animal models." *Curr Atheroscler Rep* Vol 9, No 6 (2007): 494–500.

Calabrese C, S Myer, S Munson, et al. "A cross-over study of the effect of a single oral feeding of medium-chain triglyceride oil vs. canola oil on post-ingestion plasma triglyceride levels in healthy men." *Altern Med Rev* Vol. 4, No. 1 (1999): 23–28.

Cater NB, HJ Heller, MA Denke. "Comparison of the effects of medium-chain triacylglycerols, palm oil, and high oleic acid sunflower oil on plasma triacylglycerol fatty acids and lipid and lipoprotein concentrations in humans." *Am J Clin Nutr* Vol 1 (1997): 41-45.

Covas MI. "Olive oil and the cardiovascular system." *Pharmocol Res* Vol 55, No 3 (2007): 175–186.

Diamond D. "How bad science and big business created the obesity epidemic." A video lecture available online at: www.youtube.com/watch?v=3vr-c8GeT34.

Elwood P, D Givens, A Beswick, et al. "The survival advantage of milk and dairy consumption: an overview of evidence from cohort studies of vascular diseases, diabetes and cancer." *J Am Coll Nutr* Vol 27, No 6 (2008): 723S–734S.

Engelhart MJ, MI Geerlings, A Ruitenberg, et al. "Diet and dementia: does fat matter? The Rotterdam study." *Neurology* Vol 59, No 12 (2002): 1915–1921.

Enig MG, S Fallon. "The Oiling of America." Originally published in *Nexus Magazine* in two parts Nov/Dec 1998 and Feb/Mar 1999. Available online at: http://westonaprice.org/know-your-fats/525-the-oiling-of-america.

Erickson, BA, RH Coots, FH Mattson, et al. "The effect of partial hydrogenation of dietary fats, of the ratio of polyunsaturated to saturated fatty acids, and the dietary cholesterol upon plasma lipids in man." *J Clin Investigation* Vol 43, No 11 (1964): 2017-2025.

Evans MA, BA Golomb. "Statin-associated adverse cognitive effects: survey results from 171 patients." *Pharmacotherapy* Vol 27, No 7 (2009): 800–811.

Felton CV, D Crook, MJ Davies, et al. "Dietary polyunsaturated fatty acids and composition of human aortic plaques." *Lancet* Vol 344 (1994): 1195–1196.

Goldbourt U, M Schnaider-Beeri. "Is low percent calories from saturated fat reported at midlife related to the presence of late-life dementia among survivors?" *Alzheimers Dement* Vol 4, Iss. 4 Suppl. 2 Abstract P2-112 (Jul 2008): T404.

Goldstein JL, MS Brown. "Cholesterol: a century of research." *HHMI Bulletin* Vol 16, No 3 (2003): 10–19.

Golomb BA. "Implications of statin adverse effects in the elderly." *Expert Opin Drug Saf* Vol 4, No 3 (2005): 389–397.

Golomb BA, MA Evans. "Statin adverse effects: a review of the literature and evidence for a mitochondrial mechanism." *Am J Cardiovasc Drugs* Vol 8, No 6 (2008): 373–418.

Grande F, JT Anderson, A Keys. "The influence of chain length of the saturated fatty acids on their effect on serum cholesterol concentration in man." *J Nutrition* Vol 74 (1961): 420–428.

Gu Y, JA Luchsinger, Y Stern, et al. "Mediterranean diet, inflammatory and metabolic biomarkers and risk of Alzheimer's disease." *J Alzheimers Dis* Vol 22, No 2 (2010): 483–492.

Gu Y, JW Nieves, Y Stern, et al. "Food combination and Alzheimer disease risk." *Arch Neurol* Vol 67, No 6 (2010): E1–E8.

Hashim SA, RE Clancy, DM Hegsted, et al. "Effect of mixed fat formula feeding on serum cholesterol level in man." *Am J Clin Nutri* Vol 7 (1959): 30–34.

Hegsted DM, RB McGandy, ML Myers, et al. "Quantitative effects of dietary fat on serum cholesterol in man." *Am J Clin Nutr* Vol 17 (1965): 281–295.

Jha S, R Patel. "Some observations on the spectrum of dementia." *Neurology India* Vol 52 (2004): 213–214.

Keys A. "Atherosclerosis: a problem in newer public health." *J Mt Sinai Hosp* Vol. 20 (1953): 118.

Keys A. "Coronary heart disease in seven countries." *Circulation* Vol 41, Suppl 1 (1970): 1–211.

Keys A, JT Anderson, F Grande, "Prediction of serum cholesterol responses of man to changes in fats in the diet." *Lancet* Vol 2 (1957): 959–966.

Keys A, JT Anderson, O Mickelson, et al. "Diet and serum cholesterol in man: lack of effect of of dietary cholesterol." *J Nutrition* Vol 59 (1956): 39.

Keys A, RW Parlin. "Serum cholesterol response to changes in dietary lipids." *Am J Clin Nutr* Vol 19 (1966): 175–181.

Knopp RH, BM Retzlaff. "Saturated fat prevents coronary artery disease? An American paradox." *Am J Clin Nutr* Vol 80 (2004): 1102–1103.

Kris-Etherton PM, S Innis. "Position of the American Dietetic Association and Dietitians of Canada: dietary fatty acids." *J Am Diet Assoc* Vol 107, No 9 (2007): 1599–1611.

Kris-Etherton PM, S Yu. "Individual fatty acid effects on plasma lipids and lipoproteins: human studies." *Am J Clin Nutr* Vol. 65 (1997): 1628–1644S.

Le Fanu J. "The case of the missing data." *BMJ* Vol. 325 (2002): 1490–1493.

Lütjohann D, M Stroick, T Bertsch, et al. "High doses of simvastatin, pravastatin, and cholesterol reduce brain cholesterol synthesis in guinea pigs." *Steroids* Vol 69 (2004): 431–438.

Mann GV. "Diet and coronary heart disease." *AMA Arch Intern Med* Vol. 104 (1959): 95–103.

McNamara DJ, R Kolb, TS Parker, et al. "Heterogeneity of cholesterol homeostasis in man: response to changes in dietary fat quality and cholesterol quantity." *J Clin Invest* Vol 79 (1987): 1729–1739.

Mensink RP, MB Katan. "Effects of dietary *trans* fatty acids in high-density and low-density lipoprotein cholesterol levels in health subjects." *NEJM* Vol 323 (1990): 439–445.

Mensink RP, PL Zock, ADM Kester, et al. "Effects of dietary fatty acids and carbohydrates on the ratio of serum total to HDL cholesterol and on serum lipids and apolipoproteins: a meta-analysis of 60 controlled trials." *Am J Clin Nutr* Vol 77 (2003) 1145–1155.

Morin RJ, S Bernick, RB Alfin-Slater. "Effects of essential fatty acid deficiency and supplementation of atheroma formation and regression." *J Atheroscler Res* Vol. 4 (1964): 387–396.

Morris MC, DA Evans, JL Benias, et al. "Consumption of fish and n-3 fatty acids and risk of incident Alzheimer disease." *Arch Neurol* Vol 60 (2003): 940–946.

Morris MC, DA Evans, JL Bienias, et al. "Dietary fats and the risk of incident Alzheimer disease." *Arch Neurol* Vol 60 (2003): 194–200.

Mozaffarian D, EB Rimm, DM Herrington. "Dietary fats, carbohydrate, and progression of coronary atherosclerosis in postmenopausal women." *Am J Clin Nutr* Vol 80 (2004): 1175–1184.

Mulder M, R Ravid, DF Swaab, et al. "Reduced levels of cholesterol, phospholipids, and fatty acids in cerebrospinal fluid of Alzheimer disease patients are not related to apolipoprotein E4." *Alzheimer Dis Assoc Disord* Vol. 12 (1998): 198–203.

Ng TKW, K Hassan, JB Lim, et al. "Nonhypercholesterolemic effects of a palm-oil diet in Malaysian volunteers." *Am J Clin Nutr* Vol. 53 (1991): 1552–1561.

Prior IA, F Davidson, CE Salmond, et al. "Cholesterol, coconuts, and diet on Polynesian atolls: a natural experiment: the Pukapuka and Tokelau island studies." *Am J Clin Nutr* Vol 34, No 8 (Aug 1981): 1552–1561.

Ravnskov U. "The questionable role of saturated and polyunsaturated fatty acids in cardiovascular disease." *J Clin Epidemiol* Vol 51, No 6 (Jun 1998): 443-460.

Ren J, SM Grundy, J Liu, et al. "Long-term coronary heart disease risk associated with very low-density lipoprotein cholesterol in Chinese: the result of a 15-year Chinese multi-provincial cohort study (CMCS)." *Atherosclerosis* Vol 211, No 1 (Jul 2010): 327–332.

Ridker PM, N Rifai, L Rose. "Comparison of C-reactive protein and low-density lipoprotein cholesterol levels in the prediction of first cardiovascular events." *NEJM* Vol 347, No 20 (Nov 2002): 1557–1565.

Scarmeas N, Luchsinger JA, R Mayeuax, et al. "Mediterranean diet and Alzheimer disease mortality." *Neurology* Vol. 69 (2007): 1084–1093.

Schatz IJ, K Masaki, K Yano, et al. "Cholesterol and all-cause mortality in elderly people from the Honolulu Heart Program: a cohort study." *Lancet* Vol 358 (Aug 2001): 351–355.

Schatz IJ, K Masaki, K Yano, et al. Author's reply to letter to editor. *Lancet* Vol 358 (Dec 2001): 1906.

Seneff S, G Wainwright, L Mascitelli. "Nutrition and Alzheimer's disease: the detrimental role of a high-carbohydrate diet." *EurJ Intern Med* (2011) Article in press.

Shorland FB, Z Czochanska, AM Prior. "Studies on fatty acid composition of adipose tissue and blood lipids of Polynesians." *Am J Clin Nutr* Vol 22, No 5 (1969): 594–605.

Singh-Manoux A, D Gimeno, M Kivimaki, et al. "Low HDL cholesterol is a risk factor for deficit and decline in memory in midlife: the Whitehall II study." *Arterioscler Thromb Vasc Biol* Vol 28, No 8 (Aug 2008): 1418–1420.

Siri-Tarino PW, Sun Q, Hu FB, et al. "Meta-analysis of prospective cohort studies evaluating the association of saturated fat with cardiovascular disease." *Amer J Clin Nutr* Vol 91, No 3 (Mar 2010): 535–546.

Sofi F, F Cesari, R Abbate, et al. "Adherence to Mediterranean diet and health status: meta-analysis." *BMJ* Vol 337 (2008): a1344.

Solfrizzi V, V Frisardi, C Capurso, et al. "Dietary fatty acids and predementia syndromes." *Scientific World Journal* Vol 9 (2009): 792–810.

Solomon A, M Kivipelto, B Wolozin, et al. "Midlife serum cholesterol and increased risk of Alzheimer's and vascular dementia three decades later." *Dement Geriatr Cogn Disord* Vol 28 (2009): 75–80.

St-Onge MP, A Bosarge, LLT Goree, et al. "Medium-chain triglyceride oil consumption as part of a weight loss diet does not lead to an adverse metabolic profile when compared to olive oil." *J Am Coll Nutri* Vol 27, No 5 (2008): 547–552.

Tan Z, S Seshadri, A Beiser, et al. "Plasma total cholesterol level as a risk factor for Alzheimer disease: the Framingham study." *Arch Intern Med* Vol 163 (May 2003): 1053–1057.

Tholstrup T, P Marckmann, J Jespersen, et al. "Effect on blood lipids, coagulation, and fibrinolysis of a fat high in myristic acid and a fat high in palmitic acid." *Am J Clin Nutr* Vol 60 (1994): 919–925.

Tong J, PP Borbat, JH Freed, et al. "A scissors mechanism for stimulation of SNARE-mediated lipid mixing by cholesterol." *PNAS* Vol 106, No 13 (Mar 2009): 5141–5146.

Volek JS, CE Forsythe. "The case for not restricting saturated fat on a low-carbohydrate diet." *Nutri Metab* Vol 2 (2005): 21.

Wagstaff LR, MW Mitton, B McLendon Arvik, et al. "Statin-associated memory loss: analysis of 60 case reports and review of the literature." *Pharmacotherapy* Vol 23, No 7 (2003).

Williams MA, J Tinoco, I Hicenbergs, et al. "Increased plasma triglyceride secretion in EFA-deficient rats fed diets with or without saturated fat." *Lipids* Vol 24, No 5 (1989): 448–453.

Willet WC, MJ Stamfer, JE Manson, et al. "Intake of trans fatty acids and risk of coronary heart disease among women." *Lancet* Vol 884, No 5 (1993): 581–585.

Wong A. "Incident solar radiation and coronary heart disease mortality rates in Europe." *Eur J Epidemiol* Vol 23, No 9 (2008): 609–614.

Yerushalmy J, HE Hilleboe. "Fat in the diet and mortality from heart disease." *New York State J Medicine* Vol 57 (1957): 2343–2354.

Yudkin J. "Diet and coronary thrombosis: hypothesis and fact." *Lancet* (Jul 1957): 155–162.

Zock P, J de Vries, M Katan. "Impact of myristic acid versus Palmitic acid on serum lipids and lipoprotein levels in healthy women and men." *Arterioscler Thromb* Vol 14 (1994): 567–575.

Chapter 22: Why Diet Makes a Difference

Gu Y, JW Nieves, Y Stern, et al. "Food combination and Alzheimer disease risk." *Arch Neurol* Vol 67, No 6 (2010): E1–E8.

Chapter 23: Questions and Answers about Coconut Oil

Studzinski CM, WA MacKay, TL Beckett, et al. "Induction of ketosis may improve mitochondrial function and decrease steady-state amyloid-? precursor protein (APP) levels in the aged dog." *Brain Res* Vol. 1226 (2008): 209–217

Taha AY, ST Henderson, WM Burnham. "Dietary enrichment with medium-chain triglycerides (AC-1203) elevates polyunsaturated fatty acids in the parietal cortex of aged dogs: implication for treating age-related cognitive decline." *Neurochem Res* Vol 34, No 9 (Sept 2009): 1619–1625.

Index

About the Author

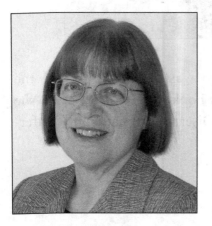

Mary T. Newport, M.D., grew up in Cincinnati, Ohio, attended Xavier University for pre-medicine and graduated from the University of Cincinnati College of Medicine in 1978. She trained in pediatrics at Children's Hospital Medical Center in Cincinnati and completed her fellowship in neonatology at the Medical University Hospital in Charleston, South Carolina. She has practiced neonatology in Florida since 1983 and has been medical director of the Newborn Intensive Care Unit at Spring Hill Regional Hospital since opening in 2003. Dr. Newport is employed by the All Children's Specialty Physicians group, which provides newborn services to Spring Hill Regional Hospital. She is also volunteer clinical faculty for the Department of Pediatrics, University of South Florida, since January 2004. She previously practiced neonatology and served as medical director at Mease Hospital Dunedin after founding the newborn intensive care unit at that hospital in 1987.

Dr. Newport has been married to Steve Newport since 1972, and they have two daughters and a grandson. In 2008, Dr. Newport wrote an article, "What If There Was a Cure for Alzheimer's

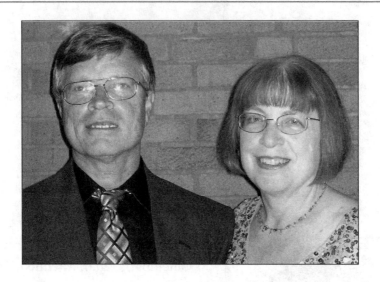

Disease and No One Knew?" which was circulated around the world and became the subject of this book as well as a lecture she presented at the 2010 Alzheimer's Disease International Conference in Thessaloniki, Greece.